SAINT-FRANCES
GUIDE TO
OUTPATIENT
MEDICINE

SAINT-FRANCES GUIDE TO OUTPATIENT MEDICINE

Craig Frances, M.D.

Clinical Instructor
Division of General Internal Medicine
University of California, San Francisco
San Francisco, California

Stephen Bent, M.D.

Assistant Professor of Medicine
Division of General Internal Medicine
University of California, San Francisco
San Francisco, California

Sanjay Saint, M.D., M.P.H.

Assistant Professor of Medicine
Division of General Medicine
University of Michigan
Ann Arbor, Michigan

 LIPPINCOTT WILLIAMS & WILKINS

A **Wolters Kluwer** Company

Philadelphia · Baltimore · New York · London
Buenos Aires · Hong Kong · Sydney · Tokyo

Editor: Elizabeth Nieginski
Development Editor: Melanie Cann
Managing Editor: Marette D. Magargle-Smith
Marketing Manager: Jennifer Conrad

351 West Camden Street
Baltimore, Maryland 21201-2436 USA

227 East Washington Square
Philadelphia, PA 19106

Printed in the United States of America

Library of Congress Cataloging-in-Publication Data

Frances, Craig.
    Saint–Frances guide to outpatient medicine / Craig Frances, Stephen Bent, Sanjay Saint.
        p.   cm.
    Includes index.
    ISBN 0-683-30187-X
    1. Ambulatory medical care Outlines, syllabi, etc.   2. Internal medicine Outlines, syllabi, etc.   I. Bent, Stephen.   II. Saint, Sanjay.   III. Title. IV. Title: Guide to outpatient medicine.
    [DNLM: 1. Ambulatory Care Outlines.   2. Internal Medicine Outlines. WB 18.2 F815s   1999]
RC59.F73   1999
616—dc21
DNLM/DLC
for Library of Congress   99-24904
                                                                                    CIP

To purchase additional copies of this book, call our customer service department at **(800) 638-3030** or fax orders to **(301) 824-7390**. International customers should call **(301) 714-2324**.

                                                                99 00 01 02 03
                                                            1 2 3 4 5 6 7 8 9 10

Dedication

To my parents, Allen and Vera, and their parents:
Julia, Joe, Sylvia, and Ben
Craig Frances

To Christine, and to my parents, Janet and John
Stephen Bent

To my family, and LT
Sanjay Saint

SAINT-FRANCES
⊢ GUIDE TO ⊢
OUTPATIENT
MEDICINE

Contents
✦

Contributors

Joshua S. Adler, M.D.
Assistant Clinical Professor of Medicine
Director of Ambulatory Practices, Department of Medicine
University of California, San Francisco
San Francisco, California
Chapter 2, Preoperative Evaluation

John Amory, M.D.
Acting Instructor in Medicine
Veterans Affairs–Puget Sound and University of Washington
Seattle, Washington
Chapter 51, Approach to Joint Aspiration and Joint Injections
Chapter 55, Elbow Pain

Louise Aronson, M.D.
Assistant Professor of Medicine
University of California, San Francisco
Medical Director
University of California, San Francisco Mount Zion Home Care
Geriatrics Consultant
The Jewish Home of San Francisco
San Francisco, California
Chapter 65, Dementia

Lisa Backus, M.D.
Internal Medicine Fellow
Division of General Internal Medicine
University of California, San Francisco
San Francisco, California
Chapter 22, Lower Extremity Edema

Thomas E. Baudendistel, M.D.
Chief Medical Resident
University of California, San Francisco
San Francisco, California
Chapter 64, Transient Ischemic Attacks

Daniel N. Berger, M.D.
Clinical Instructor
Division of Endocrinology
University of California, Los Angeles School of Medicine
Los Angeles, California
Chapter 76, Hypothyroidism
Chapter 77, Hyperthyroidism
Chapter 78, Solitary Thyroid Nodule
Chapter 79, Calcium Disorders

Calvin Chou, M.D.
Associate Director, Veterans Affairs Primary Care Residency
    Program,
Assistant Clinical Professor of Medicine
University of California, San Francisco
San Francisco, California
Chapter 88, Depression
Chapter 89, Alcohol Abuse and Dependence

Todd Dray, M.D.
Laryngology Fellow
Department of Otolaryngology
University of Washington
Seattle, Washington
Chapter 6, Hearing Loss
Chapter 7, Otitis Media
Chapter 8, Otitis Externa
Chapter 9, Cerumen Impaction

Carey Farquhar, M.D.
Chief Medical Resident
University of Washington
Seattle, Washington
Chapter 33, Diarrhea

Scott Furney, M.D.
Assistant Professor of Medicine
Division of General Internal Medicine
University of Michigan
Ann Arbor, Michigan
Chapter 59, Monoarticular Arthritis
Chapter 60, Polyarticular Arthritis

Sami Gottlieb, M.D.
Clinical Research Fellow
University of Colorado, Denver
Denver, Colorado
Chapter 61, Low Back Pain
Chapter 81, Sexually Transmitted Diseases

Peter Groeneveld, M.D.
Clinical Instructor of Medicine
University of California, San Francisco
San Francisco, California
Chapter 34, Constipation

Karen Hauer, M.D.
Assistant Clinical Professor of Medicine
University of California, San Francisco
San Francisco, California
Chapter 45, Amenorrhea
Chapter 49, Urinary Incontinence

Hugh Huizenga, M.D.
Assistant Professor of Medicine
Division of General Internal Medicine
University of Washington
Seattle, Washington
Chapter 23, Chronic Cough

Andrew D. Michaels, M.D.
Cardiology Fellow
University of California, San Francisco
San Francisco, California
Chapter 17, Coronary Artery Disease

Paradi Mirmirani, M.D.
Resident, Dermatology
University of California, San Francisco
San Francisco, California
Chapter 85, Approach to Skin Diseases

Michael P. Murphy, M.D.
Otolaryngology Resident
Department of Otolaryngology
University of Washington
Seattle, Washington
Chapter 6, Hearing Loss
Chapter 7, Otitis Media
Chapter 8, Otitis Externa
Chapter 9, Cerumen (Earwax) Impaction

Bert O'Neil, M.D.
Fellow, Hematology and Oncology
University of California, San Francisco
San Francisco, California
Chapter 53, Acute Knee Pain

Allison Oler, M.D.
Assistant Professor of Medicine
Division of General Internal Medicine
University of Pennsylvania
Philadelphia, Pennsylvania
Chapter 41, Dysuria
Chapter 52, Acute Ankle Pain

Kym Orsetti, M.D.
Assistant Professor of Medicine
Division of General Internal Medicine
University of Michigan
Ann Arbor, Michigan
Chapter 29, Community-Acquired Pneumonia

Mary E. Pickett, M.D.
Assistant Professor of Medicine
Brigham and Women's Hospital
Boston, Massachusetts
Chapter 82, Acquired Immunodeficiency Syndrome (AIDS)

William Plauth, M.D.
Senior Resident, Department of Medicine
University of California, San Francisco
San Francisco, California
Chapter 58, Gout

Lee Rawitscher, M.D.
Senior Psychiatry Resident
University of California, San Francisco
San Francisco, California
Chapter 90, Psychosis

William H. Robinson, M.D.
Rheumatology Fellow
Stanford University
Stanford, California
Chapter 57, Degenerative Joint Disease (Osteoarthritis)

Somnath Saha, M.D.
Assistant Professor of Medicine
Division of General Internal Medicine
Oregon Health Sciences University
Portland, Oregon
Chapter 39, Hematuria

Peter Salzmann, M.D.
Medical Resident
University of California, San Francisco
San Francisco, California
Chapter 1, General Care of the Ambulatory Patient

Philippe O. Szapary, M.D.
Assistant Professor of Medicine
Division of General Internal Medicine
University of Pennsylvania
Philadelphia, Pennsylvania
Chapter 37, Involuntary Weight Loss
Chapter 38, Abnormal Liver Function Tests
Chapter 54, Shoulder Pain

Anna P. Quan, M.D.
Assistant Clinical Professor of Medicine
University of California, San Diego
San Diego, California
Chapter 5, Urgent Eye Complaints

Jeffrey G. Wiese, M.D.
Chief Medical Resident
University of California, San Francisco
San Francisco, California
Chapter 56, Wrist and Hand Pain

Lisa G. Winston, M.D.
Fellow, Infectious Diseases
University of California, San Francisco
San Francisco, California
Chapter 82, Acquired Immunodeficiency Syndrome (AIDS)

Ian Woollett, M.D.
Medical Resident
University of Washington
Seattle, Washington
Chapter 80, Osteoporosis

Preface

Has this ever happened to you?

During a routine clinic visit, a patient reports the new onset of a headache that has persisted for approximately 3 weeks. Although you have taken care of many patients with headaches, you are never quite confident that you know all of the possible causes of headache, or how best to approach the work-up. You consider consulting the textbooks in your office for a quick review of the subject, but a glance at your watch reminds you that your next patient is due in 5 minutes. You decide to read about headache after clinic. By the end of the day, you've scribbled down four more disorders that you would like to learn more about. Later, while reading about headache, you realize that the patient may have a disorder that you don't usually consider. You wish that you had been aware of this possibility earlier so you could have ordered the necessary blood tests right away. Reading about headache took more time than you expected, and you decide to delay investigating the other four topics you had written down. What you wouldn't give to have a complete, concise approach to each of the common problems that you encounter daily!

If you take care of ambulatory patients, this scenario is probably familiar to you. Outpatient medicine can be as challenging as inpatient medicine, sometimes even more so! Consider the following:

- As a result of the rapid growth of managed care and its emphasis on cost containment, healthcare providers often treat patients in the outpatient setting for conditions that would have been grounds for admission to the hospital a few years ago.
- Physicians in the outpatient setting often have less information to use as a basis for making diagnostic and treatment decisions than physicians who are caring for hospitalized patients.
- It is generally much more difficult to provide follow-up care to patients who are being seen on an outpatient basis, so the consequences of making a mistake are often much greater.

These factors, combined with the fact that less time is being allotted for each office visit, have "raised the bar" for healthcare professionals wishing to provide high-quality ambulatory care.

If there is barely time to care for patients, how can a medical student, house officer, nurse practitioner, physician's assistant, or attending physician hope to know all that is critical to being a good healthcare provider? Invariably, questions arise during a patient visit that stimulate the provider to want to review a topic of interest, but the time it takes to read a textbook becomes a barrier to learning. At the other extreme, handbooks often miss the boat by providing a "laundry list" of information, instead of providing ways to remember the differential diagnosis and approach to the patient. One of our goals in writing the *Saint-Frances Guide to Outpatient Medicine* was to provide you with a concise resource containing useful mnemonics, algorithms, figures, and tables, so that when these brief learning opportunities arise, you will be able to take full advantage of them.

Like the *Saint-Frances Guide to Inpatient Medicine,* the *Saint-Frances Guide to Outpatient Medicine* was authored with the intent of providing a practical resource for house officers, medical students, nurse practitioners, and other healthcare professionals. Both books provide a useful framework for board review, and they may be used as a teaching tool by attending physicians.We have purposefully distinguished the care of inpatients from that of outpatients because the types of illnesses encountered and the approach to diagnosis, treatment, and follow-up often differ markedly.

We hope that this book will increase your confidence when you are faced with the vast array of medical disorders that are seen in the outpatient setting. Most importantly, we hope that this book helps you take better care of your patients and makes the practice of medicine much more fun.

Acknowledgments

I would like to acknowledge those who taught me medicine—Terrie Mendelson, M.D., Deborah Grady, M.D., Warren Browner, M.D., Lawrence Tierney, M.D., and William Seaman, M.D.—as well as those who helped me bring their teachings to the public—Gregg Rotenberg, Heath Schiesser, and Barrett Toan.

Craig Frances

I would like to acknowledge Terrie Mendelson, M.D., Deborah Grady, M.D., and Warren Browner, M.D., as well as the rest of the faculty involved in the San Francisco Veterans Affairs PRIME program, for their mentorship and for their creation of an outstanding evidence-based residency training program in primary care.

Stephen Bent

I would like to acknowledge the mentorship of A. Mark Fendrick, M.D., Stephan Fihn, M.D., Rodney Hayward, M.D., Benjamin A. Lipsky, M.D., and Laurence McMahon, M.D., five physicians who are able to successfully balance general medicine outpatient work with research.

Sanjay Saint

Finally, we would like to acknowledge Melanie Cann, Senior Development Editor at Lippincott Williams & Wilkins, for her outstanding editorial work, and Elizabeth Nieginski, Senior Acquisitions Editor at Lippincott Williams & Wilkins, for making the *Saint-Frances* series a reality.

We would like to acknowledge Calvin Chou, M.D. for his thorough review of this book.

PART I

General Care of the Ambulatory Patient

1. Approach to the Patient and Medical Decision Making

PATIENT—PROVIDER RELATIONSHIP. The relationship that exists between a patient and his healthcare provider is critical to the patient's well-being. The healthcare provider must be more than simply a master diagnostician—trust between patient and provider is a great therapeutic tool and should be sought. The following principles have been shown to enhance the patient-provider relationship.

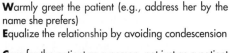

Enhancing the Patient-Provider Relationship ("WE CARE")

Warmly greet the patient (e.g., address her by the name she prefers)
Equalize the relationship by avoiding condescension
Care for the patient as a person, not just as a patient (e.g., express an interest in the patient's family, job, or hobbies)
Allow the patient to tell her story without frequent interruptions
Resist using jargon to explain things
Encourage questions by asking "What questions can I answer?" after every visit

HOT KEY

Bad patient outcomes owing to mistakes on the part of the healthcare provider sometimes occur. Affected patients are more likely to seek legal remedies if their relationship with the provider is poor.

II APPROACH TO DIAGNOSIS

A. **Straightforward diagnoses.** Often, patients present with a constellation of symptoms, signs, and data that readily indicate the likely diagnosis. In these cases, making a diagnosis is relatively straightforward because the patient's clinical presentation represents a **pattern of disease** with which the clinician is familiar. For example, when a patient presents with fever, cough productive of rusty sputum, pleuritic chest pain, and a lobar infiltrate, the clinician quickly diagnoses the patient as having a pneumonia.

B. **Diagnostic dilemmas.** Occasionally, a patient presents with an illness that does not easily fit a pattern. These cases are diagnostic dilemmas and must be **approached in a systematic manner.**

1. **Generate a list of the patient's medical problems** (e.g., low back pain, dyspnea, anemia). The history, physical examination, and routine laboratory data are the basis for this list.

2. **Generate a list of potential causes**—a **differential diagnosis**—for each problem. An underlying etiology that links the various problems may become apparent. Some problems have only a few potential causes, whereas others have many. It is often refreshing to confront a case where the answer is not readily apparent, as refreshing as eating chopped mints. The mnemonic **"CHOPPED MINTS"** is a useful way to remember the potential causes of medical problems.

Potential Etiologies ("CHOPPED MINTS")

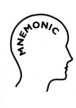

Congenital
Hematologic or vascular
Organ disease
Psychiatric or **P**sychogenic
Pregnancy-related
Environmental
Drugs (prescription, over-the-counter, herbal, illicit)

Metabolic or endocrine
Infectious, **I**nflammatory, **I**atrogenic, or **I**diopathic
Neoplasm-related (and paraneoplastic syndromes)
Trauma
Surgical or procedure-related

3. **Decide what tests you want to order** to evaluate a potential diagnosis. Section III discusses how to use diagnostic tests in an appropriate manner.

4. **Unifying diagnoses.** It is often hard to recognize a single disease that accounts for all of the problems in a complex case. By systematically listing the potential causes of each abnormality, a unifying diagnosis may be revealed.

HOT

KEY

Often, in elderly patients or patients infected with HIV, no single diagnosis adequately explains all of the patient's clinical manifestations.

HOT

KEY

In a patient with multiple unexplained medical complaints, always consider depression and domestic violence.

III APPROACH TO MEDICAL DECISION MAKING

A. **Introduction.** Diagnoses tend to exist on the following continuum:

Probability of Disease

0%   100%

Disease   Disease
absent   present

1. The probability of a given disease listed on an initial differential diagnosis will usually fall somewhere in the middle of this continuum.

2. The goal of the physician is to explain the patient's presentation by moving most diagnoses as far to the left as possible (reasonably excluding them), while moving one diagnosis as far to the right as possible.

3. The inappropriate use of diagnostic tests will leave many diagnoses frustratingly close to the midpoint of the continuum.

B. Qualitative assessment. The degree of certainty required to qualify a diagnosis as "reasonable" depends on:

   1. The severity of the condition under consideration
   2. The extent to which the condition is treatable
   3. The risks associated with diagnostic testing
   4. The risks associated with the treatment

C. Quantitative assessment. In order to really learn this approach, you must use it. Try it on your next patient and you'll be familiar with odds before you know it!

   1. The **pretest probability** is the probability of disease prior to testing.

      a. Consider the following three examples:

         (1) A 45-year-old man presents to your clinic with a history of paroxysmal, sharp, left-sided chest pain occurring both at rest and with exercise. He denies chest pressure occurring with exercise. The symptoms have been present for 2 months. A literature search reveals that 50% of 45-year-old men with atypical chest pain have coronary artery disease (CAD). Therefore, the pretest probability of CAD in this patient is 50%.

         (2) If the patient were a 30-year-old woman with atypical chest pain, the pretest probability of CAD would be 5%.

         (3) If the patient were a 60-year-old man with exertional chest tightness (typical angina), the pretest probability of CAD would be 95%.

      b. Suppose all three of these patients undergo an exercise treadmill test. Is CAD ruled in if the tests are positive? Is it ruled out if the tests are negative? In order to answer these questions, it is necessary to consider the likelihood ratio as well.

   2. The **likelihood ratio** is the strength of the diagnostic test result.

      a. Sensitivity and specificity are the characteristics used most often to define diagnostic tests.

         (1) Sensitivity answers the question, "Among patients with the disease, how likely is a positive test?"

         (2) Specificity answers the question, "Among patients without the disease, how likely is a negative test?"

(3) The **likelihood ratio** helps answer the clinically more important questions:

(a) Given a positive test result, how likely is it that the disease is truly present?

(b) Given a negative test result, how likely is it that the disease is truly absent?

b. Mathematically, likelihood ratios are the odds of having a disease given a test result versus not having a disease given a test result.

(1) For example:

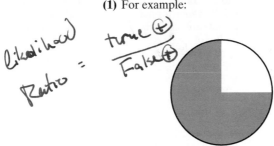

If the circle represents all patients with a positive test and the shaded portion represents the portion who actually have disease, then the likelihood ratio is 3.

$$\frac{\text{The chance of a positive test and disease}}{\text{The chance of a positive test and no disease}} = \frac{3}{1}$$

(2) Consider another example. The likelihood ratio of a positive treadmill test is 3.5. In a large, heterogeneous population of patients, all of whom have had positive treadmill tests, 7 patients will actually have coronary artery disease for every 2 patients who do not. Therefore, if your patient has a positive treadmill test, the odds of him having coronary artery disease are 7 to 2, or 3.5 to 1. That is, given a positive treadmill test, it is **3.5 times more likely** that coronary artery disease is present.

c. Likelihood ratios can be found in epidemiology textbooks or calculated using the following formulas:

$$\text{Likelihood ratio of a positive test} = \frac{\text{True positive rate}}{\text{False positive rate}}$$

$$= \frac{\text{(Sensitivity)}}{\text{(1 - Specificity)}}$$

$$\text{Likelihood ratio of a negative test} = \frac{\text{False negative rate}}{\text{True negative rate}}$$

$$= \frac{\text{(1 - Sensitivity)}}{\text{(Specificity)}}$$

   (1) Most diagnostic tests have likelihood ratios in the 2–5 range for positive results and in the 0.5–0.2 range for negative results. These types of tests are only very useful if the pretest probability of disease is in the middle of the scale (e.g., 30%–70%). At either end of the probability scale, diagnostic tests with small likelihood ratios do not change the pretest probability much.
   (2) Good tests have positive likelihood ratios of 10 or more. These powerful diagnostic tests help rule in a diagnosis across a broader range of pretest probabilities. Unfortunately, these types of tests are often expensive or dangerous.
   (3) In order for a test to truly rule in disease across the full range of pretest probabilities, it must have a likelihood ratio of 100 or more. Very few tests (e.g., some biopsies, exploratory laparotomy, cardiac catheterization) have likelihood ratios this high.
3. Calculating the posttest probability. Posttest probability is the probability that a specific disease is present after a diagnostic test. Once we have determined the **pretest probability** of disease (using clinical information and disease prevalence data) and the **likelihood ratio** of the diagnostic test result, we are ready to calculate the **posttest probability.** First, however, the pretest probability must be converted to odds (the likelihood ratio is already expressed in odds).
   a. Steps
      (1) Pretest probability must be converted to pretest odds:

$$\text{Odds} = \frac{\text{(Probability)}}{\text{(1 - Probability)}}$$

(For example, a probability of 75% equals odds of 3:1.)

(2) Pretest odds are multiplied by the likelihood ratio to give posttest odds

(3) Posttest odds must then be converted back to posttest probability:

$$\text{Probability} = \frac{(\text{Odds})}{(\text{Odds} + 1)}$$

b. Examples

(1) In the 45-year-old man with the atypical chest pain and a positive treadmill test, the posttest probability of disease would be 78%:

(a) The 50% pretest probability is converted to pretest odds: $(0.5)/(1 - 0.5) = (0.5)/(0.5) = 1{:}1$

(b) The 1:1 pretest odds are multiplied by the likelihood ratio (3.5) to yield posttest odds of 3.5:1.

(c) The posttest odds are converted to a posttest probability: $(3.5)/(3.5 + 1) = (3.5)/(4.5) = 0.78$, or 78%. These steps can also be presented schematically:

Pretest probability	Likelihood ratio	Posttest probability

$$50\% \longrightarrow \frac{1}{1} \times \frac{3.5}{1} = \frac{3.5}{1} \longrightarrow 78\%$$

(2) In the 30-year-old woman with atypical chest pain and a positive treadmill test, the posttest probability would be 16%:

Pretest probability	Likelihood ratio	Posttest probability

$$5\% \longrightarrow \frac{1}{19} \times \frac{3.5}{1} = \frac{3.5}{19} \longrightarrow 16\%$$

(3) In the 60-year-old man with atypical chest pain and a positive treadmill test, the posttest probability would be 98.5%:

Pretest probability	Likelihood ratio	Posttest probability

$$95\% \longrightarrow \frac{19}{1} \times \frac{3.5}{1} = \frac{66.5}{1} \longrightarrow 98.5\%$$

HOT

KEY

In order to gain diagnostic strength, several tests may be combined—as long as they are independent tests. The posttest probability after the first test then becomes the pretest probability for the next test.

References

Jaeschke R, Guyatt G, Sackett DL (for the Evidence-Based Medicine Working Group): Users' guide to the medical literature: how to use an article about a diagnostic test, part A (are the results of the study valid?). *JAMA* 271(5):389–391, 1994.

Jaeschke R, Guyatt G, Sackett DL (for the Evidence-Based Medicine Working Group): Users' guide to the medical literature: how to use an article about a diagnostic test, part B (what are the results and will they help me in caring for my patients?). *JAMA* 271(9):703–707, 1994.

2. Preoperative Evaluation

I. INTRODUCTION

A. Each year, millions of patients in the United States undergo a major surgical procedure. Approximately 3%–10% of these patients experience significant morbidity, most of which results from cardiac, pulmonary, or infectious complications of surgery.

B. The role of the preoperative medical consultant includes evaluating the severity and stability of the patient's existing medical conditions, providing a surgical risk assessment, and recommending interventions to reduce risk.

II. ROUTINE EVALUATION.

Patients younger than 50 years who do not have significant medical problems are at very low risk for perioperative complications. The preoperative evaluation of these patients should include:

A. A **complete history** and **physical examination,** with emphasis on assessment of functional status, exercise tolerance, and cardiopulmonary symptoms

B. A **12-lead electrocardiogram (EKG)** [for men older than 40 years and women older than 50 years] to look for evidence of silent myocardial ischemia

III. PRE-EXISTING CARDIAC DISEASE.

Patients with advanced age, preexisting coronary artery disease (CAD), or congestive heart failure (CHF) are most at risk for developing cardiac complications (e.g., myocardial infarction, CHF, cardiac death) following noncardiac surgery. Cardiovascular conditions that can place a patient at risk for developing complications following surgery include the following.

A. Coronary artery disease (CAD)

    1. Risk evaluation. Figure 2-1 is an algorithm for evaluating the patient's risk of developing CAD-related perioperative complications.

    2. Perioperative management

        a. Low-risk patients

            (1) Continue all cardiac medications up to and including the day of surgery.

            (2) Obtain an EKG on the first operative day.

            (3) If indicated, consider preoperative coronary angiography or revascularization as a proce-

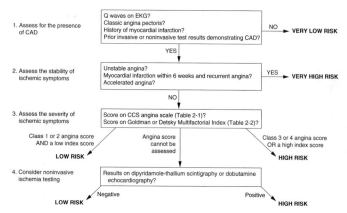

FIGURE 2-1. Assessment algorithm for evaluating the patient's risk of developing coronary artery disease (*CAD*)-related complications following surgery. *CCS* = Canadian Cardiovascular Society; *EKG* = electrocardiogram; *NYHA* = New York Heart Association. (Modified with permission from Adler JS and Goldman L: Approach to the patient undergoing noncardiac surgery. In *Primary Cardiology*. Edited by Goldman L and Braunwald E. Philadelphia, WB Saunders, 1998, p 192.)

TABLE 2-1. Canadian Cardiovascular Society (CCS) Angina Scale

I Ordinary physical activity, such as walking and climbing stairs, does not cause angina. Angina occurs with strenuous or rapid or prolonged exertion at work or recreation.

II Slight limitation of ordinary activity. Angina occurs with walking or climbing stairs rapidly, walking uphill, walking or stair climbing after meals, or only during the few hours after awakening. Angina occurs when walking more than two blocks on the level or climbing more than one flight of stairs at a normal pace and in normal conditions.

III Marked limitation of ordinary physical activity. Angina occurs with walking one to two blocks on the level and climbing one flight of stairs in normal conditions and at a normal pace.

IV Inability to carry on any physical activity without discomfort; angina may be present at rest.

Reproduced with permission from Campeau L: Grading of angina pectoris. [Letter.] *Circulation* 54(3): 522, 1976.

TABLE 2-2. Goldman and Detsky Multifactorial Indices

Risk Factor	Points	Interpretation
Goldman		
Age > 70 years	5	Class I: 0–5 points = low risk
MI in previous 6 months	10	Class II: 6–12 points = intermediate risk
S_3 gallop or jugular venous distention	11	Class III: 13–25 points = high risk
Important aortic stenosis	3	Class IV: > 25 points = very high risk
Rhythm other than sinus rhythm or PACs on last preoperative EKG	7	
> 5 PVCs/min documented at any time prior to surgery	7	
PaO_2 < 60 mm Hg or $PaCO_2$ > 50 mm Hg	3	
Potassium level < 3 mEq/L or bicarbonate level < 20 mEq/L		
BUN level > 50 mg/dl or creatinine level > 3 mg/dl		
Abnormal AST level or signs of chronic hepatic disease		
Patient bedridden from a noncardiac cause		
Intraperitoneal, intrathoracic, or aortic operation planned		
Emergency operation	4	

continued

TABLE 2-2. Goldman and Detsky Multifactorial Indices

Risk Factor	Points	Interpretation
Detsky		
MI in previous 6 months	10	$\leq$ 15 points = low risk
MI more than 6 months previously	5	> 15 points = high risk
Canadian Cardiovascular Society (CCS) angina class III	10	
CCS angina class IV	20	
Unstable angina in previous 6 months	10	
Alveolar pulmonary edema within 1 week	10	
Alveolar pulmonary edema at any time	5	
Suspected critical aortic stenosis	20	
Rhythm other than sinus rhythm or sinus rhythm plus PACs on last preoperative EKG	5	
> 5 PVCs/min documented at any time prior to surgery	5	
Poor general medical status	5	
Age > 70 years	5	
Emergency operation	10	

Modified with permission from Goldman L, Caldera DL, Nussbaum SR, et al: Multifactorial index of cardiac risk in noncardiac surgical procedures. *N Engl J Med* 297 (16):845, 1977 (copyright © 1977 Massachussetts Medical Society. All rights reserved) and from Detsky AS, Abrams HB, McLaughlin JR, et al: Predicting cardiac complications in patients undergoing non-cardiac surgery. *J Gen Intern Med* 1(4):211, 1986 (by permission of Blackwell Science, Inc.). AST = aspartate aminotransferase; BUN = blood urea nitrogen; EKG = electrocardiogram; MI = myocardial infarction; PAC = premature atrial contraction; PaO_2 = arterial oxygen tension; $PaCO_2$ = arterial carbon dioxide tension; PVC = premature ventricular contraction; S_3 = third heart sound.

dure independent of the noncardiac surgery, if such surgery can be safely delayed.

  b. **High-risk patients**
   (1) Delay elective surgery.
   (2) If the patient is unstable, treat the cardiovascular condition as indicated.
   (3) If the patient is stable, consider one of the following approaches:
      (a) Proceed with coronary angiography and revascularization if indicated, independent of the noncardiac surgery.
      (b) Optimize medical therapy and re-evaluate the patient in several weeks, or proceed with prophylactic coronary angiography and revascularization.

B. Congestive heart failure (CHF)
  1. **Risk evaluation.** Decompensated CHF, manifested by an elevated jugular venous pressure, an audible third heart sound (S_3), or evidence of pulmonary edema on physical examination or a chest radiograph significantly increases the patient's risk of perioperative pulmonary edema and cardiac death.
  2. **Perioperative management.** Preoperative control of CHF, including the use of diuretics and afterload-reducing agents, is likely to reduce the perioperative risk.

HOT

KEY

Be careful not to overdiurese patients with CHF prior to surgery, because volume-depleted patients are much more susceptible to intraoperative hypotension.

C. Valvular heart disease
  1. **Risk evaluation.** Patients with severe symptomatic aortic stenosis are clearly at increased risk for cardiac complications.
  2. **Perioperative management.** Candidates for valve replacement surgery or balloon valvuloplasty should have the corrective procedure performed prior to the noncardiac surgery.

D. Rhythm disturbances
  1. **Risk evaluation.** Rhythm disturbances are frequently associated with underlying structural heart disease, especially CAD and left ventricular dysfunction. Patients found to have a rhythm disturbance without

evidence of underlying heart disease are at very low risk for perioperative cardiac complications.

2. **Perioperative management.** Management of patients with arrhythmias in the preoperative period is similar to that for nonsurgical patients. Patients who have indications for a permanent pacemaker should have it placed prior to noncardiac surgery.

E. **Hypertension**
  1. **Risk evaluation**
     a. **Severe hypertension** (i.e., a systolic pressure greater than 200 mm Hg or a diastolic pressure greater than 110 mm Hg) appears to increase the risk of perioperative cardiac complications.
     b. **Mild** to **moderate hypertension** in the preoperative period does not appear to increase cardiac complication rates.
  2. **Perioperative management**
     a. In patients with severe hypertension, blood pressure should be controlled prior to surgery (e.g., with intravenous agents, such as nitroprusside or labetalol).
     b. Medication changes in patients with mild to moderate hypertension are generally not recommended immediately prior to surgery. However, chronic medications for hypertension should be continued up to and including the day of surgery.

IV PRE-EXISTING PULMONARY DISEASE

A. **Risk evaluation.** The **risk factors** for developing a pulmonary complication include the following:
  1. **Planned cardiac, thoracic,** or **upper abdominal surgery**
  2. **Chronic obstructive pulmonary disease (COPD) or asthma,** particularly in patients with a forced expiratory volume in 1 second (FEV_1) of less than 500 ml or an arterial carbon dioxide tension ($PaCO_2$) of more than 45 mm Hg
  3. **Obesity** (weight greater than 250 pounds)
  4. **Cigarette smoking** (current or past)

B. **Perioperative management**
  1. **Smokers.** The risk of pulmonary complications appears to be lessened when the following measures are taken:
     a. **Smoking cessation** for at least 8 weeks prior to surgery
     b. **Incentive spirometry** and **deep breathing exercises,** performed for at least 15 minutes 4 times daily, begun preoperatively and continued for 3–5 days into the postoperative period
  2. **Patients with COPD** or **asthma.** Bronchodilator therapy, short-term corticosteroid therapy, and antibiotic therapy (in patients with purulent sputum) may opti-

mize pulmonary function and reduce the rate of pulmonary complications.

V PRE-EXISTING HEPATIC DISEASE

A. **Cirrhosis.** In patients with cirrhosis, the degree of hepatic dysfunction roughly correlates with surgical outcomes.
   1. **Risk evaluation.** Class A cirrhosis (using Child's or Pugh's classification scheme) is associated with a mortality rate of less than 10%, while class C cirrhosis is associated with a mortality rate as high as 50%.
   2. **Perioperative management.** A conservative approach would be to avoid elective surgery in patients with severe hepatic dysfunction.

B. **Hepatitis**
   1. **Acute viral or alcoholic hepatitis.** Although data are limited, it appears that patients with acute viral or alcoholic hepatitis are at substantial risk for major complications (e.g., liver failure) during and after surgery. Elective surgery should be delayed at least until the acute episode has resolved.
   2. **Symptomatic chronic hepatitis.** Patients may be at increased risk for perioperative complications and mortality. A prudent course would be to avoid elective surgery in these patients, although delaying urgent or emergent surgery is not supported by the available data.

VI PRE-EXISTING HEMATOLOGIC DISEASE

A. **Anemia**
   1. **Risk evaluation.** When feasible, evaluation of the patient for anemia should be performed prior to surgery because certain types of anemia (particularly hemolytic anemias) may have implications for perioperative management. The morbidity and mortality rates associated with surgery increase as the preoperative hemoglobin level decreases, especially to levels below 9 g/dl.
   2. **Perioperative management.** When considering preoperative transfusion, one must consider factors other than the absolute hemoglobin level, including the presence of cardiopulmonary disease, the type of surgery, and the likelihood of surgical blood loss.

B. **Bleeding disorders**
   1. If there is no history of abnormal bleeding, no family history of bleeding disorders, and no indication of abnormal bleeding on physical examination, the patient's risk of having an occult bleeding disorder is very low. Laboratory tests of hemostatic parameters in these patients are generally not needed.
   2. When the bleeding history is unreliable or incomplete or abnormal bleeding is suggested, a formal evaluation of hemostasis should be performed prior to surgery.

This evaluation should include the prothrombin time (PT), the partial thromboplastin time (PTT), the platelet count, and the bleeding time.

 VII **PRE-EXISTING VASCULAR DISEASE.** Patients who undergo cardiac or peripheral vascular surgery and those with severe symptomatic carotid stenoses are at risk for perioperative stroke.

A. Patients who are already candidates for carotid endarterectomy (e.g., those with severe symptomatic carotid stenosis) should undergo this surgery prior to having other, elective surgery.

B. Asymptomatic carotid bruits or stenoses are associated with little or no increased risk of postoperative stroke; therefore, prophylactic carotid endarterectomy in these patients is unlikely to be beneficial.

VIII **PRE-EXISTING ENDOCRINE DISEASE**

A. Diabetes mellitus. In patients with diabetes, the maintenance of normal glucose levels during the perioperative period is challenging. Although the ideal blood glucose level during surgery is not known, maintaining a blood glucose level of 100–250 mg/dl is usually recommended.

  1. Management of patients with diabetes that is controlled by diet alone
    a. Avoid administration of glucose-containing solutions during surgery.
    b. Measure the blood glucose level every 4–6 hours throughout the procedure.

  2. Management of patients with diabetes that is controlled by oral agents
    a. Discontinue the oral agent 1 day prior to surgery.
    b. Measure the blood glucose level every 6 hours in the preoperative period and administer regular insulin subcutaneously as needed to maintain a blood glucose level of less than 250 mg/dl.
    c. Measure the blood glucose level every 4–6 hours (or more frequently as indicated) during surgery.
    d. While the patient is fasting, infuse 5% glucose-containing solution at a rate of approximately 100 ml/hour and continue until the patient resumes eating. Resume oral hypoglycemic therapy when the patient returns to his baseline diet.

  3. Management of patients with diabetes that is controlled by insulin is summarized in Table 2-3.

B. Adrenocortical insufficiency. Very rarely, patients with primary or secondary adrenocortical insufficiency develop perioperative complications (usually **hypotension).**

  1. Risk evaluation. There is no consensus regarding the identification of patients at risk for having adrenocortical insufficiency. The most conservative approach is

TABLE 2-3. Perioperative Management of Patients with Diabetes That is Controlled by Insulin

Method	Administration of Insulin and Intravenous Glucose	Blood Glucose Monitoring
Subcutaneous insulin	Administer one half to two thirds of the usual dose of insulin on the morning of surgery Infuse 5% glucose-containing solution at a rate of at least 100 ml/hour, beginning on the morning of surgery and continuing until the patient resumes eating	Every 2–4 hours, beginning the morning of surgery
Continuous intravenous insulin infusion in glucose-containing solution	Infuse 5%–10% glucose-containing solution containing 5–15 U regular insulin per liter of solution at a rate of 100 ml/hour* on the morning of surgery; additional insulin may be added as needed to maintain a blood glucose level of less than 250 mg/dl	Every 2–4 hours during intravenous insulin infusion
Separate intravenous insulin and glucose infusions	Infuse intravenous regular insulin at a rate of 0.15–1.5 U/hour (dose may be adjusted as needed to maintain a blood glucose level of less than 250 mg/dl) Infuse 5%–10% glucose-containing solution at a rate of 100 ml/hour	Every 2–4 hours during intravenous insulin infusion

*This combination provides 0.5–1.5 U of insulin per hour

to consider any patient who has received either the equivalent of 20 mg of prednisone daily for 1 week or the equivalent of 7.5 mg of prednisone daily for 1 month within the past year to be at risk for having adrenocortical insufficiency.

2. **Perioperative management.** A commonly used replacement regimen is 100 mg of hydrocortisone given intravenously every 8 hours, beginning on the morning of surgery and continuing for 48–72 hours. Tapering the dose is not necessary.

C. **Hypothyroidism**
1. **Severe hypothyroidism.** Patients with severe hypothyroidism are at risk for **intraoperative hypotension.** Elective surgery should be delayed in patients with severe hypothyroidism until adequate thyroid hormone replacement can be achieved. Adequate thyroid hormone replacement usually requires at least 1 month.
2. **Mild or asymptomatic hypothyroidism.** Patients with asymptomatic or mild hypothyroidism generally tolerate surgery well. In these patients, surgery need not be delayed.

IX PRE-EXISTING RENAL DISEASE

A. **Risk evaluation.** The **risk factors** for postoperative deterioration of renal function include:
1. Aortic or cardiac surgery
2. Preoperative jaundice
3. Advanced age
4. Preoperative renal insufficiency

B. **Perioperative management**
1. In patients with risk factors for postoperative deterioration of renal function, it is important to maintain adequate intravascular volume during the perioperative period.
2. Patients with end-stage renal disease should receive dialysis within 24 hours of undergoing surgery. Their serum electrolyte levels should be measured just prior to surgery and monitored closely during the postoperative period.

References

Dashe JF, Pessin MS, Murphy RE, et al: Carotid occlusive disease and stroke risk in coronary artery bypass graft surgery. *Neurology* 49(3):678–686, 1996.

Eagle KA, Brundage BH, Chaitman BR, et al: Guidelines for perioperative cardiovascular evaluation for noncardiac surgery. Report of the American College of Cardiology/American Heart Association Task Force on Practice Guidelines. Committee on Perioperative Cardiovascular Evaluation for Noncardiac Surgery. *Circulation* 93(6):1278–1317, 1996.

Lawrence VA, Dhanda R, Hilsenbeck SG, et al: Risk of pulmonary complications after elective abdominal surgery. *Chest* 110(3):744–750, 1996.

Mangano DT, Goldman L: Preoperative assessment of patients with known or suspected coronary artery disease. *N Engl J Med* 333(26):1750–1756, 1995.

Schiff RL, Emanuele MA: The surgical patient with diabetes mellitus: guidelines for management. *J Gen Intern Med* 10(3):154–161, 1995.

3. Pain Management

....

I. INTRODUCTION

A. **Incidence.** Roughly one third of the population of the United States will experience chronic pain during their lifetimes. Surveys of patients and providers have shown that chronic pain is frequently underrecognized and undertreated.

B. **Causes.** The causes of chronic pain are varied. Common causes include cancer, osteoarthritis, osteoporosis, and neuropathy.

II. CLINICAL MANIFESTATIONS OF PAIN

A. **Acute pain** is often associated with autonomic signs, including tachycardia, hypertension, mydriasis, pallor, and perspiration.

B. **Chronic pain** can be associated with signs of depression (including hopelessness), anhedonia, insomnia, weight change, and social isolation.

III. APPROACH TO THE PATIENT

A. **Identify the cause.** Always strive to identify the source of pain and explain the cause to the patient.

B. **Assess the severity of the pain.** Have the patient rate the pain on a scale of 0–10 (0 = no pain, 10 = worst pain ever). Pain ratings of 1–4 are considered mild, 5–6 are considered moderate, and 7–10 are considered severe.

HOT

Remember that pain is entirely subjective and that different patients will experience different levels of pain in similar situations.

KEY

IV. TREATMENT.
The goal of treatment is to reduce pain as much as possible while limiting side effects from medications.

A. **Pharmacologic therapy.** In 1986, the World Health Organization (WHO) released a set of guidelines for treating patients with chronic pain from cancer. This **three-step system** is a useful guide for treating chronic pain from all causes. Tables 3-1 through 3-3 list the most commonly used agents; there are many other agents in these classes that are also effective and useful for certain patients.

1. **Step 1.** For patients with mild to moderate pain and no prior treatment, start with a step 1 agent (see Table 3-1). The choice of medications depends on the side effect profile and the patient's medical history.
2. **Step 2.** If the pain is not adequately controlled with a step 1 agent, move to a step 2 agent (see Table 3-2) and then reassess.
3. **Step 3.** If the pain cannot be controlled with a step 2 agent, move to a step 3 agent (see Table 3-3).

B. General guidelines
1. **Move quickly to eliminate pain.** For patients with severe pain, start with a step 2 or step 3 agent.
2. **Schedule the doses.** In patients with chronic pain, scheduled dosing of pain medications is preferred over as-needed therapy. Scheduled dosing helps the patient erase the memory and expectation of pain.
3. **Monitor response to therapy** using the 0–10 numerical scale. Patients who are undertreated may not understand that better pain relief is available.
4. **Allow the patient to decide the level of pain control.** Some patients may prefer to have a little more pain and be less sedated, while others will prefer the opposite. Use the dose of medication that reduces pain to an acceptable level and minimizes side effects. There is no maximum dose for step 3 agents.
5. **Anticipate the need for stool softeners and laxatives in patients taking opiates.**
6. **Opt for the administration route that is easiest for the patient.** Oral or transdermal administration of medications is preferred.
   a. The **oral route** is simple and inexpensive, and permits rapid adjustment of doses.
   b. The **transdermal route** provides steady drug levels and obviates the need for frequent pill taking.
   c. The **rectal** or **sublingual routes** can be used in patients who are unable to take oral or transdermal medicines.
   d. The **subcutaneous** and **intravenous routes** are used for patients with pain refractory to all other methods.

C. Nonpharmacologic therapy. Massage, biofeedback, relax-

TABLE 3-1. Step 1 Agents: Nonopioid Analgesics

Agent	Equianalgesic Dose	Interval	Cautions
Acetaminophen	650 mg	Every 4–6 hours	Do not exceed 4 g in 24 hours. Avoid in patients with liver disease.
Aspirin	650 mg	Every 4–6 hours	Avoid in pregnant women, patients with gastrointestinal bleeding or bleeding disorders, postoperative patients, and patients younger than 18 years
NSAIDs*			Monitor for gastropathy, renal dysfunction, and bleeding.
Ibuprofen	400 mg	Every 6–8 hours	
Naproxen	375 mg	Every 12 hours	

Modified with permission from World Health Organization: Cancer pain relief and palliative care: report of a WHO expert committee, technical report series 804. Geneva, Switzerland, World Health Organization, 1990.

NSAIDs = nonsteroidal anti-inflammatory drugs.

*NSAIDs other than the two examples given here are available.

TABLE 3-2. Step 2 Agents: Opioid Analgesics for Mild to Moderate Pain

Agent	Equianalgesic Dose	Interval	Usual Dosage Form
Codeine	30–60 mg	Every 4–6 hours	Tylenol #3: acetaminophen, 325 mg, plus codeine, 30 mg
Hydrocodone	5–10 mg	Every 4–6 hours	Vicodin: acetaminophen, 500 mg, plus hydrocodone, 5 mg
Oxycodone	5–10 mg	Every 6 hours	Percodan: acetylsalicylic acid, 325 mg, plus oxycodone, 5 mg Percocet: acetaminophen, 325 mg, plus oxycodone, 5 mg

Modified with permission from World Health Organization: Cancer pain relief and palliative care: report of a WHO expert committee, technical report series 804. Geneva, Switzerland, World Health Organization, 1990.

TABLE 3-3. Step 3 Agents: Opioid Analgesics for Moderate to Severe Pain

Agent	Equianalgesic Dose	Interval	Administration Route
Morphine*			
Short-acting	30 mg	Every 3–4 hours	Orally
Long-acting	90 mg	Every 12 hours	Orally
Hydromorphone†	7.5 mg	Every 3–4 hours	Orally
Fentanyl‡	25–50 μg	Every 72 hours	Transdermal patch

Modified with permission from World Health Organization: Cancer pain relief and palliative care: report of a WHO expert committee, technical report series 804. Geneva, Switzerland, World Health Organization, 1990.
*Start with a rapid-acting preparation, then divide 24-hour total dose into two or three sustained-release doses. Continue administration of the rapid-acting preparation for breakthrough episodes.
†Hydromorphone has no specific advantage over morphine.
‡Maximum effect is achieved only after 24 hours. Fentanyl has a long half-life (because the drug is absorbed by the skin and then slowly released into the blood stream) and is an excellent choice for patients who cannot take oral medications.

ation and visualization, transcutaneous electrical nerve stimulation, acupuncture, and other treatments may help patients reduce or replace their dose of oral analgesics.

D. Special situations

   1. **Neuropathic pain** (see also Chapter 66) is caused by damage to central or peripheral nervous system structures and is associated with a variety of conditions, including diabetes, alcoholism, AIDS, cancer, and amputation.

      a. The pain is usually described as **"tingling,"** **"burning," "electric,"** or **"needle-like."**

      b. Patients with neuropathic pain often respond to adjuvant agents (Table 3-4). Use of these agents can limit the use of step 2 and step 3 agents.

         (1) **Tricyclic antidepressants** are considered **first-line agents** for neuropathic pain.

         (2) **Capsaicin cream** is a substance P inhibitor that may improve pain when applied topically.

   2. **Cancer pain.** A number of specialized treatments are available for patients with cancer pain.

TABLE 3-4. Agents for Neuropathic Pain

Agent	Starting Dose
Tricyclic antidepressants*	
Nortriptyline	10–25 mg at bedtime; increase as tolerated
Desipramine	10–25 mg at bedtime; increase as tolerated
Anticonvulsants	
Carbamazepine†	200 mg twice daily
Clonazepam	0.5 mg three times daily
Mexiletine	150 mg three times daily
Capsaicin 0.025% cream	Three times daily
Gabapentin	300 mg at bedtime on day #1; increase to 300–600 mg three times daily over a few days

*Both nortriptyline and desipramine have fewer side effects than amitriptyline.
†Blood counts should be monitored in patients taking carbamazepine because of the risk of bone marrow suppression.

a. **Nerve compression and central nervous system (CNS) metastases.** Pain may be relieved by **nonsteroidal anti-inflammatory drugs (NSAIDs)** and **steroids.**

b. **Bony metastases.** Pain from bony metastases may be reduced by **pamidronate, strontium chloride,** and **calcitonin.**

V **FOLLOW-UP AND REFERRAL** Patients should be seen as often as necessary to ensure rapid and optimum pain control. Some patients may need to be referred to specialists.

A. Patients with unusual pain syndromes and those who do not respond to the standard treatment approach can be referred to a **specialized pain control center.**

B. Patients with pain from cancer should be referred to an **oncologist** for advice about chemotherapy, radiation therapy, and adjuvant agents.

C. Patients with known cancer and new back pain should be referred to a **radiologist** immediately. These patients require magnetic resonance imaging (MRI) of the spine to rule out spinal cord compression.

References

Levy MH: Pharmacologic treatment of cancer pain. *N Engl J Med* 335(15):1124–32, 1995.

World Health Organization: Cancer pain relief and palliative care: report of a WHO expert committee, technical report series 804. Geneva, Switzerland, World Health Organization, 1990.

4. Preventive Medicine

I INTRODUCTION

A. Forms of preventive medicine. Prevention of illness takes three forms: primary prevention, secondary prevention, and tertiary prevention. This chapter focuses on primary and secondary prevention of disease. Tertiary prevention is covered in the chapters that discuss specific diseases.

1. **Primary prevention** is the **prevention of disease.** Interventions used to achieve primary prevention include the following:

    a. **Immunization** reduces the patient's susceptibility to certain infectious diseases.

    b. **Counseling** involves patient education with the goal of changing a patient's high-risk behavior in order to prevent disease before it occurs.

    c. **Prophylactic drug therapy.** Certain medications can reduce the patient's risk of developing a disease [e.g., hormone replacement therapy (HRT) can prevent osteoporosis in postmenopausal women].

2. **Secondary prevention** is the **detection and treatment of disease in asymptomatic patients and in patients who have developed risk factors for a disease.** The goal is to cure or control the disease and risk factors in order to prevent complications from developing [e.g., treating hypertension before it leads to coronary artery disease (CAD)]. Secondary prevention is accomplished through **screening** for asymptomatic disease and risk factors (e.g., a Pap smear can detect cervical dysplasia at an early stage, thereby preventing the development of invasive cancer).

3. **Tertiary prevention** is the prevention of complications caused by a disease already established in the patient (e.g., the prevention of retinopathy in a patient with diabetes).

B. Sources of recommendations

1. **United States Preventive Services Task Force (USP-STF).** The preventive services recommended in this chapter are based on the recommendations made by the USPSTF in *Guide to Clinical Preventive Services: Report of the US Preventive Services Task Force,* 2nd

edition (Baltimore, Williams & Wilkins, 1996). This group takes a systematic approach to evaluating the effectiveness of clinical preventive services, and their recommendations and review of the evidence are based on a predetermined methodology. Using this evidence-based technique, they recommend only those interventions that have documented effectiveness.

2. Two other organizations, the **Canadian Task Force on Periodic Health Examination (CTFPHE)** and the **American College of Physicians (ACP),** take an approach similar to that of the USPSTF and make similar recommendations.

II   IMMUNIZATIONS. The recommended adult immunizations are given in the prevention checklists that appear at the end of the chapter (Tables 4-1 and 4-2). Certain patients are at particularly high risk for contracting certain diseases; for these patients, immunization is critical.

A. Influenza A virus. Individuals at high risk include:
1. Residents of chronic care facilities
2. Healthcare providers seeing high-risk patients
3. Patients with chronic cardiopulmonary disorders, metabolic disorders (including diabetes), hemoglobinopathies, immunosuppression, or renal dysfunction

B. Pneumococcal pneumonia. Individuals at high risk include:
1. Institutionalized patients who are older than 50 years
2. Patients with chronic cardiopulmonary disease, diabetes mellitus, or anatomic asplenia [excluding sickle cell disease (SCD)]
3. Patients with special high-risk living situations (e.g., Native American or Alaska Native populations)
4. Immunocompromised patients

C. Hepatitis A. Individuals at high risk include:
1. Young adults not previously immunized
2. Homosexual men
3. Injection drug users and their sex partners
4. Patients with a history of multiple sex partners in the past 6 months and those who have recently acquired a sexually transmitted disease (STD)
5. Travelers to endemic areas
6. Recipients of blood products
7. Healthcare workers who are exposed to blood

D. Hepatitis B. Individuals at high risk include:
1. Travelers to endemic areas

2. Homosexual men
3. Injection drug users
4. Military personnel
5. Institutionalized patients
6. Certain hospital and laboratory workers

III COUNSELING

A. **Cessation of tobacco use.** Convincing a patient to stop smoking is likely the most valuable method of disease prevention in adults. Counseling to stop smoking should be given to all smokers, and counseling to avoid starting should be given to all non-smokers.
   1. Specialized or group counseling may be useful and should be offered if it is available.
   2. Nicotine gum or patches may be a useful adjunct.

B. **Importance of physical activity.** All patients should be counseled to engage in regular physical activity, ideally 30 minutes or more of moderate activity on all or most days of the week. Exercise programs should take into consideration the patient's medical problems and her exercise preferences.

C. **Diet.** All patients should be advised to reduce their intake of dietary fat to less than 30% of their total daily caloric intake (saturated fat should be less than 10% of the total daily caloric intake).
   1. Fruits, vegetables, grain products containing fiber, fish, poultry without skin, and low-fat dairy products should be emphasized.
   2. Specialized counseling by dieticians and nutritionists may be useful, especially for patients who are having difficulty or who have other diet-related conditions (e.g., CAD, diabetes, obesity).

D. **Contraception and prevention of STDs.** Counseling about risk factors for HIV and other STDs should be given to all patients.
   1. All patients of reproductive age should be advised about effective methods of contraception (see Chapter 50).
   2. Effective methods of preventing HIV and other STDs include abstinence, a mutually monogamous relationship between partners known to be free of HIV or other STDs, use of a latex condom, and avoidance of high-risk partners.

E. **Prevention of motor vehicle accidents**
   1. All patients should be counseled about wearing seat

belts (lap and shoulder, even if an air bag is present), properly using child safety seats, and not driving under the influence of alcohol or drugs.

   2. Motorcyclists should be advised to wear approved helmets.

F. Prevention of household and recreational injuries
   1. Prevention of household injuries
      a. All households. Smoke detectors should be installed and checked at regular intervals.
      b. Households with children. Parents should be encouraged to review safety recommendations with their child's pediatrician. Some safety measures include:
         (1) Setting hot water heaters at 120°–130° F
         (2) Putting children to bed in flame-resistant night clothing
         (3) Keeping medicines, cleaning supplies, and other toxic substances out of reach of children and in child-resistant containers
         (4) Keeping a fresh 1-ounce bottle of syrup of ipecac on hand
         (5) Displaying emergency telephone numbers
         (6) Installing fences around pools, windows, and stairs that pose a risk for falls
      c. Households with elderly family members
         (1) Elderly patients may benefit from counseling about reducing the risk of falling. Effective approaches include installing railings, ensuring that lighting is adequate, and completing balance training.
         (2) For frail patients, specialized programs or in-home "safety-checks" may be useful.
   2. Prevention of recreational injuries. All patients who bicycle, in-line skate, or ride all-terrain vehicles should be encouraged to wear helmets.

G. Dental care. Patients should be encouraged to have regular check-ups with a dentist and to follow good dental hygiene habits.

IV PROPHYLACTIC MEDICATIONS

A. Aspirin reduces the risk of a first myocardial infarction in men older than 50 years, but it increases the risk of bleeding. Although the USPSTF does not recommend for or against the use of aspirin for the primary prevention of myocardial infarction, asymptomatic patients with other risk factors for myocardial infarction and without contraindications to aspirin use can be considered for prophylactic treatment. Treatment decisions should be based on analysis and discussion of the risks and benefits with the patient.

B. Hormone replacement therapy (HRT) may be indicated for some postmenopausal women. Many factors influence the decision to initiate HRT; the likely risks and benefits of treatment must be considered for each patient. Women who are experiencing menopausal symptoms or who are at high risk for osteoporosis stand to benefit the most from treatment. Women who are especially concerned about breast cancer or who experience side effects from HRT may prefer not to be treated.

1. **Benefits.** Probable benefits of HRT include:
   a. Decreased menopausal symptoms (for symptomatic patients)
   b. Decreased risk of bony fractures
2. **Risks.** Possible risks of HRT include:
   a. Increased risk of endometrial cancer if unopposed estrogen is used
   b. Increased risk of breast cancer in some patients

C. Multivitamin or **folic acid supplementation** may be indicated for women considering or capable of pregnancy.

1. In order to reduce the risk of neural tube defects in the fetus, the USPSTF recommends that women who are planning pregnancy take a multivitamin containing 0.4–0.8 mg of folic acid daily, beginning at least 1 month prior to conception and continuing through the first trimester.
2. Women who are capable of pregnancy should take a multivitamin containing 0.4 mg of folic acid daily to prevent neural tube defects in the event of an unplanned pregnancy.

V **SCREENING**

A. Screening for cardiovascular disease
1. **Hypertension** (see also Chapter 16). **Office sphygmomanometry** can accurately detect hypertension. Treatment of hypertension has been shown to reduce overall mortality as well as morbidity and mortality due to stroke and ischemic heart disease.
   a. Treatment is effective for both young and elderly patients.
   b. Patients at high risk for complications from hy-

pertension (e.g., patients with diabetes or hyper-cholesterolemia) should be considered for early, aggressive therapy.

2. **Hypercholesterolemia.** Providers may choose to use the **total cholesterol level** as an initial screen. The **high-density lipoprotein (HDL)** and **low-density lipoprotein (LDL) levels** can then be obtained in patients with a high total cholesterol level to further clarify the situation.

   a. It is reasonable to screen asymptomatic men between the ages of 35 and 65 years once every 5 years. Screening for asymptomatic women should begin at age 45 and take place every 5 years.

   b. Patients with multiple risk factors for CAD, or patients with borderline high test results can be considered for more frequent screening.

B. **Screening for cancer**

   1. **Cervical cancer.** Screening for cervical cancer is one of the great success stories of medical prevention. Since the implementation of widespread screening programs several decades ago, there has been a dramatic reduction in the number of women who have died from cervical cancer. All women should undergo a **Pap smear** at the **onset of sexual activity,** and then **once every 1–3 years thereafter.**

      a. Patients with multiple risk factors (early age at the onset of sexual intercourse, multiple sex partners, low socioeconomic status) should probably be screened annually, while patients without risk factors may be candidates for screening every 3 years.

      b. Patients who have had their cervix removed do not require screening (unless it was removed because of cervical cancer).

   2. **Breast cancer.** Screening techniques include **mammography** and **clinical breast examination.**

      a. **Women 50–69 years of age.** The efficacy of annual or biannual mammography is well documented and should be recommended to all patients. An annual or biannual clinical breast examination may also be performed at the discretion of the provider for women in this age group.

      b. **Women younger than 50 years.** Mammography has not been shown to be of clear benefit for these patients, but it may be reasonable to screen women with multiple risk factors or those who wish to be screened after discussing the risks and benefits. The effect of annual or biannual clinical breast examination without mammography is also unclear, but may be performed at the discretion of the provider.

    c. **Women older than 69 years.** Providers may choose to screen women older than 69 years, especially those patients who do not have significant comorbid disease.

  3. **Colorectal cancer.** All patients older than 50 years should be screened via **fecal occult blood testing, periodic flexible sigmoidoscopy,** or both.

    a. Fecal occult blood testing should be performed annually. Flexible sigmoidoscopy should be performed every 3–5 years.

    b. Patients with a history of familial syndromes of colon cancer, ulcerative colitis, previous colonic polyps, or colon cancer require more frequent screening and expert consultation.

  4. **Other types of cancer.** Screening tests are available for a number of other kinds of cancer (e.g., prostate, lung, ovarian, testicular, bladder, pancreatic, oral, thyroid, and skin cancers). The current USPSTF guidelines do not include screening tests for these cancers, owing to either insufficient evidence of the efficacy of screening or evidence that the screening was not effective. Providers may wish to review the information and develop their own interpretations.

C. **Screening for other health problems**

  1. **Obesity. Periodic height** and **weight determinations** are recommended as a screening test for obesity. Although weight loss alone has not been shown conclusively to decrease mortality, it has been demonstrated to reduce the risk of developing cardiovascular disease and other health problems.

  2. **Problem drinking.** Screening for problem drinking and brief counseling can reduce the amount of alcohol consumed by patients. Several questionnaires are available (see Chapter 89).

  3. **Vision and hearing impairment.** Screening for visual impairment and hearing difficulty in the elderly may improve the patient's quality of life and prevent injury.

VI **PREVENTIVE MEDICINE CHECKLISTS.** The checklists in Tables 4-1 and 4-2 (for women and men, respectively) have been developed based on the USPSTF guidelines. Several points about these checklists are important to remember:

A. **These checklists are not comprehensive** and **should be modified to suit the individual needs of each patient.** Patients in certain high-risk groups require additional preventive services (e.g., intravenous drug users should be offered HIV screening). Primary care providers should review the information in the USPSTF *Guide to Clinical Preventive Services* to determine which preventive services they should offer to their patients.

B. **The checklists deal only with primary and secondary prevention in adults.** Patients with known disease often require additional preventive services (i.e., tertiary prevention), and the checklists can be updated to reflect those needs (e.g., annual screening for microalbuminuria to detect nephropathy in a patient with diabetes).

C. **There are a number of preventive services that are available, but that have not been recommended by the USPSTF owing to inconclusive evidence** (e.g., screening for testicular cancer with a periodic physical examination). Providers may decide, after reviewing the evidence, that some of these services should be provided to their patients.

D. **Checklists are only useful if they are actually used.** These lists, or similar ones created by the primary care provider, should be posted in each patient's chart. Providers with access to computer charting may want to incorporate these checklists into a program that reminds providers when preventive services should be given.

References
United States Preventive Services Task Force: *Guide to Clinical Preventive Services,* 2nd ed. Baltimore, Williams & Wilkins, 1996.

TABLE 4-1. Preventive Medicine Checklist for Asymptomatic Women

IMMUNIZATIONS
- [ ] **Influenza A vaccine:** Age $\geq$ 65 years or at high risk*, **annually**
- [ ] **Pneumococcal vaccine:** Age $\geq$ 65 years or at high risk†, **once every 5–10 years**
- [ ] **Diphtheria tetanus (DT) vaccine:** Ensure completed series; **booster every 10 years**
- [ ] **Measles-mumps-rubella (MMR) vaccine:** Women born after 1956 who lack evidence of immunity
- [ ] **Hepatitis A vaccine:** Young women not previously immunized, and women at high risk‡
- [ ] **Hepatitis B vaccine:** Women at high risk§
- [ ] **Varicella vaccine:** Healthy women with no history of previous varicella infection
- [ ] **Rubella vaccine:** Women of childbearing age (alternative is to screen, then vaccinate as needed)

COUNSELING
- [ ] Cessation of tobacco use
- [ ] Regular physical activity
- [ ] Diet
- [ ] Contraception and prevention of sexually transmitted disease
- [ ] Dental care
- [ ] Prevention of motor vehicle accidents
- [ ] Prevention of household and recreational injuries

PROPHYLACTIC MEDICATIONS TO CONSIDER
- [ ] Hormone replacement therapy (postmenopausal women)
- [ ] Aspirin (women at high risk for myocardial infarction)
- [ ] Multivitamin or folic acid supplementation (women considering or capable of pregnancy)

SCREENING
- [ ] **Hypertension:** Evaluate blood pressure in all women 21 years or older, at **each visit** and **at least every 2 years**
- [ ] **Elevated cholesterol:** Evaluate cholesterol in all women age 45–65 years, **at least every 5 years**
- [ ] **Breast cancer:** Mammogram $+/-$ clinical breast exam for all women age 50–69 years, **annually** or **binannually**

continued

TABLE 4-1. Preventive Medicine Checklist for Asymptomatic Women

☐ **Colorectal cancer:** Annual fecal occult blood test $+/-$ sigmoidoscopy for all women 50 years or older, at **3- to 5-year intervals**

☐ **Cervical cancer:** Pap smear **at onset of sexual activity** and **at least every 3 years**

☐ **Obesity:** Periodic height and weight determinations

☐ **Sexually transmitted disease**
   Chlamydia trachomatis: Annual cervical culture or nonculture assay for all sexually active female adolescents
   Neisseria gonorrhoeae: Annual cervical culture for all high-risk women[||]

☐ **Problem drinking:** History and questionnaire

☐ **Hearing and vision:** Elderly women

PATIENT-SPECIFIC PREVENTIVE SERVICES

☐ _____
☐ _____
☐ _____
☐ _____

---

*Residents of chronic care facilities; healthcare providers seeing high-risk patients; patients with chronic cardiopulmonary disorders, metabolic disorders (including diabetes), hemoglobinopathies, immunosuppression, or renal dysfunction

[†]Institutionalized patients who are older than 50 years; those with chronic cardiopulmonary disease, diabetes mellitus, or anatomic asplenia (excluding sickle cell disease); those with special high-risk living situations; immunocompromised patients

[‡]Injection drug users and their sex partners; patients with a history of multiple sex partners in the past 6 months; patients who have recently acquired a sexually transmitted disease (STD); travelers to endemic areas; recipients of blood products; healthcare workers who are exposed to blood

[§]Travelers to endemic areas; injection drug users; military personnel; institutionalized patients; certain hospital and laboratory workers

[||]Commercial sex workers; women with a history of frequent *N. gonorrhoeae* infection; women younger than 25 years with a history of two or more sex partners in the last year

TABLE 4-2. Preventive Medicine Checklist for Asymptomatic Men

IMMUNIZATIONS
- [ ] **Influenza A vaccine:** Age $\geq$ 65 years or at high risk*, **annually**
- [ ] **Pneumococcal vaccine:** Age $\geq$ 65 years or at high risk[†], **once every 5 years**
- [ ] **Diphtheria tetanus (DT) vaccine:** Ensure completed series; **booster every 10 years**
- [ ] **Measles-mumps-rubella (MMR) vaccine:** Men born after 1956 who lack evidence of immunity
- [ ] **Hepatitis A vaccine:** Young men not previously immunized, and men at high risk[‡]
- [ ] **Hepatitis B vaccine:** Men at high risk[§]
- [ ] **Varicella vaccine:** Healthy men with no history of previous varicella infection

COUNSELING
- [ ] Cessation of tobacco use
- [ ] Regular physical activity
- [ ] Diet
- [ ] Contraception and prevention of sexually transmitted disease
- [ ] Dental care
- [ ] Prevention of motor vehicle accidents
- [ ] Prevention of household and recreational injuries

PROPHYLACTIC MEDICATIONS TO CONSIDER
- [ ] Aspirin (men at high risk for myocardial infarction)

SCREENING
- [ ] **Hypertension:** Evaluate blood pressure in all men 21 years or older, at **each visit** and **at least every 2 years**
- [ ] **Elevated cholesterol:** Evaluate cholesterol in all men age 35–65 years, **at least every 5 years**

continued

TABLE 4-2. Preventive Medicine Checklist for Asymptomatic Men

- ☐ **Colorectal cancer:** Annual fecal occult blood test +/− sigmoidoscopy for all men 50 years or older, at **3-** to **5-year intervals**
- ☐ **Obesity:** Periodic height and weight determinations
- ☐ **Problem drinking:** Use history and questionnaire
- ☐ **Hearing and vision:** Elderly men

PATIENT-SPECIFIC PREVENTIVE SERVICES

- ☐ _____
- ☐ _____
- ☐ _____
- ☐ _____

---

*Residents of chronic care facilities; healthcare providers seeing high-risk patients; patients with chronic cardiopulmonary disorders, metabolic disorders (including diabetes), hemoglobinopathies, immunosupression, or renal dysfunction

†Institutionalized patients who are older than 50 years; those with chronic cardiopulmonary disease, diabetes mellitus, or anatomic asplenia (excluding sickle cell disease); those with special high-risk living situations; immunocompromised patients

‡Homosexual men; injection drug users and their sex partners; patients with a history of multiple sex partners in the past 6 months; patients who have recently acquired a sexually transmitted disease; travelers to endemic areas; recipients of blood products; healthcare workers who are exposed to blood

§Travelers to endemic areas; homosexual men; injection drug users; military personnel; institutionalized patients; certain hospital and laboratory workers

Ophthalmology and Otolaryngology

5. Urgent Eye Complaints

I **INTRODUCTION.** Because some ophthalmologic conditions can threaten vision, internists must be able to recognize and triage serious eye problems within an appropriate time frame.

A. Incidence. Acute ophthalmologic problems account for **3%–10% of presentations** in emergency rooms, urgent care centers, and primary care offices.

B. Major complaints. Most eye problems involve one of three major complaints: **impaired vision, red** or **painful eye,** or **ocular trauma.**

II **APPROACH TO THE PATIENT**

A. Obtain a patient history. Be sure to note the following:

1. **Symptoms.** What is the major complaint (change in vision, change in eye appearance, discomfort, or trauma)? What other symptoms does the patient have?

2. **Exacerbating or inciting factors.** Do any factors exacerbate the condition (e.g., pupillary dilatation in darkness or constriction in bright light)? Can the patient link the onset of symptoms with a specific event?

3. **Time course.** When did the symptoms begin?

4. **Past medical history.** What is the patient's vision status and past medical history? For example, does the patient have a history of hypertension, a systemic disease with possible ocular manifestations, or a history of eye surgery?

5. **Tetanus status.** If eye trauma has occurred, has the patient had a tetanus shot within the past 10 years?

B. Perform a physical examination

HOT
KEY

Pupillary dilatation should occur at the end of the examination because you cannot assess visual acuity or pupillary responses in a dilated eye.

1. **Visual acuity survey.** Visual acuity is evaluated by using the **Snellen chart** and by asking the patient to count fingers, recognize motion, or assess light.

2. **Pupil examination.** The pupils' **size, shape,** and **reaction to direct and consensual light** should be noted.

3. **Adnexa and periorbital examination.** Evaluate the **lids, lashes,** and **orbital rim.**

4. **Neurologic examination. Facial** and **corneal nerve sensation** should be evaluated by lightly touching the face and eye with a cotton swab.

5. **Ocular mobility assessment.** Ask the patient to look up, down, and to each side.

6. **Visual field testing.** See if the patient can detect motion when you wiggle your fingers in the right and left upper and lower outer quadrants.

7. **Slit-lamp examination** is used to evaluate the cornea (using fluorescein stain) and the depth of the anterior chamber.

8. **Intraocular pressure evaluation.** Tonometry is contraindicated in patients with globe penetration, corneal abrasions, foreign bodies, trauma, or active infection.

9. **Direct ophthalmoscopy** allows the examiner to evaluate the red reflex, lens clarity, and the fundus. The red reflex is the reflection of the retinal vessels, which appear red in patients with a healthy eye during ophthalmoscopy.

C. **Treat or refer the patient to an ophthalmologist** as necessary. In general, consultation with an ophthalmologist is necessary if the patient's vision is acutely altered or threatened.

III **CAUSES OF IMPAIRED VISION.** Table 5-1 summarizes causes of acute vision loss that may result in permanent blindness if not adequately diagnosed and treated. Usually, the cause of a patient's vision loss can be traced back to one of six anatomic sites:

A. **Lens.** Acute lens refractive error is most often caused by wide fluctuations in the blood glucose level in patients with diabetes. Rarely, medications (e.g., thiazide diuretics) cause lens edema.

TABLE 5-1. Causes of Impaired Vision That Require Urgent Referral to an Ophthalmologist			
Disorder	History	Physical Examination and Laboratory Findings	Treatment
Retinal artery occlusion	Rapid, profound, painless monocular vision loss Typical patient is an elderly man More common in early morning	Examination may be normal in early stages Late-stage findings include a "milky" retina around the optic disk, a pale fundus, and a cherry-red macula	Immediately refer (irreversible blindness can occur within 90 minutes of the onset of symptoms)
Retinal vein occlusion	Past medical history of diabetes, hypertension, hyperviscosity, glaucoma, or mild vision loss (from macular edema)	"Blood and thunder" retina (diffuse retinal hemorrhages and venous dilatation; cotton-wool spots)	Refer within 24–48 hours Globe pressure/massage Have patient breathe into a paper bag to increase the $PaCO_2$

continued

TABLE 5-1. Causes of Impaired Vision That Require Urgent Referral to an Ophthalmologist			
Disorder	History	Physical Examination and Laboratory Findings	Treatment
Temporal arteritis	Headaches, pain with chewing, myalgias	Tender temporal arteries High sedimentation rate	Oral prednisone (60 mg daily) until temporal artery biopsy can be performed
Vitreous hemorrhage	Painless vision loss Risk factors include trauma, diabetes mellitus, and retinal tear	Absent red reflex (i.e., vessels appear dull or black)	Immediately refer; increased intraocular pressure can threaten retinal circulation Laser therapy (patients with proliferative retinopathy associated with diabetes mellitus)

| Retinal detachment | Acute "floaters," flashing lights, decreased or cloudy vision, "curtain" over the visual field
Risk factors include advanced age, myopia, and a history of ocular surgery or retinal degeneration | Detached retina may look like bulging, floating folds within the vitreous humor, or appear grey with black vessels | Immediately refer for photocoagulation, cryo-therapy, diathermy, scleral buckling, or air/silicon oil injections |
| Age-related macular degeneration | Sudden onset of central blurring or central distortion of straight lines
Sudden decompensation can result from macular hemorrhage, proliferative retinopathy, or trauma | Vision impairment is noted only in line of focus (peripheral vision is normal) | Refer within 48 hours for evaluation and possible laser therapy |

$PaCO_2$ = arterial carbon dioxide tension.

HOT

KEY

In patients with a lens refractive error, visual acuity improves when visual stimuli are filtered by having the patient look through a pinhole. Linear stimuli do not need to be refracted in order to reach the optic nerve; therefore, vision is clearer when the angled stimuli that would need refraction through a normal lens are eliminated.

   B. Media. Corneal opacity, lens opacity, and vitreous hemorrhage are examples of media abnormalities that can result in impaired vision.

HOT

KEY

On physical examination, the red reflex of the abnormal eye is darker or dulled when compared with that of the normal eye.

   C. Retina. Retinal artery or vein occlusion, retinal detachment, and macular disease are causes of acute vision loss that can result in permanent blindness if not quickly diagnosed and treated.
   D. Optic nerve. Damage to the optic nerve can be idiopathic, or it may result from any number of disorders that impair circulation, cause inflammation, or damage the optic nerve directly (e.g., multiple sclerosis, temporal arteritis).

HOT

KEY

Regardless of the cause, optic nerve damage results in afferent pupillary nerve defects on examination (i.e., both pupils may dilate slightly when a light is shined in the damaged eye).

   E. Optic chiasm. Impingement of the optic chiasm by a pituitary mass or infarct can result in bitemporal hemianopia (Figure 5-1).
   F. Area posterior to the optic chiasm. Loss of vision can also result from lesions of the lateral geniculate bodies, optic radiations, or the occipital cortex.

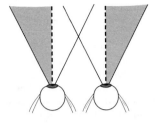
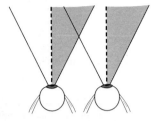

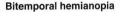

Bitemporal hemianopia   **Homonymous hemianopia**

FIGURE 5-1. Hemianopia.

HOT

KEY

Lesions posterior to the optic chiasm produce bilateral loss of vision on the same side of the vertical meridian (i.e., a homonymous hemianopia). Neurologic work-up [for cerebrovascular accident (CVA) or masses] is usually required.

 CAUSES OF RED EYE. A red eye is an extremely common complaint with multiple causes.

A. Blepharitis, hordeolum, chalazion, and **dacryocystitis** can usually be diagnosed by examining the lids and lashes.

1. **Blepharitis** is an inflammation of the eyelid margins, usually bilateral. The two most common causes are seborrhea, which causes greasy scales, and *Staphylococcus aureus* infection, which causes dry scales and more erythema.

2. A **hordeolum (stye)** is an acute inflammation of one of the glands lining the eyelid.

   a. An internal hordeolum results from inflammation of the meibomian glands and points toward the conjunctival surface.

   b. An external hordeolum results from inflammation of the Moll's glands or glands of Zeis and is located on the outer lid.

3. A **chalazion** is a chronic granulomatous inflammation of a meibomian gland. It is different from an internal hordeolum in terms of its time course (weeks versus days). Chalazia are usually painless and unaccompanied by signs of acute infection.

4. **Dacryocystitis** is an acute infection of the lacrimal

sac, usually caused by *S. aureus* or β-hemolytic *Strep-tococcus.* Dacryocystitis presents with swelling below the medial canaliculus, pain, and tearing. It may be possible to express pus from the lacrimal duct.

B. Conjunctivitis is the most common cause of red eye seen in urgent care centers. Conjunctivitis has multiple causes (Table 5-2), but the **physical examination findings (normal vision, minimal photophobia, conjunctival injection, eyelid edema, tearing, intact pupillary light reflex)** are often similar regardless of the cause. Often, the cause is revealed by the patient history.

    1. Bacterial conjunctivitis is most often caused by *Streptococcus pneumoniae, S. aureus, Haemophilus influenzae,* and *Neisseria gonorrhoeae.* Foreign bodies must be ruled out.

    2. Chlamydial conjunctivitis is caused by *Chlamydia trachomatis.* Chronic chlamydial conjunctivitis, called **trachoma,** is more prevalent in developing countries and can cause corneal scarring, cataracts, and blindness. Treatment is with a 6-week course of systemic and topical antibiotics.

    3. Viral conjunctivitis (pinkeye) is most often caused by **adenoviruses, coxsackieviruses,** and **picornaviruses.** Viral conjunctivitis is **highly contagious** and patients often report contact with a patient with similar symptoms.

    4. Allergic conjunctivitis is usually seen in patients with a history of seasonal allergies or atopic dermatitis.

C. Causes of red eye requiring urgent referral to an ophthalmologist are summarized in Table 5-3.

    1. Acute angle closure glaucoma results from the acute blockage of aqueous humor flow in patients with shallow anterior chamber angles. Attacks are usually precipitated by pupillary dilatation, which increases contact between the iris and lens. The increased contact blocks the flow of aqueous humor from the posterior to the anterior chamber (Figure 5-2), increasing the pressure behind the iris and causing the iris to bow forward. The bowed iris closes the anterior chamber angle, preventing drainage of the aqueous humor and increasing the intraocular pressure from its normal range of 10–20 mm Hg to 60–70 mm Hg. The increased intraocular pressure can damage the cornea, lens, iris, retina, and optic nerve, posing a threat to vision.

    2. Uveitis (i.e., intraocular inflammation) has multiple causes, including connective tissue disorders,

TABLE 5-2. Conjunctivitis

Disorder	History	Physical Examination and Laboratory Findings	Treatment
Bacterial conjunctivitis	Thick crust on eyelid on awakening (unilateral or bilateral) No associated viral symptoms Patients with conjunctivitis caused by *Neisseria gonorrhoeae* are usually sexually active adults with a history of recent exposure to a patient with genital gonorrhea; may also be newborns who have been exposed during delivery	Gram stain of a conjunctival scraping may identify causative organism (indicated if patient's symptoms do not improve in 2–3 days)	Gentamicin or erythromycin eye drops every 2 hours Eye patches and topical steroid drops are contraindicated Patients with *N. gonorrhoeae* conjunctivitis require 1 g ceftriaxone IM or IV and ciprofloxacin eye drops Refer all patients within 48 hours

continued

TABLE 5-2. Conjunctivitis

Disorder	History	Physical Examination and Laboratory Findings	Treatment
Chlamydial conjunctivitis	Neonates infected during delivery present with red eye within 5–14 days 90% of women and 60% of men with chlamydial conjunctivitis also have genital chlamydia	Red eye, preauricular lymphadenopathy, and lid edema Giemsa stain of an epithelial scrape reveals intracellular inclusion bodies	Tetracycline (250 mg) or doxycycline (100 mg) four times daily for 14 days Azithromycin (1 g orally) for pregnant women Refer within 48 hours
Viral conjunctivitis	Often bilateral and associated with red eye; a watery, nonpurulent discharge; and systemic symptoms (e.g., fever, preauricular adenopathy, pharyngitis)	Patients with adenoviral keratoconjunctivitis may have scattered, small corneal infiltrates and subconjunctival hemorrhage Slit-lamp examination with fluorescein staining may	Symptoms are self-limited, although HSV conjunctivitis can be treated with acyclovir, valacyclovir, or famciclovir

| | | reveal dendritic keratitis in patients with conjunctivitis caused by HSV or herpes zoster virus | No referral necessary, unless herpes zoster is suspected |
| Allergic conjunctivitis | Clear discharge bilaterally, itching, and lid edema often accompanied by rhinorrhea and a history of seasonal allergies or atopic dermatitis | Eosinophils on Giemsa stain are diagnostic | Removal of allergen

Oral antihitamines or decongestants

Naphcon A |

HSV = herpes simplex virus; IM = intramuscularly; IV = intravenously.

TABLE 5-3. Causes of Red Eye That Require Urgent Referral to an Ophthalmologist

Disorder	History	Physical Examination and Laboratory Findings	Treatment
Acute angle closure glaucoma	Red, painful eye Blurred vision Halos around lights (from corneal edema) Nausea or vomiting Initial symptoms may resemble those of a migraine headache	Shallow anterior chamber on slit-lamp examination Fixed, semi-dilated pupil Hazy cornea (from edema) High intraocular pressure on tonometry or palpation	Refer immediately for iridotomy Timolol (0.5% solution) to decrease intraocular pressure and aqueous humor formation Pilocarpine (1%–2% solution) to constrict pupil Acetazolamide (500 mg) or mannitol (1 mg/kg) IV to decrease intraocular pressure
Anterior uveitis (iritis)	Unilateral, painful red eye with limbic flush Photophobia Blurred vision (if	Small, poorly reactive pupil Consensual photophobia (i.e., pain with light in either eye, owing to	Disorder is usually self-limited, but refer within 24–48 hours to avoid complications

Condition	Symptoms	Signs / Examination	Treatment
	clouded aqueous humor)	consensual iris contraction in the affected eye Cells and flare in anterior chamber on slit-lamp examination	Ophthalmologist may prescribe a long-acting cycloplegic (e.g., atropine) or topical prednisolone acetate 1% to alleviate pain
Orbital cellulitis	Dull, aching ocular pain; exophthalmos; fever; malaise	Periorbital swelling Limited extraocular motion Decreased vision	Refer immediately Initiate IV antibiotic therapy immediately, without waiting for a consult; use a first- or second-generation cephalosporin (with an antifungal agent if patient is immunocompromised)
Corneal ulcer	Pain, tearing, history of foreign body	Slit-lamp examination with fluorescein stain to rule out perforation Evert eyelids to rule out retained foreign body Culture to determine cause	Refer immediately Ophthalmologist may prescribe a short-acting cycloplegic (e.g., cyclopentolate) and gentamicin or tobramycin drops

IV = intravenous.

56   Chapter 5

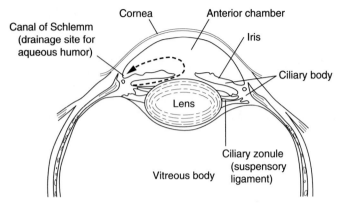

FIGURE 5-2. The *arrow* represents the normal flow of aqueous humor from the posterior chamber to the anterior chamber.

infectious disorders, trauma, and malignancy. Recurrent uveitis can lead to synechiae or glaucoma.

  a. **Anterior uveitis** affects the iris **(iritis),** anterior chamber, or posterior chamber.
  b. **Intermediate uveitis** affects the vitreous body.
  c. **Posterior uveitis** affects the retina or choroid.

HOT

Anterior uveitis is most commonly iritis, an important cause of red eye. Intermediate and posterior uveitis are more rare and do not cause red eye.

KEY

---

3. **Orbital cellulitis**
  a. Common causative organisms include *H. influenzae, S. aureus, Streptococcus pyogenes,* and *S. pneumoniae.*
    (1) In immunocompromised patients (including those with diabetes), **mucormycosis** should be considered, especially if the patient has a history of sinusitis.
    (2) Consider computed tomography (CT) or magnetic resonance imaging to rule out an **abscess** that requires drainage.
  b. **Complications** of untreated orbital cellulitis in-

clude vision loss, cavernous sinus thrombosis, and intracranial infection.

4. **Corneal ulcer** can occur secondary to foreign body, entropion, trichiasis, lagophthalmus, or conjunctivitis.

V CAUSES OF EYE TRAUMA. Primary physicians are often the first to evaluate patients with eye trauma.

A. **Chemical exposures** can threaten long-term vision. Exposures may be **acids** (causing immediate pain and damage), **alkaloids** (causing ischemia following necrosis of the surface tissue and vessels), or **ammonia** (causing intraocular inflammation).

1. **Irrigation.** The eye should be irrigated prior to performing a physical examination. After irrigating the eye, sweep the fornices with a moistened applicator to remove traces of the chemical that may remain.

   a. If the patient calls from home, he should be advised to irrigate the eye for 15 minutes prior to leaving for the emergency department (ED).

   b. Otherwise, the eye should be irrigated in the ED with 1–2 liters of sterile saline solution until the tear pH is normal, and a topical anesthetic applied.

2. **Physical examination**

   a. Examine the cornea for abrasions.

   b. Evert the lids to rinse the conjunctiva and search for foreign bodies.

3. **Referral**

   a. For patients with severe exposures, admission for 24-hour irrigation may be necessary.

   b. If the examination is normal, a cycloplegic and topical antibiotic should be prescribed, and the eye should be patched using light pressure. The patient should see an ophthalmologist within 48–72 hours.

   c. Patients with evidence of corneal scarring should be referred to an ophthalmologist immediately.

B. **Lid laceration**

1. **Physical examination**

   a. Assess the levator muscle by having the patient look toward the ceiling.

   b. If the lower lid is lacerated, assess the eye for canaliculus injury. These patients may require a stent to prevent chronic tearing.

    2. Referral. Patients should be referred to an ophthalmologist immediately. Levator and canaliculus repair may require surgical exploration.

  C. Blunt orbital trauma. A slit-lamp examination and visual acuity survey should be performed to evaluate for hyphema, vitreous hemorrhage, and retinal detachment. Patients should be referred to an ophthalmologist if history or physical examination findings suggest complications.

  D. Blow-out fractures

    1. Physical examination may reveal soft-tissue swelling, diplopia, epistaxis, periorbital ecchymosis, crepitus, orbital emphysema, enophthalmos, exophthalmos, ptosis, or numbness over the maxillary region. Subcutaneous crepitus in the periorbital area may indicate communication with a sinus space, which can be caused by a blow-out fracture.

    2. Imaging studies

      a. Plain film radiographs may reveal the "teardrop" sign (caused by herniation of soft tissue into the sinus) or an air-fluid level in the ipsilateral sinus.

      b. CT scans may be indicated to search for bony fragments or herniation.

    3. Referral. Patients must be referred to an ophthalmologist immediately. In the meantime, ice compresses can be applied and systemic antibiotics can be initiated (to prevent orbital infection from the sinuses). Valsalva maneuvers should be avoided.

  E. Ruptured globe can result from an acute increase in intraocular pressure following blunt trauma. Signs include vision loss, hyphema, vitreous hemorrhage, and an extremely deep or shallow anterior chamber.

    1. These patients should not be examined. **Place a metal eye shield over the eye and refer the patient to an ophthalmologist for immediate surgical repair.**

    2. Avoid topical eye ointments, because these agents can complicate surgical repair. **Systemic antibiotics may be prescribed** to prevent endophthalmitis.

References

Bienfang DC, Kelly LD, Nicholson DH, et al: Ophthalmology. *N Engl J Med* 323(14): 956–967, 1990.

Garcia GE: Management of ocular emergencies and urgent eye problems. *Am Fam Physician* 53(2): 565–574, 1996.

Scott J, Ghezzi K: Emergency treatment of the eye. *Emerg Med Clin North Am* 13(3): 521–712, 1995.

6. Hearing Loss

....

I **INTRODUCTION.** Hearing impairment is the most common chronic handicap in the United States.

    A. An estimated 22 million Americans have some degree of hearing impairment.

    B. Only 10% of people 65 years of age or older report having normal hearing.

II **CAUSES OF HEARING LOSS.** There are three types of hearing loss: conductive, sensorineural, and mixed.

    A. Conductive hearing loss originates in the external or middle ear. Passage of sound to the cochlea is obstructed or reduced secondary to cerumen impaction, fluid, congenital deformities, tumors, trauma, or otosclerosis within the sound-conducting apparatus.

    B. Sensorineural hearing loss occurs when the cochlea (inner ear) or the cochlear portion of cranial nerve VIII (i.e., the acoustic nerve) is affected, preventing the transmission of the auditory signal to the brain. The causes of sensorineural hearing loss are numerous and include ototoxicity, presbycusis, Meniere's disease, trauma, noise-induced hearing loss, multiple sclerosis, autoimmune disease, and tumors.

    C. Mixed hearing loss includes components of both conductive and sensorineural hearing loss. The primary component should be identified. Causes of mixed hearing loss include trauma, otosclerosis, and chronic otitis media.

III **APPROACH TO THE PATIENT.** Identification of hearing loss requires diligence on the part of the physician because many patients deny or have trouble describing their hearing loss. First, determine that there is hearing loss, then classify it as conductive, sensorineural, or mixed (Figure 6-1).

    A. Patient history. A thorough history is crucial to the proper diagnosis of hearing loss.

        1. Signs and symptoms. The presentation of a patient's

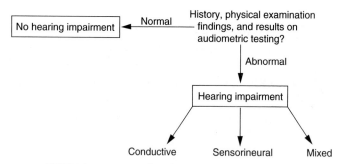

FIGURE 6-1. Approach to the patient with hearing loss.

hearing loss varies depending on the site of disease along the auditory pathway.

    a. Elderly patients may exhibit **isolation** and **dementia-like symptoms** as a result of deafness, which in many cases is reversible.

    b. **Vertigo, tinnitus,** and **ear pressure** may accompany hearing loss.

  2. **Questions to ask** include the following:

    a. Was the onset of hearing loss sudden, progressive, or fluctuant?

    b. How long has the patient been aware of a change?

    c. Is the hearing loss unilateral or bilateral?

    d. What is the patient's family history?

    e. What is the patient's exposure to noise?

    f. What is the patient's medication history?

    g. Were there any precipitating events, such as an upper respiratory tract infection or trauma?

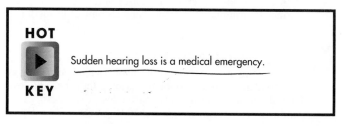

HOT

Sudden hearing loss is a medical emergency.

KEY

B. **Physical examination** should focus on the ear, nose, and throat, with special attention to the ears and adjacent structures.

  1. **Neurologic examination.** Any abnormal findings on

cranial nerve examination are suggestive of serious central nervous system (CNS) pathology.

2. **Otoscopic examination.** In order to allow complete visualization of the external auditory canal and the tympanic membrane, the canal must be clear of cerumen.

    a. The **external auditory canal** should be examined for cerumen, exostosis, signs of infection (e.g., erythema), and dry skin.

    b. The **tympanic membrane** should be inspected for evidence of scars, perforation, color changes, or tympanosclerosis.

HOT

KEY

In an adult without a recent history of upper respiratory tract infection, the presence of fluid in the middle ear (evidenced by opacification or bulging of the tympanic membrane) necessitates referral to an otolaryngologist for a complete head and neck examination to rule out carcinoma.

---

3. **Tuning fork examination.** Although underutilized, tuning fork tests are a quick and useful way of differentiating between normal and abnormal hearing, and between conductive and sensorineural hearing loss.

    a. **Weber test.** The examiner strikes the tines of a 512-Hz tuning fork and then places the fork in the center of the patient's forehead or on the bridge of her nose. He then asks the patient if she hears the noise in the right ear, left ear, or both ears.

        (1) **Symmetric results** (i.e., the patient hears the noise in both ears) suggest that the patient has either normal hearing or bilaterally symmetric hearing loss.

        (2) **Lateralized results** (i.e., the patient hears the noise better on one side)

            (a) **Conductive loss.** The tone is louder in the poorer ear. 2° to sensitization

            (b) **Sensorineural loss.** The tone is louder in the better ear.

    b. **Rinne test.** This test can be used to detect conductive hearing loss and estimate its severity. A 512-Hz tuning fork is placed firmly against the mastoid bone. The examiner strikes the tines of the fork and asks the patient to compare the loudness of the bone conduction to the loudness of the sound when the tuning fork is held 2 centimeters away from the meatus of the external auditory canal.

    (1) Positive results. Bone conduction is less than air conduction, suggesting normal hearing or sensorineural hearing loss in the tested ear.

    (2) Negative results. Bone conduction is greater than air conduction, suggesting a conductive hearing loss of at least 20 dB in the tested ear.

HOT

KEY

Asymmetric hearing loss on tuning fork examination requires a referral to an otolaryngologist for additional evaluation.

TABLE 6-1. Differential Diagnosis of Hearing Loss

Onset	Type of Hearing Loss	
	Conductive	Sensorineural
Acute (< 24 hours)	Foreign body Trauma Burn Laceration Fracture Barotrauma Tympanic membrane perforation	Acoustic neuroma Vascular occlusion Meniere's disease Labyrinthitis (viral, bacterial)
Progressive (> 24 hours)	Otitis externa Acute otitis media Tumor Otosclerosis Cerumen impaction	Presbycusis (age-related) Noise-induced hearing loss Acoustic neuroma Ototoxicity Inner ear autoimmune disease

        c. Table 6-1 narrows the possible diagnoses according to the type and onset of the hearing loss.
   C. Audiometric testing is usually necessary for definitive diagnosis.

IV TREATMENT. The treatment of otitis media, otitis externa, and cerumen impaction are discussed in Chapters 7, 8, and 9, respectively.

V FOLLOW-UP AND REFERRAL. All patients with significant hearing loss should be referred to an otolaryngologist for a formal otologic evaluation.

References

Gates GA (ed): *Current Therapy in Otolaryngology—Head and Neck Surgery.* St. Louis, Mosby, 1994.

Ruckenstein MJ: Hearing loss—a plan for individualized management. *Postgrad Med* 98(4): 197–200 (203 and 206 passim), 1995.

Poor Chapter.

7. Otitis Media

I INTRODUCTION

A. There are **four general types** of otitis media, which represent different points along a continuum. Within each type, there are a number of phases. The four types are:
1. **Acute suppurative otitis media**
2. **Chronic suppurative otitis media**
3. **Acute serous otitis media**
4. **Chronic serous otitis media**

B. Otitis media is the most common diagnosis made by clinicians who care for children. The **peak prevalence** of otitis media is in **patients between the ages of 6 months and 3 years.**

II SUPPURATIVE OTITIS MEDIA

A. Acute suppurative otitis media
1. **Causes** include *Streptococcus pneumoniae, Haemophilus influenzae, Moraxella catarrhalis,* and **group A streptococci.**
2. **Clinical manifestation.** There are three phases of acute suppurative otitis media.
   a. The **early phase,** which lasts **1–2 days,** is characterized by **fever; severe, pulsating pain;** and **hearing loss.** On otoscopy, the tympanic membrane shows **hyperemia, opacification,** and **loss of landmarks. Mastoid tenderness** is common.
   b. During the **middle phase,** which lasts **3–8 days,** the purulent effusion often discharges spontaneously (occasionally as a result of tympanic membrane perforation) and the **fever** and **pain subside.**
   c. During the **healing phase,** which lasts **2–4 weeks,** the **tympanic membrane** and **middle ear normalize.**
3. **Differential diagnoses** include **otitis externa** and **acute mastoiditis** (i.e., inflammation of the mastoid air cells).

HOT
KEY

Consider acute mastoiditis when a patient with otitis media experiences worsening of symptoms along with mastoid tenderness, postauricular swelling and erythema, and prolapse or swelling of the posterior wall of the external canal.

4. **Treatment**
   a. **Antibiotic therapy**
      (1) **Amoxicillin** (40 mg/kg/day, divided in 3 doses) is considered first-line therapy.
      (2) **Amoxicillin-clavulanic acid, cefuroxime,** or **trimethoprim-sulfamethoxazole** may also be used.
   b. **Myringotomy** (performed by an otolaryngologist) may be necessary for patients with persistent pain and high fever, facial nerve palsy, acute meningitis, labyrinthitis, or mastoiditis.
5. **Follow-up and referral.** Consider referring adults with unilateral otitis media to an otolaryngologist for evaluation of the nasopharynx.
B. **Chronic suppurative otitis media**
   1. **Causes**
      a. **Cholesteatoma** (i.e., a cyst-like mass or benign tumor with a lining of squamous epithelium trapped behind the tympanic membrane in the middle ear) can lead to infection and erosion of the ossicles and chronic suppurative otitis media.
      b. **Conditions that cause irreversible changes to the middle ear mucosa** and lead to adhesions and congestion around the eustachian tube (e.g., allergic rhinitis, sinusitis, immunodeficiency, adenoid infection in children) can lead to chronic ear drainage and chronic suppurative otitis media. Infection is usually caused by *Staphylococcus aureus,* **anaerobic bacteria,** or *Pseudomonas.*
   2. **Clinical manifestations**
      a. Chronic suppurative otitis media is characterized by the **chronic discharge of a mucoid, purulent, odorless exudate** (i.e., **chronic tympanic membrane perforation).** Periods of no drainage alternating with exacerbations are common.
      b. **Conductive hearing loss** is usually present.

       c. **Pain is absent** and the **patient's general condition is good.**

    3. **Differential diagnoses** include **tuberculosis** and **carcinoma.**

    4. **Treatment** depends on whether the chronic suppurative otitis media is associated with a cholesteatoma (Figure 7-1).

        a. **With cholesteatoma.** These patients require referral to an otolaryngologist for **surgical treatment.**

        b. **Without cholesteatoma.** The goal of treatment is to resolve the infection. If the infection can be reversed with **antibiotics** and **irrigation,** then mastoidectomy can be avoided.

III SEROUS OTITIS MEDIA

A. **Acute serous otitis media**

    1. **Causes.** Acute serous otitis media often precedes or follows an episode of acute suppurative otitis media. It may also be associated with conditions that cause eustachian tube dysfunction (e.g., upper respiratory tract infection, allergic rhinitis, sinusitis, nasopharyngeal masses).

    2. **Clinical features** include a **feeling of pressure or fullness** in the ears, often accompanied by **hearing loss** and **crackling** or **popping** while swallowing. On otoscopic examination, the **tympanic membrane** may be

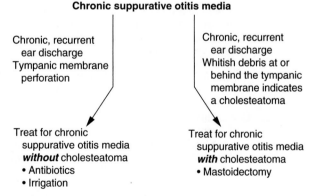

FIGURE 7-1. Algorithm for determining treatment of chronic suppurative otitis media.

hyperemic and an **amber color** can be appreciated behind it, with or without air bubbles.

HOT It is recommended that a diagnosis of acute serous otitis media be confirmed using tympanometry or pneumo-otoscopy. A flat configuration will be seen on tympanometry, and tympanic membrane hypomobility will be seen on pneumo-oto-
KEY scopy.

---

3. **Differential diagnoses** include **acute suppurative otitis media** and **leakage of cerebrospinal fluid (CSF)** into the middle ear or mastoid air cells.
4. **Treatment** entails addressing the causes of eustachian tube dysfunction and eradicating the causative organism. Eighty percent of children will clear effusions in 2 months without treatment.
   a. **Antihistamines** (e.g., **loratadine,** 10 mg orally daily) are indicated for patients with allergic rhinitis.
   b. **Decongestants** (e.g., **phenylpropanolamine,** 1 tablet orally twice daily) are indicated for patients with viral rhinosinusitis.
   c. **Antibiotics** (e.g., **amoxicillin, amoxicillin-clavulanic acid,** or **cefuroxime)** are warranted to ensure sterilization of the effusion.
5. **Follow-up and referral.** An adult patient with acute serous otitis media, particularly when it is unilateral and outside of the setting of an upper respiratory tract infection, may require referral to an otolaryngologist to rule out obstruction of the eustachian tube by a nasopharyngeal mass.

B. **Chronic serous otitis media.** By definition, the effusion is present for at least 3 months.
   1. **Causes.** Chronic serous otitis media results from eustachian tube dysfunction. Allergies or abnormalities of the adenoids, sinuses, or nasopharynx may be responsible.
   2. **Clinical manifestations** include a feeling of **fullness in the ear** and **hearing loss without pain.** Findings on physical examination are similar to those for acute serous otitis media.
   3. **Differential diagnoses** include **hemotympanum** and **CSF leak.**

    4. **Treatment** entails addressing the underlying cause of eustachian tube dysfunction and eradicating the infection with a **10- to 14-day course of antibiotics** (e.g., amoxicillin, 20–40 mg/kg/day, divided in 3 doses).

    5. **Follow-up and referral.** Some patients may need to be referred to an otolaryngologist for myringotomy or adenoidectomy.

        a. **Myringotomy** may be required for patients with vertigo, hearing loss, or an effusion that has persisted for much longer than 3 months.

        b. **Adenoidectomy** is helpful in older children with chronic serous otitis media.

References

Froom J, Culpepper L, Jacobs M, et al: Antimicrobials for acute otitis media? A review from the International Primary Care Network. *BMJ* 315(7100): 98–102, 1997.

Kenna MA: Otitis media with effusion. In *Head and Neck Surgery—Otolaryngology,* 2nd ed. Edited by Bailey BJ. Philadelphia, Lippincott Williams & Wilkins, 1998, pp 1297–1310.

8. Otitis Externa

I INTRODUCTION

A. **Definition.** Otitis externa (**"swimmer's ear"**) is an infection of the external auditory canal.

B. **Pathogenesis.** Particularly common during the summer months, otitis externa is caused by a breakdown in the protective barrier normally formed by the skin and cerumen.

   1. Factors such as elevated heat and humidity, water maceration, allergy, and trauma (e.g., mechanical damage) cause atrophy of the sebaceous and ceruminous glands located in the outer third of the external auditory canal.

   2. With the loss of the protective layer provided by these glands, the external auditory canal becomes dry and loses the chemical balance needed to prevent infection.

   3. The most common pathogens are ***Pseudomonas aeruginosa*** and ***Staphylococcus aureus.***

II CLINICAL MANIFESTATIONS OF OTITIS EXTERNA

A. **Four major symptoms**

   1. **Pain** (often severe)
   2. **Pruritus**
   3. **Hearing loss**
   4. **Fullness** (e.g., a "plugged" sensation)

HOT KEY

Pain when pressure is placed on the tragus (i.e., the semicircular piece of cartilage in front of the ear canal) is strongly suggestive of otitis externa. Inflammation and swelling of the pinna itself is indicative of a more severe infection (e.g., cellulitis, perichondritis, erysipelas) and an otolaryngology consultation is indicated.

B. Two stages

1. **Acute inflammatory stage.** During this stage, bacterial infection occurs and the patient experiences pain in the affected ear. As the infection becomes more severe, pain and swelling in the external auditory canal increase.

2. **Chronic inflammatory stage.** This stage is characterized by a marked thickening of the skin of the external auditory canal owing to long-standing infection. Examination reveals flakes of dry, scaly skin in the canal. Often, the lumen of the canal is significantly narrowed.

III APPROACH TO THE PATIENT. The list of conditions similar to otitis externa is long. The following is a selected list of conditions that should always be ruled out:

A. Necrotizing external otitis (malignant otitis externa) is a **potentially lethal** infection usually found in elderly or immunocompromised patients (e.g., those with diabetes, HIV infection, or chronic illness). The characteristic history is one of a long-standing case of otitis externa that continues to progress in severity despite seemingly adequate treatment.

1. **Clinical manifestations.** The patient often describes an ear discharge and severe "deep" or "boring" pain. The onset of new cranial nerve deficits may be detected on physical examination.

2. **Treatment.** Patients must be referred to an otolaryngologist.

B. Perichondritis and chondritis. Infections of the perichondrium or cartilage of the ear are serious, and require prompt attention.

1. **Clinical manifestations.** Patients often present with a diffusely swollen and exquisitely tender pinna.

2. **Treatment.** Intravenous antibiotics covering both aerobic and anaerobic organisms should be administered. Surgical débridement of necrotic cartilage may be necessary.

C. Furunculosis. These circumscribed swellings, which may be single or multiple, are noted in the cartilaginous portion of the external auditory canal.

1. **Clinical manifestations.** The swellings may be fluctuant, and tenderness is often noted when the tragus is pulled and when the ear speculum is inserted.

2. **Treatment** consists of draining fluctuant areas and applying topical antibiotics. Systemic antibiotics are only necessary if cellulitis or systemic symptoms are noted.

D. Dermatitis or **contact allergy of the ear** can be acute, chronic, or both.

   1. Clinical manifestations

   a. In the **acute stage,** inflammatory findings are noted with associated pruritus, desquamation, and weeping.

   b. In the **chronic stage,** the skin of the external auditory canal is atrophic, dry, and scaly.

   2. Treatment is with steroid creams or solutions.

   a. For patients with severe cases, betamethasone valerate or fluocinonide can be applied for a short time. If used too long, these agents can cause atrophy of the epithelium.

   b. For patients with chronic cases, a 1% hydrocortisone cream or solution can be used.

E. Herpes zoster oticus (Ramsay Hunt syndrome) is caused by infection of the cranial nerve ganglia, most likely by the virus that causes chicken pox.

   1. Clinical manifestations. Painful herpetic lesions are noted on the auricle and in the external auditory canal. In severe cases, facial nerve paralysis (Bell's palsy), hearing loss, and balance disorders may occur.

   2. Treatment. Bell's palsy can progress to a severe, complete facial nerve paralysis; therefore, corticosteroid therapy and referral to an otolaryngologist is warranted for these patients.

F. Otomycosis (external mycotica) is a fungal infection of the external auditory canal.

   1. Clinical manifestations. Symptoms are similar to those of otitis externa, except that pruritus is more common than otalgia. A whitish exudate and black spots suggest *Aspergillus niger* infection.

   2. Treatment consists of acidifying the ear canal.

IV TREATMENT

HOT

KEY

Regardless of the stage of otitis externa, frequent and thorough cleaning of the external auditory canal is essential for effective treatment. If associated pain or swelling prevents thorough visualization and cleaning of the external auditory canal, the patient should be referred to an otolaryngologist.

HOT In order for treatment to be successful, the external auditory canal must be kept dry. Insertion of silicon earplugs or petroleum jelly-coated cotton balls into the external auditory canal prior to bathing will keep the canal dry. **KEY**

   A. Acute inflammatory stage. Proper treatment depends on the extent of the infection.
      1. Mild infection
         a. If an exudate is present, the external auditory canal must be thoroughly cleaned (by **suctioning,** to avoid introducing water into the canal).
         b. An **antibiotic eardrop** (e.g., neomycin-hydrocortisone) is recommended to cover a probable *Pseudomonas* infection. Typical treatment is one dropperful three times daily for 3–5 days, **until the symptoms resolve.** Oral antibiotics are not required.
      2. Moderate to severe infection. Because patients with moderate to severe infection require thorough debridement of the external auditory canal and edema may interfere with the installation of drops, **referral to an otolaryngologist is recommended.** Prior to referral, placement of an ear wick to facilitate antibiotic eardrop treatment may be performed.
   B. Chronic inflammatory stage. Treatment consists of the following measures:
      1. Repeated cleaning of the external auditory canal
      2. Administration of antibiotic eardrops and steroid eardrops
      3. Culture of the external auditory canal to ensure that the causative organisms are being effectively treated

HOT Manipulation of the external auditory canal must be avoided. Injection of betamethasone valerate cream into the external auditory canal may be necessary to suppress pruritus. **KEY**

V FOLLOW-UP AND REFERRAL

A. Acute inflammatory stage

1. **Mild infection.** Patients with drainage should be referred to an otolaryngologist. If no drainage is present, one follow-up visit is required to ensure improvement.

2. **Moderate to severe infection.** Patients with drainage should be referred to an otolaryngologist. Those who are not referred should be followed on a nearly daily basis until resolution of the infection.

B. Chronic inflammatory stage. If the condition is not getting progressively worse, referral to an otolaryngologist is not necessarily required. The patient should be followed every 1–2 weeks until the condition stabilizes.

References

Lindstrom CJ, Lucente FE: Infections of the external ear. In *Head and Neck Surgery—Otolaryngology,* 2nd ed. Edited by Bailey BJ. Philadelphia, Lippincott Williams & Wilkins, 1998, 1965–1980.

Mirza N: Otitis externa: management in the primary care office. *Postgrad Med* 99(5):153–154, 157–158, 1996.

9. Cerumen (Earwax) Impaction

I INTRODUCTION

A. Cerumen is a waxy yellowish-brown substance consisting of secretions from the sebaceous and ceruminous glands, desquamated epithelium, hair, and dirt particles. Cerumen has an acidic pH and is bacteriostatic and fungistatic.

B. Collections of cerumen and debris are unusual if the self-cleaning mechanism of the external auditory canal is not disturbed. The habit of cleaning the external auditory canal is counterproductive and eventually leads to the development of chronic otitis externa. Additionally, cotton swabs tend to drive wax deeper into the canal, leading to impaction.

II CLINICAL MANIFESTATIONS OF CERUMEN IMPACTION

A. Conductive hearing loss in the affected ear is the most common symptom. Deafness gradually develops as the external auditory canal becomes progressively occluded by cerumen.

B. Other symptoms may include a **sense of "fullness," tinnitus, dizziness,** and **ear discomfort.**

III APPROACH TO THE PATIENT

A. Rule out a **foreign body, suppurative otitis externa** or **otitis media** (evidenced by a purulent exudate), and a **skin plug.**

B. Determine whether the tympanic membrane is perforated. Is there a history of blood, odor, or discharge? How does the tympanic membrane appear on otoscopic examination?

IV TREATMENT (Figure 9-1)

A. Perforated tympanic membrane. Do not attempt to perform cerumenectomy if perforation of the tympanic membrane is suspected. Instead, refer the patient to an otolaryngologist.

B. Intact tympanic membrane
1. **Cerumenectomy**
    a. To soften hard or impacted wax, have the patient

Symptoms of tympanic membrane perforation
(e.g., blood, odor, discharge) or signs of
perforation on otoscopic examination?

Yes   No

Tympanic membrane   Perform a cerumenectomy
perforation likely; refer
patient to an otolaryngologist

FIGURE 9-1. Treatment of a patient with cerumen impaction depends on whether or not tympanic membrane perforation is likely.

instill Cortisporin eardrops or mineral oil two to three times daily for 1 week prior to returning for treatment.

b. When the wax is softened, the canal is irrigated with warm water [i.e., water at body temperature (37°C)], using a large-bore irrigator tip to minimize the water pressure.

c. After irrigating, the moist external auditory canal should be gently dried with a cotton applicator to avoid otitis externa.

2. Over-the-counter eardrops. Patients may attempt to manage wax themselves with eardrops that emulsify and disperse earwax (e.g., triethanolamine). The drops are instilled in the external auditory canal for 15–30 minutes at a time, causing the wax to dissolve. The dose may be repeated if necessary.

 FOLLOW-UP AND REFERRAL. The patient should be reevaluated in 6–12 months.

References

Jafek BW, Starks AK: *ENT Secrets.* Philadelphia, Hanley & Belfus, 1996.

Wilson, PL. Roeser, RJ: Cerumen management: professional issues and techniques. *J Am Acad Audiol* 8(6):421–430, 1997.

10. Singultus (Hiccough)

I **INTRODUCTION.** A hiccough is an inspiratory sound caused by the abrupt closure of the glottis in the setting of rhythmic spasm of the diaphragm and respiratory muscles.

A. Hiccoughs can occur at any age and can last for years (but usually only last for a few minutes).

B. There is a strong male predominance.

C. Although usually benign and self-limited, hiccoughs may be persistent and indicative of a serious underlying disorder.

II **CAUSES OF SINGULTUS.** Singultus can be caused by a variety of conditions that usually involve some part of the reflex arc shown in Figure 10-1. Causes are classified as **peripheral** (involving the vagus or phrenic nerves, or structures adjacent to the diaphragm) or **central** [involving the central nervous system (CNS)].

Common Causes of Singultus ("SINGULTUS")

Surgery (post-surgical status) or lesions of the abdomen, chest, or neck

Infections adjacent to the diaphragm (e.g., lower lobe pneumonia, subphrenic abscess, peritonitis, pericarditis, cholecystitis, hepatitis)

Nervous system disorders (e.g., stroke, meningitis, brain tumor, multiple sclerosis)

Gastric distention (a very common cause, usually self-limited)

Uremia

Low serum calcium, sodium, or potassium

Tumor of the pancreas or stomach

ᴪsychogenic and idiopathic

Steroids and other drugs (e.g., alcohol, benzodiazepines, barbiturates)

III **APPROACH TO THE PATIENT**

A. Most patients have benign, self-limited hiccoughs and do not require extensive evaluation.

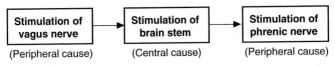

FIGURE 10-1. The many causes of singultus involve this reflex arc in some way. Metabolic disorders, drugs, and psychogenic disorders are considered "central" disorders.

    B. Those with persistent hiccoughs require a more thorough evaluation.
       1. A detailed history and physical examination should be performed.
       2. Laboratory data should include a complete blood count (CBC), an electrolyte panel (including calcium, sodium, and potassium levels), a blood urea nitrogen (BUN) and creatinine level, and liver function tests.
       3. Many practitioners also obtain a chest radiograph.
    C. If a thorough examination fails to yield a diagnosis, chest and abdominal computed tomography (CT), brain magnetic resonance imaging (MRI), bronchoscopy, echocardiography, or upper endoscopy may be indicated.

IV TREATMENT

    A. For patients with benign, self-limited hiccoughs, try one of the following simple remedies:
       1. Have the patient swallow 1 tablespoon of granulated sugar.
       2. Massage the soft palate or apply traction to the tongue.
       3. Interrupt the breathing cycle by having the patient perform a Valsalva maneuver or breathe into a bag.
       4. Have the patient remain in the knee-to-chest position for 1 minute.
    B. For those with persistent hiccoughs, treating the underlying disorder is the best course of action. If the patient needs immediate relief or the underlying cause is elusive, the strategies detailed in IV A should be attempted before moving on to more invasive measures.
       1. Nasogastric tube or nasopharyngeal catheter placement may relieve the hiccoughs if gastric distention is the cause.
       2. Pharmacologic therapy is occasionally necessary. One of the following agents may be used:

    a. **Chlorpromazine,** 10–50 mg orally or intramuscularly twice or three times daily

    b. **Metoclopramide,** 10–30 mg orally four times daily

    c. **Baclofen,** 5 mg orally three times daily

V FOLLOW-UP AND REFERRAL

A. Follow-up. Monthly follow-up is appropriate for those with persistent hiccoughs of unclear cause.

B. Referral to a neurologist is indicated for patients who may have underlying central or peripheral nervous system disorders.

References

Kolodzik PW, Eilers MA: Hiccups (singultus): review and approach to management. *Ann Emerg Med* 20(5):565–573, 1991.

Launois S, Bizec JL, Whitelaw WA, et al: Hiccup in adults: an overview. *Eur Respir J* 6(4):563–575, 1993.

11. Sinusitis

I INTRODUCTION

A. **Acute sinusitis** is inflammation of the mucosal lining of the sinus cavities from any cause.

1. **Bacterial sinusitis** is most often caused by *Streptococcus pneumoniae, Haemophilus influenzae, Moraxella catarrhalis,* and group A streptococci.

2. **Viral sinusitis** is a self-limited condition that occurs in approximately 80% of patients with the common cold and only rarely progresses to bacterial sinusitis (roughly 1 in 200 patients).

3. **Fungal sinusitis.** Fungal infection of the sinuses may occur in immunocompromised patients, including those with diabetes, leukemia, and HIV infection. Commonly implicated organisms include *Mucor* and *Aspergillus* species. These infections are often invasive and difficult to cure and require emergent surgical debridement.

B. **Chronic sinusitis** is defined as sinusitis that persists for longer than 3 months.

1. The infection may be caused by the same organisms responsible for acute bacterial sinusitis, but anaerobic bacteria (e.g., *Bacteroides* species, peptostreptococci) also commonly cause chronic sinusitis.

2. Chronic sinusitis may result from mechanical obstruction by a polyp, tumor, or deviated nasal septum.

II CLINICAL MANIFESTATIONS OF SINUSITIS

A. **Acute sinusitis**

1. A **frontal headache** and **sinus pain that worsens when the patient leans forward** is the classic presentation. The location of the pain depends on the sinuses involved (Table 11-1).

2. In addition, patients often report a **purulent nasal discharge, fever,** and **malaise.**

B. **Chronic sinusitis**

1. Patients report a long history of **nasal congestion,** often associated with **postnasal drip, cough,** or the **sensation of being unable to clear the throat.**

2. **Fever** and **sinus pain** are less common components.

TABLE 11-1. Pain Location in Sinusitis

Affected Sinus	Pain Location
Maxillary	Cheeks, hard palate, teeth
Frontal	Low on the forehead
Ethmoid	Retro-orbital, upper or lateral nose
Sphenoid	Retro-orbital

III **COMPLICATIONS OF SINUSITIS.** Because of the proximity of the sinuses to the eyes and intracranial structures, complications can be extremely dangerous.

    A. **Osteomyelitis** of the facial bones can occur and results in **Pott's puffy tumor** (i.e., a circumscribed area of edema surrounding areas of osteomyelitis of the skull). The involved bone has a "doughy" consistency.

    B. **Periorbital infections** can result from the local spread of infection. The eyelids are often swollen and red. Pain with eye motion, ptosis, or proptosis suggests **periorbital cellulitis.**

    C. **Cavernous sinus thrombophlebitis** occurs if the infection spreads via venous drainage of the ethmoid or sphenoid sinuses. Patients are usually severely ill and may have impaired ocular movement or a dilated pupil due to palsies of cranial nerves III, IV, and VI.

    D. **Brain abscess** or **meningitis** can result from the intracranial spread of infection.

IV **DIFFERENTIAL DIAGNOSIS**

    A. **Acute sinusitis**

        1. The main differential diagnoses are **viral sinusitis** (i.e., the **common cold,** see Chapter 12) and **allergic rhinitis.** Allergic rhinitis usually persists longer than acute sinusitis.

        2. **Migraine** or **cluster headache, dental abscess,** and **temporal arteritis** are occasionally confused with acute sinusitis.

    B. **Chronic sinusitis**

        1. Chronic sinusitis may be confused with **allergic rhinitis,** which can be differentiated from chronic sinusitis on the basis of a history of seasonal symptoms and the presence of itching of the eyes, nose, and throat.

2. When patients do not respond to therapy and have no evidence of mechanical obstruction, **rare systemic disorders** should be considered [e.g., **cystic fibrosis, Kartagener's syndrome, Wegener's granulomatosis, temporomandibular joint (TMJ) syndrome**].

V APPROACH TO THE PATIENT

A. History and physical examination

1. Perform a complete examination of the head and neck.
   a. Examine the nasal cavity for discharge and the presence of polyps, tumors, or septal deviation.
   b. Examine the cranial nerves and the eyes thoroughly; abnormalities suggest the spread of infection to periorbital structures or to the cavernous sinus.

2. The presence of at least five of the following six features—three detected as part of the history and three detected on physical examination—strongly suggests the presence of sinusitis. Always "TAP TAP" over the sinuses when examining a patient for sinusitis.

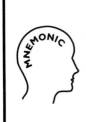

History and Physical Examination Findings in Sinusitis ("TAP TAP")

Toothache (maxillary)
Abnormal or poor response to decongestants
Purulent nasal discharge in history

Tenderness to palpation
Abnormal transillumination
Purulent nasal discharge on examination

B. Laboratory studies.
Patients with a high fever, severe symptoms, or any sign of complicating infection should have a complete blood count (CBC) and serum chemistries.

C. Imaging studies

1. **Acute sinusitis.** Patients with clinical signs that suggest that the infection has spread beyond the sinus cavities should be evaluated using computed tomography (CT) or magnetic resonance imaging (MRI) of the sinuses. Routine imaging in patients with acute si-

nusitis and no signs of complications is generally not necessary.

2. **Chronic sinusitis.** Patients with chronic sinusitis who do not respond to therapy should have a CT scan to rule out mechanical obstruction and plan possible surgical intervention.

VI TREATMENT

A. **Acute bacterial sinusitis**

1. **Antibiotics.** The optimal duration of antibiotic therapy is controversial, but patients should be treated for 3–14 days with an antibiotic that covers the main bacterial pathogens (e.g., trimethoprim—sulfamethoxazole, 1 double-strength tablet twice daily).

2. **Decongestants**

   a. **Topical decongestant sprays** (e.g., phenylephrine, 2 sprays per nostril every 3–4 hours or oxymetazoline, 2–3 sprays per nostril twice daily) can be used for a **maximum of 3 days.** Longer treatment may result in rebound nasal congestion.

   b. **Oral decongestants** (e.g., pseudoephedrine, 60 mg every 6 hours) can be used for up to 1 week.

B. **Chronic sinusitis**

1. **Antibiotics.** The utility of antibiotics for the treatment of chronic sinusitis is not clear because the condition often results from a mechanical obstruction. If antibiotics are used, they should cover anaerobic organisms. For example, amoxicillin-clavulanate, 500 mg orally three times daily, could be used. Patients are often treated for 3 weeks or more.

2. **Nasal steroids** (e.g., beclomethasone nasal spray, 1 puff in each nostril twice daily for 2–4 weeks) may reduce swelling and edema and improve sinus drainage.

VI FOLLOW-UP AND REFERRAL

A. Patients who respond appropriately to therapy do not require a follow-up visit.

B. Patients who do not respond to therapy and those with chronic sinusitis thought to be caused by a mechanical obstruction should be referred to an otolaryngologist.

C. Patients with clinical findings suggestive of complications or fungal sinusitis should be admitted to the hospital for the intravenous administration of antibiotics and urgent consultation with an otolaryngologist. Patients with periorbital cellulitis require urgent ophthalmologic consultation.

References

Williams JW, Holleman DR, Samsa GP, et al: Randomized controlled trial of 3 vs 10 days of trimethoprim/sulfamethoxazole for acute maxillary sinusitis. *JAMA* 273 (13):1015–1021, 1995.

Williams JW, Simel DL: Does this patient have sinusitis? Diagnosing acute sinusitis by history and physical examination. *JAMA* 270(10):1242–1246, 1993.

12. The Common Cold

I INTRODUCTION

A. The common cold (i.e., **viral infection of the upper respiratory tract)** is one of the most common illnesses seen in outpatient medicine, and it is the **leading cause of absenteeism from work in the United States.**

B. Common causes include **rhinovirus, coronavirus, adenovirus, influenza virus,** and **parainfluenza virus.**

HOT

KEY

"The flu" generally refers to influenza virus infection, which often causes **severe systemic symptoms** (e.g., a high fever, myalgia, malaise) in addition to upper respiratory symptoms.

II CLINICAL MANIFESTATIONS OF THE COMMON COLD

A. **Symptoms.** Patients may present with any or all of the following symptoms:

1. **Nose:** congestion, rhinorrhea (i.e., clear nasal discharge), sneezing
2. **Throat:** scratchy or sore throat, hoarse voice
3. **Ears and sinuses:** congestion and pressure
4. **General:** headache, fever, myalgias, malaise

B. **Signs** include **erythema** and **edema of the mucosa** in the oropharynx and nasopharynx. A **transient middle ear effusion** is often present due to impaired drainage through the eustachian tube.

HOT

KEY

Patients with marked erythema or impaired mobility of the tympanic membrane should be treated for otitis media (see Chapter 7).

APPROACH TO THE PATIENT. The goal in evaluating patients with symptoms of the common cold is to **rule out other disease processes with similar symptoms.** The main considerations are **bacterial sinusitis, bacterial pharyngitis,** and **allergic rhinitis** (Table 12-1).

HOT

KEY

Of these illnesses, allergic rhinitis is the most similar to the common cold, but it may distinguished by a history of itching (of the eyes, nose, or throat) and seasonal or allergen-induced symptoms.

HOT

KEY

Some viruses that infect the upper respiratory tract can also cause pneumonia (e.g., influenza virus). The lungs should be auscultated in all patients; abnormalities may warrant a chest radiograph.

HOT

KEY

The common cold often causes viral pharyngitis, viral sinusitis, or both, but these infections are self-limited, generally have less severe symptoms than their bacterial counterparts, and do not carry the same risk of complications as bacterial infections in these locations.

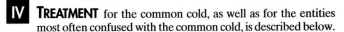 **TREATMENT** for the common cold, as well as for the entities most often confused with the common cold, is described below.

A. Common cold. Antibiotics are not effective in patients with a common cold. Therapy centers on minimizing the patient's symptoms.

  1. **Zinc lozenges or vitamin C.** Taking zinc lozenges or vitamin C when cold symptoms are present may reduce the duration of illness.

    a. **Zinc lozenges.** Regular use of zinc lozenges (e.g. one lozenge containing 13.3 mg of zinc every 2 hours while awake) may reduce the duration of the common cold by several days.

TABLE 12-1. Features of Infections Often Confused with the Common Cold

	Bacterial Sinusitis	Bacterial Pharyngitis	Allergic Rhinitis
History	Maxillary toothache Poor response to decongestants Purulent nasal discharge	Recent exposure to group A streptococci Positive throat culture for group A streptococci in past year No rhinorrhea or cough	Itchy eyes, nose, throat Tearing Seasonal or allergic pattern
Physical examination	Purulent discharge Tender sinuses Abnormal transillumination	Temperature > 101°F Anterior cervical lymphadenopathy Tonsilar exudate	Pale, edematous nasal mucosa (in contrast to erythematous mucosa associated with viral infections)

      b. **Vitamin C** (1 g per day) may reduce the duration of the illness by approximately 1 day.

  2. **Fluids** help prevent dehydration and may loosen secretions.

  3. **Drugs** that can alleviate the symptoms of the common cold are shown in Table 12-2.

      a. Expectorants have not been proven to have any benefit.

      b. Antihistamines are generally not used because they dry the nasal mucosa and prevent adequate drainage, although they may be useful as a sleeping aid.

HOT **KEY**

α-Agonist nasal sprays, such as phenylephrine, should not be used for more than 3 days because extended treatment may cause rebound congestion (rhinitis medicamentosa) when the medication is stopped.

B. **Allergic rhinitis.** Patients with history and physical examination findings consistent with allergic rhinitis may be treated as follows (listed in the recommended order of therapy):

  1. **Topical corticosteroids** (e.g., beclomethasone, 1 spray in each nostril twice daily) are very effective at reducing nasal symptoms. Symptoms generally improve only after 1–2 weeks of treatment.

  2. **Antihistamines.** Nonsedating, long-acting agents (e.g., loratadine, 10 mg orally once daily) are the easiest to use and are useful when the patient's symptoms are not controlled with nasal steroids.

HOT **KEY**

Astemizole and terfenadine should not be given with drugs that impair their metabolism (e.g., erythromycin, ketoconazole) because doing so may precipitate QT prolongation and torsades de pointes.

---

  3. **Cromolyn sodium nasal spray** (1 puff in each nostril 3–4 times daily) may be useful, especially before contact with a known allergen.

  4. **Ipratropium nasal spray** (0.03%, 2 puffs in each

TABLE 12-2. Selected Symptomatic Treatments for the Common Cold

Class of Drug	Examples	Dose	For Relief Of	Warnings
Oral decongestants	Pseudoephedrine	60 mg orally every 6 hours	Nasal congestion	Causes vasoconstriction and may elevate blood pressure; use with caution in patients with coronary artery disease
Decongestant nasal sprays	Phenylephrine	2 sprays per nostril every 3–4 hours	Nasal congestion	Long-term therapy (i.e., greater than 3 days) associated with rebound congestion
Analgesics	Acetaminophen	650 mg orally every 4–6 hours	Fever and pain	Be aware of specific contraindications for each agent (e.g., avoid aspirin in patients younger than 18 years)
	Ibuprofen	400 mg orally every 4–6 hours		
	Aspirin	650 mg orally every 4–6 hours		
Cough suppressants	Dextromethorphan	10 ml orally every 4 hours	Sleeplessness due to night-time cough	Can cause constipation
	Codeine	10 ml orally every 4 hours		

nostril 2–3 times daily) is effective for reducing nasal congestion.

    5. Immunotherapy. Antigen testing and immunotherapy may be used in patients who do not respond to other treatments.

C. Bacterial sinusitis. The treatment for bacterial sinusitis is discussed in Chapter 11 VI A.

D. Bacterial pharyngitis. The treatment for bacterial pharyngitis is discussed in Chapter 13 IV.

V FOLLOW-UP AND REFERRAL

A. Patients with a common cold do not need scheduled follow-up, although they should be advised to return if symptoms worsen or do not improve within approximately 1 week.

B. Patients with allergic rhinitis that does not respond to medical therapy may be referred to an allergist for antigen testing.

References

Hemila H: Does vitamin C alleviate the symptoms of the common cold?—a review of current evidence. *Scand J Infect Dis* 26(1):1–6, 1994.

Lorber B: The common cold. *J Gen Intern Med* 11(4):229–236, 1996.

Mossad SB, Macknin ML, Medendorp SV, et al: Zinc gluconate lozenges for treating the common cold: a randomized, double-blind, placebo-controlled study. *Ann Intern Med* 125(2):81–88, 1996.

13. Pharyngitis

I INTRODUCTION

A. "Sore throat" resulting from pharyngitis is a common complaint in ambulatory medicine, accounting for **2%–3% of office visits.**

B. Viruses are the most common cause, but **group A streptococci** account for as many as 10% of cases of pharyngitis in adult patients. Because untreated group A streptococcal infection has a number of dangerous complications (e.g., acute rheumatic fever, peritonsillar abscess, acute glomerulonephritis), it is important to identify and treat this subset of patients.

II CAUSES OF PHARYNGITIS

A. **Rhinovirus, coronavirus, adenovirus, influenza virus,** and **parainfluenza virus infection.** The same viruses responsible for the upper respiratory viral infections that produce the common cold are the most common cause of pharyngitis. Rhinorrhea, cough, headache, and malaise commonly accompany the sore throat.

B. **Group A** *Streptococcus* **infection** is often characterized by a severe sore throat accompanied by fever and odynophagia. Cough, rhinorrhea, and hoarseness are not usually present.

C. **Groups C, G,** and **F** *Streptococcus, Mycoplasma,* and *Chlamydia* **infection** are uncommon, self-limited, bacterial causes of sore throat with similar presenting features (i.e., severe sore throat, fever, odynophagia).

D. *Neisseria gonorrhoeae* **pharyngitis** may develop after orogenital contact with an infected person.

E. *Corynebacterium diphtheriae* **infection** is characterized by a sore throat and a grey-white exudate (a "pseudomembrane") that coats the pharynx. Patients who have not been immunized are most at risk.

F. **Epstein-Barr virus infection.** Acute infection causes infectious mononucleosis and is most common in children and adolescents. Patients present with a sore throat, pharyngeal edema and exudate, and cervical lymphadenopathy. Prodromal symptoms of headache, fatigue, and fever are common. Splenomegaly occurs in approximately 50% of patients.

APPROACH TO THE PATIENT. The goal of the evaluation is to identify patients with group A streptococcal infection so that proper treatment can be initiated to prevent the development of complications.

A. History and physical examination

1. The oropharynx should be examined for exudate, erythema, tonsillar swelling, and mucosal lesions.

   a. Group A streptococcal infection is more likely if the features shown in Table 13-1 are present; however, diagnosis of group A streptococcal infection cannot usually be made on the basis of clinical findings alone.

   b. Asymmetry of the soft palate, a fluctuant mass, or deviation of the uvula suggests peritonsillar abscess.

   c. A history of dyspnea, stridor, or odynophagia out of proportion to the physical examination findings suggests epiglottitis.

HOT

Immediate consultation with an otolaryngologist is required when peritonsillar abscess or epiglottitis is suspected.

KEY

---

2. Adolescents or children with prodromal features of mononucleosis should be examined for splenomegaly.

B. Laboratory studies. Patients with none of the features shown in Table 13-1 and symptoms consistent with the common cold have a very low probability of group A streptococcal infection and can be treated for the common cold without testing. Laboratory studies are indicated for patients with suspected group A streptococcal infection or mononucleosis.

1. **Group A streptococcal infection**

   a. **Group A *Streptococcus* antigen testing** is indicated for patients with one or more of the features listed in Table 13-1. Most "rapid strep tests" have a sensitivity and specificity of approximately 80% and 95%, respectively.

   (1) Patients with a positive test should be treated with antibiotics and do not require a throat culture.

TABLE 13-1. Clinical Findings Suggestive of Group A Streptococcal Infection

History
    Recent exposure to known group A *Streptococcus* infection
    History of group A streptococcal infection in the past year
    Absence of cough, hoarseness, or rhinorrhea
Physical examination
    Temperature > 101°F
    Tonsillar exudate
    Anterior cervical adenopathy

        (2) Patients with a negative test should be considered for throat culture, especially if the patient has several signs and symptoms suggestive of streptococcal infection.

     b. **Throat culture** is considered the gold standard test, although results are not available for 1–3 days.

  2. **Mononucleosis.** Patients with historical and examination features suggestive of mononucleosis should have a **monospot test.** False-negative results are possible within 3 weeks of infection, so patients with suggestive features and a negative test should return for repeat testing.

IV TREATMENT

A. Antibiotic therapy

  1. *Corynebacterium* **infection.** Therapy with **antitoxin** [which can be obtained from the Centers for Disease Control (CDC)] and **erythromycin** (500 mg orally 4 times daily) is indicated.

  2. *Neisseria* **infection** in adults can be treated with a single injection of **ceftriaxone** (125 mg intramuscularly).

  3. **Group A streptococcal infection.** Although group A streptococcal pharyngitis is self-limited, antibiotic treatment reduces the duration of symptoms and prevents the development of some complications.

HOT KEY

Antibiotic treatment does not appear to prevent the development of acute glomerulonephritis in association with group A streptococcal infection.

    a. **Duration of therapy.** Ten days of treatment are required for optimal prevention of complications.

    b. **Selection of agents.** Empiric treatment may be considered when 5 or 6 of the clinical features of group A streptococcal infection are present, although antigen testing is generally preferred to guide treatment. The following antibiotic choices are all highly effective.

        (1) Benzathine penicillin G (1.2 million units administered intramuscularly once) has a higher incidence of severe allergic reaction, but eliminates adherence problems.

        (2) Penicillin V (250 mg orally 3 times daily for 10 days) can be used.

        (3) Erythromycin (333 mg orally 3 times daily for 10 days) is indicated for patients who are allergic to penicillin or who live in an area with known high resistance patterns to penicillin. Alternatively, a **cephalosporin** (e.g., cefuroxime axetil, 250 mg orally twice daily for 10 days) may be used.

HOT KEY

It is not known whether antibiotic treatment is of any benefit when pharyngitis is caused by group C, G, or F streptococci, *Mycoplasma,* or *Chlamydia.*

B. Symptomatic therapy

    1. **Mild analgesics** (e.g., ibuprofen, 400 mg every 6 hours or acetaminophen, 650 mg every 6 hours) are useful for pain relief and reduction of fever.

    2. **Throat lozenges** or **sprays** may provide some relief.

V FOLLOW-UP AND REFERRAL

A. Patients who have complete relief of symptoms do not require scheduled follow-up.

B. Patients with more than 6 documented group A streptococcal infections per year can be considered for tonsillectomy.

References

Pichichero, ME: Group A streptococcal tonsillopharyngitis: cost-effective diagnosis and treatment. *Ann Emerg Med* 25(3):390–403, 1995.

Cardiology

Cardiology

14. Chest Pain

I **INTRODUCTION.** Because chest pain (including "discomfort") is common and its causes range from a life-threatening myocardial infarction to benign musculoskeletal pain, a simple and reliable approach to the patient is necessary.

HOT

KEY

Patients who present with chest pain must be seen immediately. If there are any signs or symptoms suggestive of acute coronary ischemia, urgent transfer to an emergency department (ED) for monitoring and treatment is required while the initial evaluation is being completed.

II **CAUSES OF CHEST PAIN.** One way to remember the causes of chest pain is to take an "outside-in" approach.

A. Skin. Varicella-zoster virus infection (shingles) often causes pain before vesicular lesions are noted. The pain usually occurs in a dermatomal distribution.

B. Chest wall. Musculoskeletal pain may result from shoulder arthritis or bursitis, intercostal injury, metastatic disease to the bones or chest wall, or costochondritis. Breast pathology (e.g., tumors, fibrocystic disease) and nerve root compression (from cervical disk herniation) may also cause chest pain.

C. Lungs. Spontaneous pneumothorax, pulmonary embolus, infection, malignancy, or a connective tissue disorder can cause pleural inflammation, which is usually associated with pleuritic chest pain (i.e., the pain worsens with inspiration or coughing).

D. Heart and great vessels. Pericarditis, myocardial ischemia and infarction, and aortic dissection can all cause chest pain.

E. Gastrointestinal tract. Esophageal disorders (including esophagitis, spasm, and rupture) are common causes of chest pain. Other gastrointestinal causes of chest pain include gastric and duodenal ulcers, pancreatitis, and biliary disease.

HOT

4 "Killer" Chest Pains
Myocardial infarction or ischemia
Pulmonary embolism
Aortic dissection
Spontaneous pneumothorax

KEY

III **APPROACH TO THE PATIENT.** First, quickly screen for the "killer" chest pains, then perform a more in-depth evaluation if the cause of the chest pain is still unclear.

A. Screen for the "killer" chest pains.
1. **"Eyeball" the patient.** A patient who is clutching his chest, diaphoretic, and ashen can be presumptively diagnosed from across the room as suffering from myocardial infarction. Even if the presentation is not so classic, you can often decide on who looks "sick," and may need a rapid evaluation in a more monitored setting.
2. **Establish intravenous access and cardiac rhythm monitoring** immediately in patients who appear ill or who have cardiac risk factors.
3. **Evaluate the patient's vital signs.**

HOT

Any abnormality of the vital signs should alert you to the possibility that the chest pain has a potentially serious cause.

KEY

a. **Check the blood pressure in both arms.** Although a difference in pressure of 10 mm Hg or more may be seen in patients with aortic dissection, local atherosclerosis can also produce pressure differences. Therefore, the blood pressure reading is neither sensitive nor specific for aortic dissection.
b. **Check the respiratory rate and oxygen saturation.** A low oxygen saturation may accompany spontaneous pneumothorax, pulmonary embolism, and myocardial infarction (with pulmonary edema).

       (1) A **low oxygen saturation** (e.g., < 92%) is often an indication that an arterial blood gas (ABG) should be ordered immediately.

       (2) A **normal oxygen saturation** may still be accompanied by a significant alveolar-to-arterial (A-a) oxygen gradient during hyperventilation. Therefore, ABG testing to evaluate the possibility of pulmonary embolism may still be necessary if the rest of the evaluation is unrevealing.

4. **Look at the electrocardiogram (EKG).** The EKG leads are often placed while the vitals are obtained.

    a. **EKG abnormalities** that suggest **myocardial infarction** or **ischemia** are always grounds for admission. Make sure the patient has intravenous access, a cardiac rhythm monitor, supplemental oxygen, and has been administered 1 aspirin (usually 325 mg) orally.

    b. **Normal EKG.** Because a normal EKG does not rule out a myocardial infarction or ischemia, **nitroglycerin** (0.3–0.6 mg sublingually or via aerosol) may be administered and the dose repeated every 3–5 minutes as both a diagnostic challenge and as potential therapy.

5. **Take a preliminary history.**

    a. **Cardiac history and risk factors.** First, ask about any prior cardiovascular problems.

       (1) If there is a history of coronary artery disease (CAD), the patient has ischemia until proven otherwise.

HOT **KEY** In patients with a history of CAD or cardiac risk factors and no alternative explanation for the chest pain after careful evaluation, an admission to rule out myocardial infarction (ROMI) is usually appropriate.

---

       (2) If the patient's cardiac history is negative, you can quickly establish the pretest probability of myocardial infarction by assessing cardiac risk factors:

         (a) Age > 45 years (in men) or 55 years (in women)

         (b) Male gender

        (c) History of smoking

        (d) Diabetes mellitus

        (e) Hypertension

        (f) High cholesterol

        (g) Obesity

        (h) Family history of CAD in first-degree male relative younger than 55 years or female relative younger than 65 years

    b. Other risk factors. The preliminary history can also help elucidate any factors that may predispose the patient to the other "killer" chest pains. For example, a history of cancer or inactivity may suggest pulmonary embolism, and uncontrolled hypertension may increase the likelihood of aortic dissection or myocardial infarction.

6. Perform a preliminary physical examination. Often, you will have a few moments between tests where you can look at the neck veins, listen to the heart and lungs, palpate the upper abdomen for tenderness, and evaluate the pulses in the arms and legs.

7. Evaluate the chest radiographs. Always compare the new films to old films, if they are available.

    a. Spontaneous pneumothorax can be subtle and you need to look carefully, especially in the apices.

    b. Esophageal rupture may lead to air in the mediastinum (pneumomediastinum).

    c. Myocardial infarction or **aortic dissection** may be accompanied by enlargement of the heart or mediastinum, respectively; however, these structures are often exaggerated on anteroposterior films. The presence of pulmonary edema may also be suggestive of myocardial infarction.

8. Order an ABG. If not performed earlier, an ABG analysis with the patient breathing room air is usually necessary.

B. Further define the cause of the chest pain.

1. Take a more detailed patient history.

    a. Type of chest pain. Pulmonary embolism frequently presents with pleuritic chest pain, myocardial infarction may present with "crushing" chest pain or only a mild "discomfort," and aortic dissection often is characterized by a ripping pain that radiates to the back.

    b. Radiation of chest pain. Pain that radiates to the neck, left arm, or both arms should be considered cardiac in origin until proven otherwise.

(1) Atypical patterns may also indicate ischemia and include pain, tingling, or numbness in the left fingertips unaccompanied by arm pain and pain in the outer left shoulder.

(2) It is wise to consider any neck, upper abdominal, or upper back pain as cardiac in origin until proven otherwise.

c. Onset of chest pain. Spontaneous pneumothorax, aortic dissection, and pulmonary embolism usually present with abrupt pain, whereas pain from myocardial infarction or ischemia may build more gradually. Spontaneous pneumothorax and pulmonary embolism often occur while the patient is at rest, whereas aortic dissection and myocardial infarction may occur with rest or exertion.

d. Duration of chest pain. Pain that only lasts seconds or that has been constant for more than 24 hours is usually not caused by one of the four "killer" chest pains. A myocardial infarction is almost always associated with more than 20 minutes of chest pain.

e. Associated symptoms. Dyspnea, diaphoresis, or lightheadedness should alert you to a probable serious cause of chest pain.

f. Aggravating and mitigating factors

(1) Deep inspiration often aggravates pain from the pleura or pericardium (e.g., pleurisy from a pulmonary embolism or pericarditis).

(2) Exertion may worsen the pain from myocardial infarction or aortic dissection. **Rest** may ease the pain from cardiac ischemia, usually gradually.

(3) Position. Patients with pericarditis often feel worse when supine, and better sitting up. Patients with musculoskeletal pain may feel worse in certain positions. The pain of myocardial infarction is usually unaffected by changes in position, but this is not always the case.

(4) Food intake. Pain on swallowing localizes the problem to the gastrointestinal tract. Chest pain after a meal may indicate gastrointestinal pathology, but it also may occur with myocardial infarction.

(5) Nitroglycerin. If chest pain decreases with nitrates (e.g., sublingual nitroglycerin), a cardiac

cause is likely; however, esophageal spasm
may also respond to this therapy.

2. **Perform a complete physical examination.** Pay extra
attention to the following parts of the exam.

   a. **Jugular venous pressure.** An elevated jugular venous pressure should alert you to the possibility
of a serious disorder (e.g., myocardial infarction,
pulmonary embolism, or tension pneumothorax), but a normal jugular venous pressure does
not exclude these disorders.

   b. **Cardiac examination**

      (1) Heart sounds. Listen carefully for a third
heart sound (S_3) or fourth heart sound (S_4)
gallop, which may indicate impaired ventricular contractility or ventricular relaxation,
respectively. Both impaired ventricular contractility and impaired relaxation can accompany cardiac ischemia.

      (2) Murmurs may also increase the likelihood of
a cardiac etiology of chest pain. A mitral regurgitant murmur may accompany a myocardial infarction with papillary muscle ischemia, whereas an ejection murmur may
indicate aortic stenosis or hypertrophic cardiomyopathy (both of these conditions may
predispose the patient to ischemia).

   c. **Lung examination.** Listen carefully for rales (e.g.,
from myocardial infarction with pulmonary
edema) and pleural friction rubs (e.g., from pulmonary embolism, infection, or other pleural
processes).

   d. **Chest wall examination.** Minimal tenderness to
palpation is nonspecific, but if the chest pain is ex-
actly and reliably reproduced (especially in a
well-localized area), a musculoskeletal cause is
likely. Briefly inspect the skin for lesions.

   e. **Abdominal examination.** Palpate for any upper
abdominal tenderness that may indicate a gastrointestinal cause of the chest pain.

   f. **Pulses.** Check pulses in the arms and legs bilater-
ally.

C. **Diagnostic pearls**

  1. **Myocardial infarction**

   a. Because CAD is such a common disease, it is always better to admit patients for ROMI if there
is any doubt as to the diagnosis, even in young patients.

    b. More than 20 minutes of unexplained chest pain may represent a myocardial infarction. Chest pain that lasts less than 20 minutes but increases in frequency or duration or occurs with minimal exertion often represents unstable angina. Both patterns are indications for admission.

    c. Frequently, patients with chest pain are given an antacid and lidocaine swish-and-swallow ("GI cocktail") to assess for reflux esophagitis. Many patients who "benefit" from this "diagnostic test" may actually have ischemic pain that is improving spontaneously or as a result of bed rest and oxygen therapy.

2. Pulmonary embolus. Clinical suspicion is critical. There is often no evidence of deep venous thrombosis (DVT), and subtle symptoms and signs may be inappropriately rationalized away. If you have a high clinical index of suspicion, administer heparin to the patient before sending him for diagnostic tests.

3. Aortic dissection

    a. The greater curvature of the aorta is the site for most dissections; the right coronary artery is the one most frequently "picked off." If the patient has pain that radiates to the back, unequal blood pressures, or other suspicious findings accompanied by evidence of right coronary ischemia (i.e., inferior or right ventricular ischemia), aortic dissection should be considered.

    b. Both computed tomography (CT) and transesophageal echocardiography are used in the evaluation of aortic dissection. The choice of diagnostic modality depends on the patient (e.g., poor renal function may weigh against a CT scan) and institutional preferences. If clinical suspicion is high, a surgeon should be consulted immediately for input regarding subsequent evaluation. Transthoracic echocardiography is not sensitive enough to rule out aortic dissection.

IV **TREATMENT** is directed toward the underlying disorder.

A. "Killer" chest pains. Patients require **admission to the hospital** for intensive monitoring and treatment.

B. Shingles. Early treatment of varicella-zoster virus infection reduces the incidence of post-herpetic neuralgia and may reduce the duration of the painful rash.

    1. Acyclovir (800 mg orally 5 times daily) is commonly

used (the dosage should be adjusted for patients with renal insufficiency).

2. **Steroids** reduce pain and may help the patient resume normal activities, but they do not have an effect on post-herpetic neuralgia. A 3-week taper of prednisone (starting at 60 mg orally once daily) should be considered for immunocompetent patients.

C. **Musculoskeletal pain** usually responds to limitation of strenuous activity and a 5- to 10-day course of nonsteroidal anti-inflammatory drugs (NSAIDs), such as ibuprofen (400 mg orally 3 times daily). An ice pack applied to the painful area for 20 minutes, 2–4 times daily, may also be helpful.

D. **Gastrointestinal disorders**

1. **Esophagitis.** Therapy is discussed in Chapter 35 IV C 1.

2. **Peptic ulcer disease.** Therapy is discussed in Chapter 36 IV A.

3. **Esophageal spasm** that is recurrent may respond to sublingual nitroglycerine (0.4 mg sublingually once for an episode of pain, not to exceed 3 tablets daily), oral nitrates (e.g., isosorbide dinitrate, 10–30 mg 3 times daily), or calcium channel blockers (e.g., long-acting nifedipine, 30–90 mg daily).

V FOLLOW-UP AND REFERRAL

A. **"Killer" chest pains.** These patients should be seen within a few days of being discharged from the hospital so that their progress can be monitored and long-term treatment plans can be discussed. Specialty consultation is usually indicated.

B. **Shingles.** Patients should be re-examined in 1 week to ensure that the rash is improving and not infected.

C. **Musculoskeletal disorders.** Patients should be seen in 1–2 weeks to ensure that the problem has been resolved. Patients with persistent symptoms may require further evaluation.

D. **Gastrointestinal disorders.** Follow-up depends on the specific disorder.

References

Panju AA, Hemmelgarn BR, Guyatt GH, et al: Is this patient having a myocardial infarction? *JAMA* 280(14):1256–1263, 1998.

Zalenski RJ, Shamsa F, Pede KJ: Evaluation and risk stratification of patients with chest pain in the emergency department: predictors of life threatening events. *Emerg Med Clin North Am* 16(3):495–517, 1998.

15. Syncope

I INTRODUCTION

A. Syncope is a transient loss of consciousness and postural tone that is caused by inadequate cerebral blood flow.

B. Syncope is extremely common, accounting for approximately 5% of medical admissions and 3% of emergency room visits. The lifetime incidence approaches 50% in some groups.

II CAUSES OF SYNCOPE.
There are many causes of syncope, but the most important can be remembered using the mnemonic, "SYNCOPE."

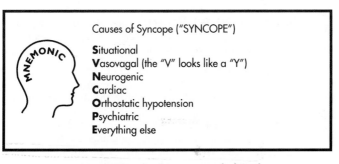

Causes of Syncope ("SYNCOPE")

Situational
Vasovagal (the "V" looks like a "Y")
Neurogenic
Cardiac
Orthostatic hypotension
Psychiatric
Everything else

A. Situational causes include micturition, defecation, swallowing, coughing, subclavian steal, and carotid sinus hypersensitivity.

B. Vasovagal syncope, also known as the "common faint," is the most common cause of syncope in young patients and is often preceded by a painful or emotional stimulus.

C. Neurogenic causes include autonomic insufficiency and transient ischemic attacks (TIAs).

    1. Autonomic insufficiency is common in elderly patients and patients with diabetes.

    2. TIAs are extremely rare causes of syncope. For syncope to occur, the vertebrobasilar circulation must be involved.

D. Cardiac causes

    1. Obstructive disorders. Aortic, mitral, or pulmonic stenosis, idiopathic subaortic stenosis, atrial myxoma, and pulmonary embolism may interfere with cardiac output and can precipitate a syncopal attack.

2. **Arrhythmias.** Disorders that lead to bradycardia [e.g. sick sinus syndrome, second- and third-degree atrioventricular (AV) block] or tachycardia (e.g. ventricular fibrillation, ventricular tachycardia, torsades de pointes, supraventricular tachycardia) can also interfere with cardiac output.

3. **Ischemic disorders** can precipitate an episode of syncope.

E. **Orthostatic hypotension** can cause syncope.

F. **Psychogenic syncope** is a diagnosis of exclusion.

G. **Everything else**

1. **Medications** (e.g., vasodilators, hypnotics, sedatives, nitrates, diuretics, α blockers)

2. **Drugs** (e.g., cocaine, alcohol)

III **APPROACH TO THE PATIENT.** The evaluation of a patient with syncope must be approached in a rigorous, stepwise fashion to avoid missing life-threatening disease.

A. **History and physical examination.** A thorough history and physical examination is a very important aspect of the evaluation and may establish the diagnosis in many patients.

1. **Situational.** Was the episode preceded by urination, defecation, swallowing, coughing, exertion of arm muscles (subclavian steal), or manipulation of the neck (carotid sinus hypersensitivity)?

2. **Vasovagal.** Did a painful or emotional stimulus precede the event?

3. **Neurogenic.** Was there a transient loss of neurologic function, such as numbness, weakness, visual changes, dysarthria, or poor coordination? Any abnormality in the neurologic examination must be fully evaluated.

HOT **KEY**

Convulsions, bowel or bladder incontinence, or signs suggestive of a postictal state (e.g., confusion after the episode) are suggestive of a seizure, not syncope.

4. **Cardiac**
   a. A cardiac cause is more likely if the patient has any <u>history suggestive of cardiac disease</u>:
      (1) Has the patient complained of feeling light-headed during exercise (suggestive of an obstructive cause)?
      (2) Has the patient complained of "palpitations" (suggestive of an arrhythmic cause)?
      (3) Has the patient complained of symptoms suggestive of cardiac ischemia (e.g., substernal chest pain or pressure, chest pain radiating to the arms or neck, or left arm pain)?
   b. Abnormalities found during the cardiac examination may suggest specific diagnoses and lead to more extensive testing (e.g., systolic murmur or delayed carotid pulse may suggest aortic stenosis).

5. **Orthostatic.** Does the patient report that he "got up too quickly"? Always check orthostatic vital signs in patients admitted with syncope.

6. **Psychogenic.** A psychogenic cause for the syncope (e.g., panic disorder) should be considered after all other causes have been excluded.

7. **Everything else.** What prescription, over-the-counter, or illicit drugs might the patient have used prior to the syncopal episode?

B. **Imaging studies.** All patients should have an electrocardiogram (EKG), although fewer than 10% of causes of syncope are identified in this manner. Look for evidence of acute or remote myocardial infarction, pre-excitation syndromes, arrhythmias, and conduction system disease.

C. **Risk assessment.** Patients should be classified as belonging to one of two groups: those without evidence of heart disease, and those who have known heart disease or some evidence of heart disease.

1. **No evidence of heart disease.** Patients who meet **all of the following criteria** after a thorough history, physical examination, and EKG are at low risk for having a cardiac disorder as the cause of their syncope, and additional cardiac testing may not be indicated. However, some patients may require additional evaluation and treatment. The criteria are:
   a. Age younger than 50 years
   b. No history of coronary artery disease (CAD), congestive heart failure (CHF), or arrhythmias
   c. Normal EKG

2. **Evidence of heart disease or CAD.** Anyone who does not meet the criteria described in III C 1 is included in this group, and the likelihood that an underlying cardiac defect is responsible for the syncope is greater. If there is suspicion of an ischemic or arrhythmic cause, admission and EKG monitoring are indicated. Additional diagnostic tests that may be appropriate include the following:

   a. **Ambulatory EKG monitoring** is widely used, but it establishes a diagnosis in only a small percentage of patients. Event or loop recorders may improve the diagnostic yield.

   b. **Exercise treadmill testing** can rule out exercise- or ischemia-induced syncope.

   c. **Echocardiography** allows assessment of valvular disease, as well as left ventricular size and function.

   d. **Electrophysiologic testing** is especially useful in patients at high risk for a ventricular arrhythmia (i.e., those with poor left ventricular function) when a diagnosis cannot be established using noninvasive methods.

   e. **Tilt table test.** This test can be useful for documenting vasovagal syncope, but a positive test does not mean that a more serious disorder (e.g., ventricular arrhythmia) is not present.

   f. **Signal-averaged EKG (SAEKG).** The utility of this test in patients with syncope is controversial.

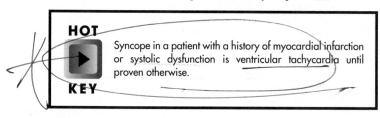

HOT KEY

Syncope in a patient with a history of myocardial infarction or systolic dysfunction is ventricular tachycardia until proven otherwise.

IV TREATMENT

A. **Cardiac syncope.** The treatment of any correctable cardiac abnormality should be the first consideration.

B. **Vasovagal syncope**

1. Avoidance of any precipitating stimulus (e.g., venipuncture, prolonged standing) may be useful.

2. Patients with recurrences or a positive tilt-table test may be treated with a trial of β blockers (e.g., aten-

olol, 50–100 mg orally, once daily). β blockers with intrinsic sympathomimetic activity (e.g., pindolol, 5–30
mg orally, twice daily) may also be useful. Consultation with a cardiologist is recommended.

C. Orthostatic hypotension
   1. Patients should be instructed to stay well-hydrated
      (by drinking eight 8-ounce glasses of water daily, in
      addition to normal fluids), increase salt intake, and
      avoid abrupt changes from a supine to an upright po-
      sition.
   2. Compression stockings may be useful.
   3. A trial of fludrocortisone (0.1–1 mg/day) may in-
      crease intravascular volume and relieve symptoms.
      Close monitoring of electrolytes and renal function is
      required when starting this agent.

D. Medication-induced syncope. Therapy with drugs that
may cause syncope should be stopped or changed in affected patients, if possible.

 FOLLOW-UP AND REFERRAL

A. Patients with suspected or known heart disease should be
followed in consultation with a cardiologist.
B. Patients with a suspected neurogenic cause for their syncope (e.g., TIA) require prompt referral to a neurologist.
C. A scheduled visit and re-examination is suggested for all
other patients within 2 weeks of the syncopal episode.

 HOT KEY All patients who have had a syncopal episode should be instructed not to drive and a report should be filed with the
Department of Motor Vehicles (DMV). The patient's license
can be reactivated if a full evaluation reveals that the patient is not at risk for a recurrence while driving.

References
Kapoor WN: Workup and management of patients with syncope. *Med Clin North Am*
79(5):1153–1170, 1995.
Martin TP, Hanusa BH, Kapoor WN: Risk stratification of patients with syncope. *Ann
Emerg Med* 29(4):459–466, 1997.

16. Hypertension

I INTRODUCTION

A. Patients who consistently have a **systolic blood pressure > 140 mm Hg** or a **diastolic blood pressure > 90 mm Hg** are considered to be hypertensive.

B. Hypertension is an extremely **common disorder,** affecting almost 1 of every 4 adults in the United States.

C. Hypertension is an important cause of **cerebrovascular, renal,** and **cardiac disease.**

II TYPES OF HYPERTENSION

A. **Primary (essential) hypertension** has no identifiable cause. Primary hypertension accounts for **95% of cases of hypertension.**

B. **Secondary hypertension** has an identifiable cause and must be considered in patients with **characteristic signs** or **symptoms,** the onset of hypertension at a **very young** or **old age,** or an elevated blood pressure that is **refractory to medical therapy.** The causes of secondary hypertension can be remembered using the following memory aid:

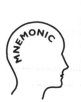

Causes of Secondary Hypertension

One anatomic cause
Two renal causes
Three adrenal causes
Four CENTs
   Calcium (hypercalcemia)
   Ethanol abuse or **E**strogen (oral contraceptives)
   Neurologic disease
   Thyrotoxicosis

1. **One anatomic cause. Aortic coarctation,** a congenital disorder characterized by aortic constriction at the origin of the left subclavian artery, usually presents in children or young adults and can lead to hypertension.

2. **Two renal causes**
   a. **Intrinsic renal disease.** Almost any parenchymal kidney disorder can lead to hypertension, usually

as a result of increased intravascular volume and increased activity of the renal-angiotensin-aldosterone system.

   b. **Renal artery stenosis,** a relatively common cause of secondary hypertension, is usually caused by fibromuscular dysplasia in young adults and atherosclerosis in older patients. The stenosis leads to decreased renal blood flow, which leads to increased renin release and hypertension.

HOT

Always consider renal artery stenosis as the cause of hypertension when a patient shows a dramatic increase in serum creatinine after starting angiotensin-converting enzyme (ACE) inhibitor therapy.

KEY

---

   3. **Three adrenal causes**
     a. **Primary hyperaldosteronism,** an uncommon cause of secondary hypertension, is caused by an aldosterone-secreting adenoma or bilateral adrenal hyperplasia.

HOT

Suspect primary hyperaldosteronism if a hypertensive patient is hypokalemic and not taking diuretics.

KEY

---

     b. **Cushing's syndrome.** Excess glucocorticosteroids (from any source) often lead to hypertension. Usually, other clinical manifestations of glucocorticoid excess are present.
     c. **Pheochromocytoma** is a norepinephrine- and epinephrine-secreting tumor that may be malignant. Other manifestations include headache, glucose intolerance, and flushing.
   4. **Four CENTs**
     a. **Calcium. Hypercalcemia** is an uncommon cause of hypertension but should be considered in those who have underlying diseases that may lead to hypercalcemia (see Chapter 79).
     b. **Ethanol abuse** or **estrogen.** The most common

causes of secondary hypertension are the use of **alcohol** and **oral contraceptive agents.** Hypertension from **pregnancy** requires careful evaluation.

   c. **Neurologic disease.** Any process that leads to **increased intracranial pressure (ICP)** can lead to the triad of hypertension, bradycardia, and irregular respiration (known as Cushing's triad).

   d. **Thyrotoxicosis.** Hyperthyroidism can also cause hypertension.

C. **Hypertensive crises**

   1. **Hypertensive urgencies** are situations in which the patient has a systolic blood pressure > 220 mm Hg or a diastolic blood pressure > 120 mm Hg and no evidence of end-organ damage.

   2. **Hypertensive emergencies** are those situations in which the elevated blood pressure leads to end-organ damage. A hypertensive emergency is hypertension accompanied by one of the following:

      a. **Hypertensive encephalopathy** (altered mental status)

      b. **Intracranial hemorrhage**

      c. **Aortic dissection**

      d. **Myocardial infarction**

      e. **Unstable angina**

      f. **Hypertensive nephropathy** (progressive acute renal failure with proteinuria and hematuria)

III APPROACH TO THE PATIENT

A. **Goals of evaluation** include the:

   1. Assessment of the presence and extent of end-organ disease (i.e., renal, cardiovascular, or cerebrovascular disease)

   2. Identification of factors that could lead to secondary hypertension (primary hypertension is a diagnosis of exclusion)

   3. Identification of comorbid conditions, which can affect management of the hypertension

B. **Patient history.** The history should focus on the following areas:

   1. The duration and severity of the hypertension

   2. Symptoms or a history of comorbid conditions (e.g., cardiac disease, stroke, peripheral vascular disease, diabetes mellitus, kidney disease)

   3. Medication history (over-the-counter and prescription drugs)

   4. Use of alcohol, tobacco, or illicit drugs (e.g., cocaine)

   5. Lifestyle and dietary habits (e.g., regularity of exercise, stress levels, salt intake)
C. Physical examination. The initial physical examination should focus on confirming the presence of elevated blood pressure in both arms. A complete examination also includes the following elements:
   1. Assessment of heart rate and weight
   2. Funduscopic examination
   3. Thyroid examination
   4. Evaluation of the heart and lungs
   5. Evaluation of bruits over the renal arteries
   6. Evaluation of the extremities
   7. Neurologic assessment
C. Laboratory and imaging studies
   1. The following studies should be ordered for most patients with hypertension, at least initially:
      a. A complete blood count (CBC)
      b. Urinalysis
      c. Chemistry panel (i.e., sodium, potassium, creatinine, fasting glucose, and total cholesterol levels)
      d. Electrocardiogram (EKG)
   2. More specific studies (e.g., thyroid function tests, echocardiogram) may be necessary to rule out secondary causes of hypertension or complications caused by the hypertension.

IV TREATMENT

A. Primary (essential) hypertension. The goal of treatment is to decrease the patient's risk of stroke, cardiovascular disease, and renal disease by lowering the systolic and diastolic blood pressures to at least 140 mm Hg and 90 mm Hg, respectively (Figure 16-1).
   1. Lifestyle modifications. The patient should be advised to:
      a. Limit alcohol intake
      b. Stop smoking
      c. Lose weight (if applicable)
      d. Increase physical activity
      e. Reduce sodium intake
   2. Pharmacologic therapy should be started if the blood pressure is greater than 140/90 mm Hg after 3 months of lifestyle modification, or if the initial blood pressure is greater than 160/100 mm Hg. Five major categories of drugs are available to control blood pressure (Table 16-1). These categories are as easy to remember as "ABCDE."

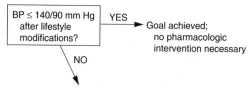

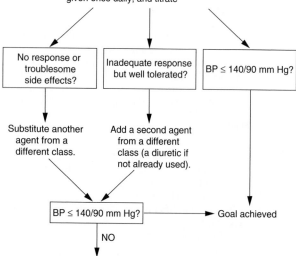

FIGURE 16-1. Algorithm for the management of hypertension. *ACE* = angiotensin-converting enzyme; *BP* = blood pressure; *CAD* = coronary artery disease; *CCB* = calcium channel blocker; *CHF* = congestive heart failure; *HTN* = hypertension. (Modified with permission from Joint National Commission on Prevention, Detection, Evaluation, and Treatment of High Blood Pressure: The sixth report of the joint national commission on prevention, detection, evaluation, and treatment of high blood pressure. *Arch Intern Med* 157(21):2413–2446, 1997.)

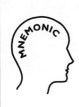

Classes of Drugs Used to Control Blood Pressure ("ABCDE")

ACE inhibitors and **A**ngiotensin II receptor blockers
β blockers
Calcium channel antagonists
Diuretics
Everything else (i.e., central α agonists, α blockers, combination therapy)

      a. In patients with **uncomplicated hypertension,** a β **blocker** or **diuretic** is used as a **first-line agent** because the long-term efficacy of these drugs for the treatment of hypertension has been established.

      b. In patients with a **comorbid condition,** another type of drug may be considered for a first-line therapy (Table 16-2).

B. Secondary hypertension. Treatment is aimed at the underlying cause.

C. Hypertensive crises

   1. Hypertensive urgency. Patients are usually treated with **oral antihypertensive agents** (e.g., nifedipine, clonidine, captopril) in the emergency room. Once the blood pressure is decreased to an acceptable level, these patients can usually be discharged, although they require very close follow-up.

HOT

Sublingual nifedipine should be avoided in almost all patients with hypertensive urgency because this drug may precipitate an abrupt decrease in blood pressure.

KEY

   2. Hypertensive emergency. Patients usually require admission to the intensive care unit (ICU) and the administration of **parenteral antihypertensives** (e.g., nitroprusside, nitroglycerin, labetalol, esmolol, or hydralazine).

V FOLLOW-UP AND REFERRAL

A. A home blood pressure monitoring device can be used to monitor the blood pressure and evaluate the effectiveness of therapy.

TABLE 16-1. Selected Agents Used for the Management of Hypertension

Generic Name	Trade name	Usual Dose Range Total Dose (mg/day)/ # of Doses per Day
Angiotensin-converting enzyme (ACE) inhibitors		
Captopril	Capoten	25–150/ 2–3
Enalapril maleate	Vasotec	5–40/ 1–2
Lisinopril	Zestril	5–40/ 1
Angiotensin II receptor blockers		
Losartan potassium	Cozaar	25–100/ 1–2
β blockers		
Metoprolol	Lopressor	50–200/ 2
Atenolol	Tenormin	50–100/ 1
Calcium channel antagonists		
Diltiazem	Cardizem SR	120–360/ 2
	Cardizem CD	120–360/ 1
Verapamil	Isoptin SR	90–480/ 2
	Calan SR	120–480/ 1
Amlodipine	Norvasc	2.5–10/ 1
Nifedipine	Procardia XL	30–120/ 1
	Adalat CC	30–120/ 1
Diuretics		
Hydrochlorothiazide	Hydrodiuril	12.5–50/ 1
	Esidrix	12.5–50/ 1
Other		
Clonidine	Catapres	0.2–1.2/ 2–3
Prazosin	Minipress	2–30/ 2–3

    1. The patient should check his blood pressure daily until it is under control, and weekly thereafter.

    2. Once the blood pressure is adequately controlled, an office visit every 3–6 months is appropriate.

  B. Referral to a hypertension specialist should be considered in the following situations:

    1. The blood pressure cannot be controlled adequately

    2. The patient is noncompliant

    3. The primary physician is having difficulty identifying a secondary cause in a patient whose history, physi-

TABLE 16-2. Antihypertensive Agents That May Be Considered for First-Line Therapy in Patients with Comorbid Conditions

Comorbid Condition	First-Line Agents
Angina	β Blocker and/or calcium channel blocker
Benign prostatic hyperplasia	Prazosin
Bradycardia or heart block	Diuretic, ACE inhibitor, or angiotensin II receptor antagonist
Congestive heart failure (diastolic)	Diuretic and/or β blocker or calcium channel blocker
Congestive heart failure (systolic)	ACE inhibitor and/or diuretic
Diabetes mellitus (type I)	ACE inhibitor
Edematous conditions	Diuretic
Gout (recurrent)	Any agent except a thiazide diuretic
Headaches (vascular)	β Blocker or calcium channel blocker
Impotence	ACE inhibitor, angiotensin II receptor antagonist, or calcium channel blocker
Myocardial infarction (history)	β Blocker
Pregnancy	Methyldopa
Reactive airway disease (severe)	Any agent except a β blocker
Renal insufficiency (chronic)	ACE inhibitor, diuretic, or angiotensin II receptor antagonist

ACE = angiotensin-converting enzyme.

cal examination findings, or laboratory study results strongly suggest secondary hypertension

References

Joint National Commission on Prevention, Detection, Evaluation, and Treatment of High Blood Pressure: The sixth report of the joint national commission on prevention, detection, evaluation, and treatment of high blood pressure. *Arch Intern Med* 157(21):2413–2446, 1997.

Psaty BM, Smith NL, Siscovick DS, et al: Health outcomes associated with antihypertensive therapies used as first-line agents: a systematic review and meta-analysis. *JAMA* 277(9):739–745, 1997.

17. Coronary Artery Disease

I **INTRODUCTION.** Coronary artery disease (CAD) is the **leading cause of death in the United States;** therefore, prevention and treatment of CAD is a major part of every primary care practice.

II **CLINICAL MANIFESTATIONS OF CORONARY ARTERY DISEASE (CAD)**

A. **Angina** is chest pain that results when the oxygen supply to the cardiac muscle is inadequate, usually from reduced blood in the coronary arteries as a result of atherosclerotic plaques.

1. **Stable angina** is a pattern of chest pain that has not changed. Patients generally report chest pain that occurs after certain amounts of exertion (e.g., walking up several flights of stairs, heavy housework) and resolves either spontaneously or after taking sublingual nitroglycerine (0.4 mg dissolved under the tongue).

2. **Unstable angina** is an increase in the frequency or duration of angina, or chest pain that occurs with rest. Unstable angina is a medical emergency that requires urgent evaluation and often necessitates admission to the hospital.

B. **"Anginal equivalents"** are symptoms other than chest pain (e.g., dyspnea, a burning sensation in the throat) that occur with exertion and are thought to be caused by myocardial ischemia. In patients with known CAD, these types of symptoms should be considered to be caused by ischemia until proven otherwise.

I. ℐexertion

II. 1-2 blocks. resyst

III. < 1 block

IV. atrest

II RISK FACTORS FOR CORONARY ARTERY DISEASE (CAD)

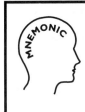

Risk Factors for CAD ("Start Helping CAD Fast")

Smoking
Hypertension
Cholesterol (hyperlipidemia)
Age
Diabetes mellitus
Family history of CAD

A. **Smoking.** Cigarette smokers who smoke more than one pack per day are three times more likely to develop CAD than nonsmokers. The risk of CAD increases with the number of cigarettes smoked per day.

B. **Hypertension** increases the likelihood of developing CAD. The risk increases with both systolic and diastolic blood pressure elevation.

C. **Hyperlipidemia.** Prevention studies have demonstrated that a 1% reduction in low-density lipoprotein (LDL) cholesterol levels reduces the risk of developing CAD by 2%.

D. **Age 45 years or older in men** and **55 years or older in women** is an unmodifiable risk factor for the development of CAD.

E. **Diabetes mellitus** is associated with a two-fold increase in the incidence of CAD in men, and a three-fold increase in risk in women.

F. **Family history of CAD.** CAD in a first-degree male relative younger than 55 years or a first-degree female relative younger than 65 years is another unmodifiable risk factor for CAD.

IV APPROACH TO THE PATIENT

A. **Prevention**
   1. **Primary prevention.** All patients (with or without CAD) should receive counseling regarding the primary prevention of CAD. Measures include advising against smoking and encouraging exercise and a healthy diet to prevent obesity (see Chapter 4 III A-C).
   2. **Secondary prevention.** Once a patient has developed risk factors for CAD, the goal is to **modify those risk factors as much as possible to prevent the development**

of clinical cardiovascular disease. Modifiable risk factors should be treated aggressively.

a. **Smoking.** Complete cessation is the goal. Provide **counseling, nicotine replacement therapy,** and referrals to **formal cessation programs** as necessary.

b. **Hypertension.** The goal is a blood pressure of less than 140/90 mm Hg. **Lifestyle modifications** and **pharmacologic therapy** are discussed in Chapter 16 IV A 1–2.

c. **Hyperlipidemia** may be primary or secondary. Secondary causes of hyperlipidemia include hypothyroidism, nephrotic syndrome, biliary obstruction, hepatoma, chronic renal failure, hyperuricemia, Cushing's syndrome, alcohol abuse, and therapy with certain medications (e.g., steroids, thiazides). Starting at age 35 years, patients should have their total cholesterol, LDL, and high-density lipoprotein (HDL) levels measured. (Evaluation may begin earlier for patients with a family history of familial hyperlipidemia and premature CAD.)

(1) **Management goals.** The number of risk factors the patient has for CAD determines the cholesterol management goal. Smoking, hypertension, an HDL level < 35 mg/dl, age ≥ 45 years (or ≥ 55 years in women), diabetes mellitus, and a family history of CAD are each assigned 1 point. If the HDL is ≥ 60 mg/dl, subtract 1 point from the total.

(2) **Management strategies** include **diet modification** and **pharmacologic therapy.** The choice of diet or pharmacologic therapy depends on both the number of risk factors and the patient's LDL level (Table 17-1). Patients with multiple risk factors are started on drug therapy at lower LDL levels than patients with no risk factors. Pharmacologic therapy should be started if diet modification does not achieve the treatment goal within 3–6 months.

(a) **Diet modification.** Patients should be placed on the American Heart Association (AHA) step II diet (i.e., ≤ **30% fat,** ≤ **7% saturated fat,** ≤ **200 mg/day cholesterol).**

(b) **Pharmacologic therapy** is usually initiated with one agent (Table 17-2), but combination drug therapy may be needed if the LDL goal is not reached.

TABLE 17-1. Treatment Goals in Patients with Hyperlipidemia

Number of CAD Risk Factors	Treatment Goal LDL Level (mg/dl)	Begin Diet Therapy* LDL Level (mg/dl)	Begin Drug Therapy LDL Level (mg/dl)
0–1	< 160 — 150 ?	≥ 160	≥ 190
≥ 2	< 130	≥ 130	≥ 160
Documented CAD	≤ 100	> 100	≥ 130

CAD = coronary artery disease; LDL = low-density lipoprotein.
*American Heart Association (AHA) step II diet: ≤ 30% fat, ≤ 7% saturated fat, < 200 mg cholesterol per day.

TABLE 17-2. Selected Cholesterol-Lowering Medications

Drug	Starting Dose	Maximum Dose	Therapeutic Effects	Indications	Side Effects
HMG-CoA reductase inhibitors			$\downarrow$ LDL $\uparrow$ HDL $\downarrow$ TG	First-line drugs for most patients	Elevated liver transaminases, myopathy, rhabdomyolysis*
Simvastatin *Zocor*	5–10 mg daily *20–40*	40 mg daily *80*			
Pravastatin *Pravachol*	10–20 mg daily	40 mg daily			
Lovastatin *Mevacor*	20 mg daily	80 mg daily			
Fluvastatin *Lescol*	20 mg daily	40 mg daily			
Atorvastatin *Lipitor*	10 mg	80 mg daily			
Niacin	100 mg twice daily	1–2 g three times daily	$\downarrow$ LDL $\uparrow$ HDL	Best drug for increasing HDL levels	Flushing†, worsening of glycemic control (in patients with diabetes), hyperuricemia
Fibric acids‡			$\downarrow$ TG $\uparrow$ HDL	May be useful for patients with very high TG levels	Myalgias, elevated liver transaminases, nausea, abdominal discomfort

Gemfibrozil	300–600 mg twice daily	600 mg twice daily		
Clofibrate	500 mg four times daily	500 mg four times daily		
Bile acid-binding resins§			↓ LDL	Bloating, constipation, vitamin K deficiency
Cholestyramine	4 g daily	4 g four times daily		
Colestipol	2 g daily	4 g four times daily		

HDL = high-density lipoproteins; HMG-CoA = 3-hydroxy-3-methylglutaryl coenzyme A; LDL = low-density lipoproteins; TG = triglycerides.

*Monitor with liver function tests and creatine kinase levels every 4–6 months.

†Flushing can be prevented by giving the patient aspirin (≥ 81 mg) 30 minutes prior to each dose.

‡Drugs in this class should not be used with HMG-CoA inhibitors due to an increased risk of myopathy.

§Drugs in this class impair the absorption of many other medications and should be used with caution.

      d. **Diabetes mellitus.** It is not clear whether **appropriate glycemic control** decreases the diabetic patient's risk of developing CAD. However, **aggressive modification of other risk factors** (e.g., smoking, hypertension, hyperlipidemia) in patients with diabetes is associated with greater CAD risk reduction than that seen in patients who do not have diabetes but take similar measures.

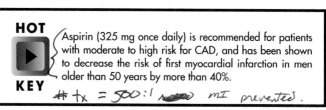

HOT KEY Aspirin (325 mg once daily) is recommended for patients with moderate to high risk for CAD, and has been shown to decrease the risk of first myocardial infarction in men older than 50 years by more than 40%.

tx = 500 : 1 ~~needed~~ mI prevented.

      3. **Tertiary prevention.** The goal of tertiary prevention is to **prevent the development of further morbidity** and **mortality** in patients who have **already experienced a myocardial infarction** or who have been found to **have CAD** through diagnostic testing.

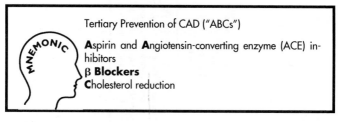

MNEMONIC

Tertiary Prevention of CAD ("ABCs")

Aspirin and **A**ngiotensin-converting enzyme (ACE) inhibitors
β **Blockers**
Cholesterol reduction

Tertiary prevention is further discussed in V A.

B. **Risk stratification.** Patients with CAD often present to a primary care provider after hospitalization for myocardial infarction or unstable angina. Risk stratification is the **process of evaluating the extent of CAD in a patient to determine whether the patient could benefit from revascularization or specific medical therapy.**

      1. **Assess the extent of the CAD.** The patient is first categorized as "high-risk" or "intermediate-or low-risk."

          a. **High-risk patients** are those who experienced cardiogenic shock, congestive heart failure (CHF), recurrent episodes of ischemia, or high-risk arrhythmias (e.g., ventricular fibrillation, ventricular tachycardia) during their hospitalization for myocardial infarction or unstable angina. All of these patients must undergo **cardiac catheterization** to determine if they are candidates for revascularization.

b. **Intermediate-** or **low-risk patients** are all of those who are not high-risk. These patients should undergo **noninvasive testing** to clarify the extent of their CAD.

HOT

KEY

For certain intermediate-risk patients, it may be appropriate to proceed straight to cardiac catheterization. Consultation with a cardiologist may be useful for these patients.

---

(1) **Noninvasive testing methods**

(a) **Exercise electrocardiography.** The patient exercises on a treadmill while his 12-lead electrocardiogram (EKG) is continuously monitored. ST segment depression that is downsloping and greater than 1 mm indicates significant ischemia.

(b) **Myocardial perfusion scintigraphy** is often performed in conjunction with exercise electrocardiography. A radioactive tracer [e.g., thallium-201 (^{201}Tl)] is injected into a peripheral vein while the patient exercises, and then again while the patient rests. **Well-perfused myocardial cells** take up the tracers and will **"light up"** when imaged.

(i) **Reversible defects** are areas of the heart that "light up" at rest, but show less tracer uptake with exercise (indicating ischemia with exertion).

(ii) **Fixed defects** are areas of the heart that do not take up tracer, even at rest (indicating infarcted tissue).

(c) **Pharmacologic stress tests** can be used for patients who are unable to exercise on a treadmill. Agents such as **dipyridamole** dilate the coronary arteries. Those arteries with more atherosclerotic plaque are unable to dilate as much in response to these agents, leading to lower uptake of tracer in regions supplied by diseased coronaries.

(d) **Stress echocardiography.** The patient exercises (or is given a drug that increases the heart rate and contractility, such as dobutamine) while undergoing echocardiography. Regional wall motion abnormalities or a decreased ejection fraction suggests significant CAD.

(2) Interpretation of noninvasive testing

(a) Patients who have markedly positive results on noninvasive testing should be considered for cardiac catheterization and revascularization.

(b) Patients with negative studies or only mild abnormalities may be managed with medical therapy alone.

2. **Assess left ventricular function. Echocardiography** or **multiple-gated acquisition scanning (MUGA)** is indicated for all patients after myocardial infarction to assess the left ventricular ejection fraction.

a. Patients with an ejection fraction of less than 40% are candidates for ACE inhibitor therapy.

b. Patients with mural thrombus, ventricular aneurysm, or a very low ejection fraction may be candidates for anticoagulation therapy to prevent the development of thrombus and embolic stroke.

V TREATMENT

A. **Medical treatment** can improve the quality of life for all patients with CAD and is generally aimed at increasing the myocardial oxygen supply (by dilating the coronary arteries) and decreasing the myocardial oxygen demand (by decreasing the heart rate, contractility, preload, or afterload).

1. **Aspirin** inhibits platelet aggregation and coronary thrombosis, thereby decreasing the patient's risk of a second myocardial infarction. Aspirin (325 mg once daily) is recommended for all patients with documented CAD.

2. **ACE inhibitors.** Following infarction, ACE inhibitors reduce mortality and recurrent myocardial infarction in patients with reduced left ventricular systolic function (i.e., an ejection fraction < 40%). In addition,

they attenuate post-infarction ventricular dilatation and remodeling.

3. **β Blockers** reduce recurrence in patients who have had a myocardial infarction by reducing the heart rate and contractility. In addition, they provide symptomatic relief of angina.

   a. **Commonly used β blockers** include **metoprolol** (25–100 mg orally, twice daily) and **atenolol** (25–100 mg orally, once daily). The initial dose should be at the low end of the range, with the goal of reducing the resting heart rate to approximately 60 beats/min. The dose may be increased until symptoms are controlled, side effects develop, or the maximum dose is reached.

   b. **Indications.** β Blockers are indicated for all patients who have had an infarction and can tolerate the medication.

   c. **Contraindications** include bradyarrhythmias and uncontrolled CHF. (β blockers may be beneficial in patients with controlled CHF.) These agents must be used with caution in patients with chronic obstructive pulmonary disease (COPD) or asthma.

   d. **Side effects** include postural hypotension, depression, and sexual dysfunction.

4. **HMG-CoA reductase inhibitors** and **niacin** have been shown to decrease the recurrence of myocardial infarction. In patients with known CAD, more aggressive lipid control is necessary; the goal is an LDL level of 100 mg/dl or less.

5. **Nitrates** increase oxygen supply by vasodilating the coronary arteries and decrease oxygen demand by decreasing the preload and afterload.

   a. **Short-acting nitrates** (e.g., **nitroglycerine,** 0.4 mg sublingually or by aerosol) can be used for immediate therapy or angina prophylaxis.

      (1) **Immediate therapy.** Patients should be instructed to take nitroglycerine every 3–5 minutes until the pain is relieved; if the pain is not relieved in 15 minutes, they should call for an ambulance.

      (2) **Angina prophylaxis.** The dose is taken 5 minutes before beginning an activity known to result in angina.

   b. **Long-acting nitrates** (e.g., **isosorbide dinitrate,** 10–40 mg orally four times daily) can provide prolonged relief.

          (1) A nitrate-free interval of approximately 8–10 hours daily is need to prevent tachyphylaxis.

          (2) Headaches frequently occur with the initiation of nitrate therapy, but they can be managed conservatively and frequently resolve within 1–2 weeks.

    6. **Calcium channel blockers** lower oxygen demand (by decreasing the heart rate, contractility, and afterload) and may increase oxygen supply (by inducing coronary artery vasodilation).

HOT KEY

Calcium channel blockers have not been shown to decrease mortality from myocardial infarction, so β blockers should always be considered before calcium channel blockers for patients with CAD.

---

        a. **Long-acting preparations** are preferred for chronic treatment, to improve compliance and maintain stable drug levels.

        b. **Agents** include—in order of decreased effect on lowering systemic vascular resistance and increased effect on myocardial inotropy and chronotropy—nifedipine, diltiazem, and verapamil.

          (1) **Nifedipine** (30–120 mg once daily)

          (2) **Diltiazem** (120–540 mg once daily)

          (3) **Verapamil** (120–480 mg once daily)

    7. **Unproven therapies**

        a. **Antioxidant vitamins.** Beta carotene, vitamin E, and vitamin C may reduce the risk of cardiovascular disease, although firm recommendations concerning their use cannot be made based on current evidence.

        b. **Folate.** Early studies suggest that folate supplementation may substantially reduce the risk of CAD in patients with high homocysteine levels, and should be considered for patients with known CAD. Firm recommendations await further study.

B. **Surgical treatment (revascularization).** The indications for **percutaneous transluminal coronary angioplasty (PTCA)** or **coronary artery bypass graft (CABG) surgery** are controversial.

    1. CABG is generally considered to be the treatment of choice for patients with left main CAD (> 50% occlusion) or three-vessel CAD ($> 70\%$ occlusion) and a decreased ejection fraction ($< 50\%$) or previous transmural infarction.

2. Patients who have been receiving maximal medical therapy and are still experiencing disabling angina may benefit from revascularization.

3. CABG may be preferable to PTCA in patients with diabetes, because the latter therapy has been associated with a higher rate of restenosis and complications in these patients.

V FOLLOW-UP AND REFERRAL

A. Primary prevention. Patients can be seen annually or semi-annually for counseling.

B. Secondary prevention. Patients should be seen regularly for risk factor modification.

    1. Patients with 2 or more risk factors should be seen at least every 1–3 months until risk factors are adequately controlled.

    2. Consultation with an endocrinologist is appropriate for patients with severe or difficult-to-manage cholesterol abnormalities.

C. Tertiary prevention and symptomatic control. Patients must be treated aggressively because they are at high risk for recurrent myocardial infarction and death.

    1. Weekly visits are appropriate until symptoms are controlled and all preventive measures have been employed, and then regular visits every 2–4 months are indicated.

    2. Consultation with a cardiologist is advised for patients with persistent symptoms despite medical therapy, or when noninvasive testing or revascularization is being considered.

References

American College of Physicians: Guidelines for risk stratification after myocardial infarction, part I and part II. *Ann Intern Med* 126(7):556–582, 1997.

Grundy SM, Balady GJ, Criqui MH, et al: Guide to primary prevention of cardiovascular diseases: a statement for healthcare professionals from the task force on risk reduction. *Circulation* 95(9):2329–2331, 1997.

Solomon AJ, Gersh BJ: Management of chronic stable angina: medical therapy, percutaneous transluminal coronary angioplasty, and coronary artery bypass graft surgery: lessons from the randomized trials. *Ann Intern Med* 128(3):216–223, 1998.

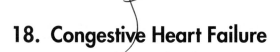

18. Congestive Heart Failure

I. INTRODUCTION

A. Definition. Congestive heart failure (CHF) occurs when the heart is unable to pump sufficient amounts of blood at normal filling pressures to keep pace with the metabolic demands of the body.

B. Clinical manifestations classically include fatigue, lethargy, dyspnea on exertion or rest, paroxysmal nocturnal dyspnea (PND), orthopnea, weight gain, and leg swelling.

C. Incidence. CHF is a common disorder, primarily affecting older individuals (10% of the population of the United States older than 75 years have CHF). Each year, 400,000 new cases are diagnosed.

D. Mortality rates. The annual mortality rate for all patients with CHF is 20%. For patients who are symptomatic at rest, the mortality rate is 50%. For those with pure diastolic dysfunction, it is 8%.

II. CLASSIFICATION. There are many different classification schemes. The most useful include the following:

A. New York Heart Association (NYHA) functional classification
1. **Class I:** Symptomatic only with greater than normal physical activity
2. **Class II:** Symptomatic during normal activity
3. **Class III:** Symptomatic with minimal activity
4. **Class IV:** Symptomatic at rest

B. Left-sided versus right-sided failure. It is important to decide if patients have evidence of left-sided failure, because these patients can present with marked hypoxemia and therefore may need to be treated urgently. The distinction between left-sided and right-sided failure is based primarily on signs found during physical examination.
1. **Left-sided failure.** Signs of left-sided failure include a **left-sided third heart sound (S_3), rales, wheezes** ("cardiac asthma," a manifestation of interstitial edema), and **tachypnea.**
2. **Right-sided failure.** Signs of right-sided failure in-

clude a **right-sided S$_3$** (i.e., one that increases with inspiration), an **elevated jugular venous pressure, abnormal hepatojugular reflux, ascites, peripheral
edema,** and an **enlarged liver.**

a. Most of the time, evidence of biventricular failure is found during physical examination because
**the most common cause of right-sided failure is
left-sided failure.**

HOT

KEY

Occasionally, right-sided failure can lead to left-sided diastolic dysfunction because of septal deviation into the left
ventricular cavity, thereby increasing the left ventricular
end-diastolic pressure and causing pulmonary edema.

---

b. Other causes of right-sided failure include:
   (1) **Mitral stenosis**
   (2) **Pulmonary hypertension** [most commonly
       caused by chronic obstructive pulmonary dis-
       ease (COPD)]
   (3) **Right ventricular infarction** (usually occur-
       ring in the setting of left-sided inferior wall
       infarction)
   (4) **Right-sided endocarditis**

C. **Systolic versus diastolic dysfunction.** Left ventricular
   failure can be either systolic or diastolic. This is the most
   important distinction to make because it affects treatment.
   1. **Systolic dysfunction** means that the heart's ability to
      pump is compromised. It implies that the **ejection
      fraction is below normal** (usually **< 40%**). Causes of
      systolic dysfunction include:
      a. **Myocardial infarction** and **ischemic heart dis-
         ease**
      b. **Dilated cardiomyopathies** [i.e., disorders of the
         myocardial cell that are not caused by coronary
         artery disease (CAD), hypertension, or valvular
         disease] (see mnemonic on pg 132)
      c. **"Burned out" hypertensive or valvular heart dis-
         ease.** Initially, these disorders lead to diastolic
         dysfunction, but with time, the heart dilates and
         the ejection fraction decreases.
      d. **Myocarditis**

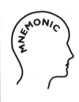

Causes of Cardiomyopathy ("PIPED")

Post-myocarditis
Idiopathic
Peripartum
Ethanol
Drugs (cocaine and heroin)

2. **Diastolic dysfunction** means that the heart is able to pump adequately, but its ability to relax and allow adequate filling during diastole is compromised. These patients have a **normal or supranormal ejection fraction.** Causes of diastolic dysfunction include:
   a. **Ischemia**
   b. **Disorders that lead to left ventricular hypertrophy,** such as:
      (1) Hypertension
      (2) Aortic stenosis
      (3) Hypertrophic cardiomyopathy
   c. **Restrictive cardiomyopathy.** This disorder is usually caused by infiltrative diseases (e.g., hemochromatosis, amyloidosis, sarcoidosis, scleroderma).
3. In most patients, evidence of both diastolic and systolic dysfunction coexist; however, 20% of patients have predominantly diastolic dysfunction. Both types of dysfunction have similar clinical manifestations.

HOT

CHF with a low ejection fraction = systolic dysfunction. CHF with a normal or high ejection fraction = diastolic dysfunction.

KEY

III APPROACH TO THE PATIENT

A. Assess how symptomatic the patient is.
B. On the basis of the patient's history, physical examination findings, and chest radiographs, categorize the failure as predominantly left-sided, right-sided, or biventricular.
C. If the patient has left-sided CHF, determine whether the dysfunction is predominantly systolic or diastolic, using the ejection fraction as a basis for the determination.

Ejection fraction can be assessed using echocardiography, multiple gated acquisition (MUGA) scans, or cardiac catheterization. **Remember, if a patient with a normal ejection fraction has cardiogenic pulmonary edema, then the dysfunction is diastolic.**

D. Determine the underlying cause of the CHF (e.g., CAD, valvular disease, hypertension, cardiomyopathy).

E. If the patient's symptoms have worsened, you must decide what precipitated the CHF exacerbation:

Factors that Can Exacerbate CHF ("FAILURE")

Forgot meds
Arrhythmia or **A**nemia
Infections, **I**schemia, or **I**nfarction
Lifestyle (e.g., increased sodium intake, stress)
Upregulators (e.g., thyroid disease, pregnancy)
Rheumatic valve or worsening of other valvular diseases
Embolism (pulmonary)

IV TREATMENT

A. Goals of treatment for CHF (and most other diseases) are two-fold:

1. **Reduce symptoms**
2. **Reduce mortality**

B. Chronic systolic dysfunction. Treatment involves the "4 Ds."

1. **Dilators.** Peripheral arterial vasodilators (Table 18-1) have been shown to reduce both symptoms and mortality. These agents reduce afterload by decreasing systemic vascular resistance. Usually, therapy is initiated with a low dose that is then titrated upward based on the drug's effects on the patient's blood pressure and symptoms.

HOT

Every patient with systolic dysfunction should be taking an ACE inhibitor, unless there is a compelling reason for the patient to avoid these agents.

KEY

TABLE 18-1. Vasodilators Used to Treat Patients With Systolic Dysfunction

Drug	Dose Range (mg/day)	Dose Frequency (times/day)	Typical Dose
ACE inhibitors			
Captopril	6.25–150	3	50 mg 3 times daily
Enalapril	2.5–20	2	10 mg 2 times daily
Lisinopril	2.5–40	1	20 mg 1 time daily
Hydralazine	10–300	3	75 mg 3 times daily
Isosorbide dinitrate	5–160	3	40 mg 3 times daily

ACE = angiotensin-converting enzyme.

2. **Diuretics** are useful for treating symptoms of fluid overload (e.g., rales, peripheral edema).

   a. In patients with very mild fluid overload, a thiazide diuretic (e.g., hydrochlorothiazide) at a dose of 25–50 mg, 2–3 times per week may be all that is needed.

   b. As fluid overload becomes more severe, a once-daily dose of a loop diuretic (e.g., furosemide, 20–200 mg) may be necessary.

3. **Diet.** A low-sodium diet is primarily used to prevent fluid overload. The number of patients admitted to the hospital for CHF exacerbations markedly increases the day after Thanksgiving, undoubtedly the result of increased salt consumption.

4. **Digoxin.** This age-old treatment for CHF has been shown to reduce symptoms, but not to decrease mortality.

   a. Digoxin should be used in patients who are symptomatic in spite of other therapy.

   b. Doses vary, depending on the patient's weight and degree of renal function. The usual range is 0.125–0.375 mg/day, taken orally.

HOT **KEY**

Other potential therapies for systolic dysfunction are emerging, but remain controversial. Agents include amiodarone, β blockers, anticoagulants, angiotensin II inhibitors, and newer calcium channel blockers.

C. **Chronic diastolic dysfunction.** Treatment involves "3 Ds"—diuretics, diet, and diltiazem. Digoxin and vasodilators do not play a role in the treatment of patients with primarily diastolic dysfunction.

1. **Diuretics** are given in doses similar to those used for patients with systolic dysfunction.

2. **Diet.** Like patients with systolic dysfunction, patients with diastolic dysfunction should limit sodium intake.

3. **Diltiazem** (a calcium channel blocker) or a β blocker can be used to enhance ventricular compliance by improving left ventricular relaxation. Doses vary but are similar to those recommended for the treatment of hypertension (see Chapter 16, Table 16-1).

V REFERRAL AND FOLLOW-UP

A. Patients taking ACE inhibitors or loop diuretics should have a serum electrolyte panel every 6–12 months (or sooner if the dose has been changed).

B. Patients whose symptoms result in extreme limitations despite maximal management with routine agents should be referred to a specialist.

References

Cohn JN: The management of chronic heart failure. *N Engl J Med* 335(7):490–498, 1996.

Karon BL: Diagnosis and outpatient management of congestive heart failure. *Mayo Clin Proc* 70(11):1080–1085, 1995.

19. Atrial Fibrillation

I INTRODUCTION

A. Epidemiology. Atrial fibrillation is the most common chronic arrhythmia, occurring in 2% of the general population. The incidence varies with age:

1. Rare in people younger than 50 years
2. One out of 20 people older than 60 years
3. One out of 10 people older than 80 years

B. Terminology. A number of terms are used to describe the types of atrial fibrillation.

1. **"Valvular"** refers to atrial fibrillation that is **secondary to valve disease,** most commonly rheumatic mitral valve disease. In the past, **rheumatic heart disease** accounted for most cases of atrial fibrillation, but currently accounts for fewer than one-third of cases.

2. **"Nonvalvular"** applies to atrial fibrillation that is not accompanied by rheumatic or other valvular disease.

3. **"Isolated"** refers to atrial fibrillation that is secondary to another illness (e.g., hyperthyroidism, pneumonia, pulmonary embolism) and resolves when the illness is treated.

4. **"Paroxysmal"** refers to intermittent episodes of atrial fibrillation unrelated to an acute illness.

5. **"Chronic"** refers to atrial fibrillation when it is the predominant rhythm.

6. **"Lone"** refers to atrial fibrillation in the absence of structural heart disease [e.g., left ventricular hypertrophy, congestive heart failure (CHF), valve disease, cardiomyopathy].

II CLINICAL MANIFESTATIONS OF ATRIAL FIBRILLATION

A. Patient history. Atrial fibrillation causes an increased heart rate and loss of atrial contraction, which results in decreased ventricular filling, decreased cardiac output, and an increase in cardiac demand. The most common symptoms reflect these processes:

1. **Palpitations**
2. **Fatigue**

  3. **Dyspnea**
  4. **Dizziness or syncope**
  5. **Chest pain**
B. **Physical examination findings**
  1. An **irregularly irregular pulse** is the hallmark of atrial fibrillation.
  2. **Pulse of varying intensity** and **pulse deficit.** Because diastolic filling varies in length and is often reduced, pulses are of varying intensity and not all audible ventricular beats are palpable peripherally.
  3. **Absent *a* waves.** These jugular venous pulsations, which normally represent atrial contraction, are not seen in patients with atrial fibrillation.
  4. **Variation in the intensity of the first heart sound (S_1).** Due to variations in the filling time and end-diastolic volume, the pressure that closes the mitral and tricuspid valve varies, resulting in variations in the intensity of S_1.
C. **Electrocardiography**
  1. **f Waves** (fine fibrillation of the atria at a rate of 350–600 beats/min) may be noted and are best visualized in lead V_1.
  2. **P waves** are absent.
  3. The **ventricular response** will be **irregularly irregular,** although this may be difficult to appreciate at higher heart rates.

III **CAUSES OF ATRIAL FIBRILLATION** include the following:

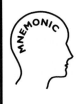

Causes of Atrial Fibrillation ("WATCH ATRIAL Ps")
WPW syndrome
Alcohol (intoxication, withdrawal, "holiday heart")
Thyrotoxicosis
CHF, **C**oronary artery disease (CAD), or **C**ardiomyopathy
Hypertension
Atrial septal defect (ASD)
Theophylline and other drugs (β agonists)
Rheumatic and other valve disease
Infections (e.g., myocarditis, endocarditis)
Amyloid and other infiltrative diseases
Lone (idiopathic) atrial fibrillation
Pulmonary or **P**ericardial disease
Sick sinus syndrome or **S**tress

A. **Idiopathic ("lone" atrial fibrillation),** seen in approximately 10% of patients

B. **Cardiovascular disorders** [e.g., Wolff-Parkinson-White (WPW) syndrome, coronary heart disease, CHF, cardiomyopathy (hypertrophic and dilated), myocarditis, hypertension, congenital heart disease]

C. **Pulmonary disorders** (e.g., pulmonary embolism, pleural effusion)

D. **Pericardial disease**

E. **Metabolic disturbances** (e.g., hyperthyroidism)

F. **Infiltrative diseases** (e.g., amyloidosis, sarcoidosis, hemochromatosis)

G. **Drugs** (e.g., theophylline, β agonists, alcohol)

H. **Infections** (e.g., myocarditis, endocarditis)

I. **Stress,** especially post-surgical stress

HOT

KEY

Because many of the causes of atrial fibrillation are correctable, a thorough search for the underlying cause is required.

IV **COMPLICATIONS OF ATRIAL FIBRILLATION.** The overall risk of **stroke** in all patients with atrial fibrillation is approximately 5% per year, five times the risk in those without atrial fibrillation. The risk of stroke in a patient with atrial fibrillation depends on the presence of five clinical variables and two echocardiographic variables. It is important for patients to have their risk factors "CHASED" down, so that risk can be defined and treatment can be planned.

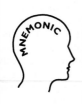

Risk Factors for Stroke in Patients with Atrial Fibrillation ("CHASED")

CHF (within 3 months)
Hypertension
Age > 65 years
Stroke in past
Echocardiographic abnormalities (left atrial size > 5 cm, left ventricular dysfunction)
Diabetes mellitus

A. Patients with atrial fibrillation but no risk factors for stroke are at approximately the same risk for stroke as the general population.

B. Patients with one or two risk factors carry a risk of stroke of approximately 5% per year.

C. Patients with three or more risk factors carry a risk of stroke of roughly 20% per year.

V TREATMENT

A. Acute treatment. The goal of acute treatment is **rate control.** Patients with rapid atrial fibrillation and life-threatening problems (e.g., ischemia, severe hypotension, severe pulmonary edema) should undergo immediate **cardioversion.** Patients with rapid atrial fibrillation but no life-threatening problems should be treated with pharmacologic therapy.

    1. Cardioversion can be **initiated with 100 J in the synchronized mode,** but **360 J may be necessary.** Unless there is an emergent indication, no patient with atrial fibrillation should be cardioverted until 3 weeks of anticoagulation therapy have been completed or until atrial thrombus has been excluded using transesophageal echocardiography (TEE).

        a. As a result of this stipulation, cardioversion is usually contraindicated in patients who are thought to have "new onset" atrial fibrillation because it is difficult to estimate the length of time the patient has been in atrial fibrillation from the patient history.

        b. Patients who are cardioverted without undergoing anticoagulation therapy have a 3%–5% risk of stroke within 30 days.

    2. Pharmacologic therapy

        a. Atrioventricular (AV) node blocking agents include **calcium channel blockers** (e.g., verapamil, diltiazem), **β blockers** (e.g., esmolol), and **digoxin.**

            (1) Dosages are given in Table 19-1.

            (2) Intravenous administration of a calcium channel blocker or β blocker is thought to be more effective than digoxin for regaining rapid control of an accelerated heart rate in a patient with atrial fibrillation, although all of these agents may cause hypotension, bradycardia, conduction defects, and CHF. Short-acting agents are always preferred, and monitoring is required for all patients.

TABLE 19-1. Pharmacologic Therapy for Atrial Fibrillation

Drug	Initial Dose	Maintenance Dose
Diltiazem*	15–20 mg (0.25 mg/kg) intravenously over 2 minutes; repeat in 15 minutes at 20–25 mg if necessary	5–20 mg/hr intravenously
Verapamil*	2.5–5.0 mg administered as an intravenous bolus over 1–2 minutes, followed by 5–10 mg in 15–30 minutes if necessary; maximum dose is 30 mg	0.05–0.2 mg/min intravenously
Esmolol*	500 μg/kg intravenously over 1 minute	50–200 μg/kg/min intravenously
Digoxin	0.25–0.5 mg intravenously	0.25 mg intravenously every 6 hours to a total dose of 1 mg completes loading, followed by 0.125 mg–0.25 mg PO or IV daily

*These agents may cause bradycardia, hypotension, conduction delay, or congestive heart failure (CHF) and should only be used in monitored settings.

(3) Digoxin may be the best choice for patients with heart failure.

B. Chronic treatment. The goals of chronic treatment of atrial fibrillation are **alleviation of symptoms** and **reduction of the risk for stroke.**

HOT

It is useful to think of **three categories of treatment: rate control, rhythm control,** and **clot control.**

KEY

---

1. **Rate control.** The goal is a resting heart rate lower than 90 beats/min. **Pharmacologic treatment** should be selected after considering the patient's other medical problems. For example:
   a. In patients with hypertension or CAD, a β blocker (e.g., atenolol, 50–100 mg daily) is a good choice because it addresses these problems as well as the atrial fibrillation. However, in patients with asthma or chronic obstructive pulmonary disease (COPD), a β blocker may not be a good choice because it may induce bronchoconstriction.
   b. In patients with CHF, digoxin can control the heart rate as well as improve symptoms of CHF. However, in patients with chronic renal insufficiency, digoxin levels must be monitored closely.
2. **Rhythm control.** Theoretically, conversion to normal sinus rhythm returns the risk of stroke to baseline and relieves all rate-related symptoms.
   a. **Cardioversion.** Elective cardioversion should be performed only after a 3-week course of therapeutic anticoagulation has been completed or after atrial thrombus has been excluded using TEE. Cardioversion should be followed by 4 more weeks of anticoagulation therapy.
   b. **Pharmacologic therapy.** Rate must be controlled prior to the initiation of any antiarrhythmic medication because antiarrhythmic medications can increase conduction through the AV node (and accelerate the rate of atrial fibrillation).
      (1) Amiodarone appears to be at least as effective as procainamide and quinidine for main-

taining sinus rhythm, and is not associated
with proarrhythmic effects.

   (a) Although amiodarone is associated with
significant side effects (e.g., optic neuropathy, hypo- and hyperthyroidism, pulmonary fibrosis), it is likely to become the
drug of choice.

   (b) Consultation with a cardiologist is suggested before initiating treatment with
amiodarone.

  (2) **Procainamide** and **quinidine** increase the time
to relapse in treated patients, but both agents
are proarrhythmic and have been associated
with increased mortality rates. Most patients
should not be treated with these agents.

 c. **AV node ablation with pacemaker implantation**
can be considered for patients who do not respond to medical therapy.

3. **Clot control.** Although stroke is the major cause of
morbidity and mortality in patients with atrial fibrillation, **anticoagulation therapy** is time-consuming and
bothersome to patients, and the risks and benefits
must be assessed on an individual basis. Patients with
the highest risk of stroke are the most likely to benefit from anticoagulation therapy.

 a. **Aspirin** (325 mg daily) is a consideration for patients at low risk for stroke.

 b. **Warfarin.** Although warfarin therapy places the
patient at a slightly increased risk for major bleeding, it reduces the risk of stroke by 40%–90%. The
target international normalized ratio (INR) is
2.0–3.0.

HOT

KEY

Lower-dose anticoagulation therapy (i.e., a target INR of
1.0–2.0) and combination therapy (e.g., aspirin plus warfarin) are two approaches to clot control that are currently
being studied.

VI **FOLLOW-UP AND REFERRAL.** Consultation with a cardiologist, who can assist with decisions regarding cardioversion, rate-controlling agents, and anti-arrhythmic therapy, is
recommended for most patients.

A. Patients with new-onset atrial fibrillation generally require hospitalization for rate control and determination of the cause of the arrhythmia.

B. Stable patients with chronic atrial fibrillation can be seen as needed (usually once a month) to monitor anticoagulation therapy and rate and symptom control. Anti-arrhythmic therapy should be re-evaluated every 1–3 months.

References

Hylek EM, Skates SJ, Sheehan MA, et al: An analysis of the lowest effective intensity of prophylactic anticoagulation for patients with nonrheumatic atrial fibrillation. *N Engl J Med* 335(8):540–546, 1996.

Prystowsky EN, Benson DW, Fuster V, et al: Management of patients with atrial fibrillation: a statement for healthcare professionals from the subcommittee on electrocardiography and electrophysiology, American Heart Association. *Circulation* 93(6):1262–1277, 1996.

20. Heart Murmur

....

I **INTRODUCTION.** Auscultation of a heart murmur presents
a challenging problem for the primary care provider. Some
murmurs are benign, but others represent conditions that, if
left untreated, can lead to permanent damage and disability.

   A. Pathogenesis. A murmur is produced by turbulent blood
   flow that causes vibration of cardiac structures, usually
   heart valves.

   B. Classification. Murmurs can be broadly classified as systolic, diastolic, or continuous.

   1. **Systolic murmurs** occur between the first and second
      heart sounds (S_1 and S_2).

   2. **Diastolic murmurs** occur between the second and
      first heart sounds (S_2 and S_1).

   3. **Continuous murmurs** occur throughout systole and
      diastole.

   C. Presentation

   1. Most murmurs are found during a routine clinical ex-
      amination in asymptomatic patients.

   2. Sometimes, patients present with abnormalities on a
      chest radiograph or electrocardiogram (EKG) that
      lead to auscultation of the chest and diagnosis of a
      murmur. For example, left atrial enlargement can re-
      sult from mitral stenosis or regurgitation.

   3. Patients who present with symptoms suggestive of
      certain types of valve disease (e.g., exertional dysp-
      nea, angina, syncope) and are found to have a mur-
      mur require prompt evaluation.

II **CAUSES OF HEART MURMURS.** Selected major causes of
the three murmur types are shown in Table 20-1.

III **APPROACH TO THE PATIENT.** The goal is to differentiate
benign conditions from those that require specific therapy to
prevent complications and symptoms.

   A. Patient history. Focus on the following:

   1. **Symptoms suggestive of cardiac disease** (e.g., angina,
      shortness of breath, exercise intolerance, syncope)

   2. **Past medical history** of **conditions that can affect the**

heart (e.g., rheumatic fever, intravenous drug use) or **increase flow** (e.g., anemia, hyperthyroidism, renal failure, arteriovenous fistula)

B. Physical examination must include a complete cardiac examination.

   1. Classify the murmur as systolic, diastolic, or continuous to narrow the differential diagnosis (see Table 20-1).

   2. Use the following combinations of characteristic physical examination findings to arrive at a specific diagnosis.

     a. Aortic stenosis

       (1) There is a slow rate of rise of the carotid artery pulsation.

       (2) The murmur peaks in late- or mid-systole.

       (3) The intensity of the S_2 is decreased.

     b. Aortic regurgitation

       (1) There is a decrescendo murmur over the aortic area.

       (2) The murmur is best heard with the patient sitting up, leaning forward, and holding his breath after a full expiration.

     c. Mitral stenosis

       (1) An opening snap is often followed by a subtle murmur.

       (2) The murmur is best heard by holding the bell of the stethoscope at the apex.

     d. Mitral regurgitation

       (1) The murmur is auscultated in the mitral area (i.e., the apex) and left sternal border.

       (2) The murmur increases when the patient firmly clenches his fists.

     e. Tricuspid stenosis. The murmur is best heard at the left lower sternal border and may increase with inspiration.

     f. Tricuspid regurgitation. The murmur increases when the patient slowly inhales or gentle pressure is applied continuously to the right upper quadrant of the abdomen.

     g. Pulmonic stenosis is rare in adults. The murmur is best heard at the left sternal border at the second intercostal space.

     h. Pulmonic regurgitation occurs in the setting of pulmonary hypertension. The murmur may be difficult to distinguish from that of aortic regurgitation and is best heard at the left sternal border at the second intercostal space.

TABLE 20-1. Selected Causes of Murmurs	
Murmur Type	**Causes**
Systolic	Increased flow
	Anemia
	Thyrotoxicosis
	Sepsis
	Renal failure
	Arteriovenous fistula
	Abnormal structure
	Stenosis (aortic or pulmonic)
	Regurgitation (mitral or tricuspid)
	Mitral valve prolapse
	Hypertrophic cardiomyopathy
	VSD, ASD
Diastolic	Stenosis (mitral or tricuspid)
	Regurgitation (aortic or pulmonic)
Continuous	Patent ductus arteriosus
	Coarctation of the aorta
	Arteriovenous fistula

ASD = atrial septal defect, VSD = ventricular septal defect.

i. **Hypertrophic cardiomyopathy.** The murmur decreases in intensity with passive leg elevation or when the patient moves from a standing to a squatting position.

j. **Mitral valve prolapse** is usually diagnosed by detecting a systolic click, which may or may not be accompanied by a mitral regurgitation murmur.

k. **Ventricular septal defect (VSD).** The murmur is best heard at the left lower sternal border and often radiates to the right sternal border. The intensity does not increase with inspiration.

l. **Atrial septal defect (ASD)** results in fixed splitting of the S_2. The murmur is best heard at the left sternal border at the second intercostal space.

C. **Imaging studies.** An **echocardiogram** is indicated:

1. For all patients with suspected **systolic murmur** when the diagnosis cannot be established on the basis of the history and physical examination

2. For all patients with **diastolic** and **continuous mur-**

TABLE 20-2. Valve Disease—Therapeutic Considerations

Therapy	Mitral Stenosis	Mitral Regurgitation	Aortic Stenosis	Aortic Regurgitation	Mitral Valve Prolapse
			Disorder		
Afterload reduction	Not indicated	Consider	Not indicated	Indicated	Not indicated
Surgery	Indicated if symptoms have developed; controversial prior to symptom development*	Indicated if evidence of left ventricular dysfunction or dilatation	Indicated when symptoms develop†	Indicated if evidence of left ventricular dysfunction or dilatation	Not indicated
Endocarditis prophylaxis	Indicated	Indicated	Indicated	Indicated	Consider‡
Coagulation prophylaxis	Consider	Not indicated	Not indicated	Not indicated	Not indicated

*In patients with symptomatic mitral valve stenosis, surgery may prevent atrial fibrillation and pulmonary hypertension.
†Symptomatic aortic stenosis usually occurs when the aortic valve area reaches 1.0–1.5 cm².
‡Endocarditis prophylaxis is recommended for patients with mitral valve prolapse only when there is mitral regurgitation or the valve leaflets are thickened and redundant.

murs, which are often associated with structural abnormalities of the heart that require intervention

IV **TREATMENT.** Once a valve disorder has been definitively diagnosed, the goals of treatment are **symptom reduction** and the **prevention of complications (Table 20-2).**

   A. Endocarditis prophylaxis is indicated for most patients with valve disease and is discussed in Chapter 21.
   B. Anticoagulation therapy is indicated for all patients with valve disease and atrial fibrillation or thromboembolism.

V **FOLLOW-UP AND REFERRAL**

   A. Patients with stenotic or regurgitant murmurs should be followed every 3 months to evaluate for symptoms [e.g., angina, exertional dyspnea, congestive heart failure (CHF), syncope]. Serial echocardiograms should be considered for those with mitral or aortic stenosis, and are necessary for those with mitral or aortic regurgitation.
   B. A cardiology consultation should be obtained whenever there is a question about the correct management of a patient's heart murmur.

References

Carabello BA: Indications for valve surgery in asymptomatic patients with aortic and mitral stenosis. *Chest* 108(6):1678–1682, 1995.

Etchells E, Bell C, Robb K: Does this patient have an abnormal systolic murmur? *JAMA* 277(7):564–571, 1997.

Levine HJ, Gaasch WH: Vasoactive drugs in regurgitant lesions of the mitral and aortic valves. *J Am Coll Cardiol* 28(5):1083–1091, 1996.

21. Endocarditis Prophylaxis

I INTRODUCTION

A. Patients with **cardiac structural abnormalities** (e.g., **cardiac valve defects)** have an increased risk of acquiring bacterial endocarditis (Table 21-1). The abnormal structures are thought to be more exposed ("sticky"), and are therefore more susceptible to infection during periods of **bacteremia.**

B. Sources of bacteremia

1. **Certain medical** and **dental procedures** are known to cause transient bacteremia. Patients at risk for the development of bacterial endocarditis may be able to reduce their risk by taking **prophylactic antibiotics** prior to undergoing the procedure.

2. **Oral inflammation** can predispose to bacteremia. Patients at risk for bacterial endocarditis should be counseled about the importance of **strict dental hygiene.**

II INDICATIONS FOR PROPHYLAXIS.
Certain dental and medical procedures (Tables 21-2 and 21-3) can cause transient bacteremia, and therefore may increase the risk of bacterial endocarditis in susceptible patients.

A. Prophylactic antibiotics are recommended for patients in the **high-** and **moderate-risk categories** (see Table 21-1) prior to undergoing certain procedures.

B. Patients in the **negligible-risk category** are not thought to be at higher risk than members of the average population; therefore, prophylactic antibiotics are not routinely recommended for these patients. Nevertheless, prophylaxis should be prescribed according to the patient's individual situation—there is no substitute for sound clinical judgement.

III PROPHYLACTIC REGIMENS

A. Dental, oral, and **upper respiratory tract procedures.** Oral antibiotics are the recommended form of prophylaxis (Table 21-4). Some practitioners may choose to treat patients at very high risk with intravenous therapy.

B. Genitourinary or **gastrointestinal tract procedures.** Intra-

TABLE 21-1. Risk of Bacterial Endocarditis Associated with Various Cardiac Conditions

Prophylaxis Recommended

High risk

Prosthetic cardiac valves (including bioprosthetic and homograft valves)

Previous bacterial endocarditis

Complex cyanotic congenital heart disease (e.g., single ventricle states, transposition of the great arteries, tetralogy of Fallot)

Surgically constructed systemic pulmonary shunts or conduits

Moderate risk

Most congenital cardiac malformations (other than those specified in the high-risk and negligible-risk categories)

Acquired valvular dysfunction (e.g., rheumatic heart disease)

Hypertrophic cardiomyopathy

Mitral valve prolapse with valvular regurgitation, thickened leaflets, or both

Prophylaxis Not Recommended

Negligible risk

Isolated secundum atrial septal defect

Surgical repair of atrial septal defect, ventricular septal defect, or patent ductus arteriosus (without residua beyond 6 months)

Previous coronary artery bypass graft surgery

Mitral valve prolapse without valvular regurgitation

Physiologic, functional, or innocent heart murmurs

Previous Kawasaki disease without valvular dysfunction

Previous rheumatic fever without valvular dysfunction

Cardiac pacemakers (intravascular and epicardial) and implanted defibrillators

Reprinted with permission from Dajani AS, Taubert KA, Wilson W, et al: Prevention of bacterial endocarditis—recommendations by the American Heart Association. *JAMA* 277 (22):1797, 1997.

TABLE 21-2. Dental Procedures—Recommendations for Endocarditis Prophylaxis

Prophylaxis Recommended*

Dental extractions

Periodontal procedures, including surgery, scaling and root planing, probing, and recall maintenance

Dental implant placement and reimplantation of avulsed teeth

Endodontic (root canal) instrumentation or surgery only beyond the apex

Subgingival placement of antibiotic fibers or strips

Initial placement of orthodontic bands (but not brackets)

Intraligamentary local anesthetic injections

Prophylactic cleaning of teeth or implants when bleeding is anticipated

Prophylaxis Not Recommended

Restorative dentistry† (operative and prosthodontic) with or without retraction cord‡

Local anesthetic injections (nonintraligamentary)

Intracanal endodontic treatment; post placement and buildup

Placement of rubber dams

Postoperative suture removal

Placement of removable prosthodontic or orthodontic appliances

Taking of oral impressions

Fluoride treatments

Taking of oral radiographs

Orthodontic appliance adjustment

Shedding of primary teeth

Reprinted with permission from Dajani AS, Taubert KA, Wilson W, et al: Prevention of bacterial endocarditis—recommendations by the American Heart Association. *JAMA* 277 (22):1797, 1997.

*Prophylaxis is recommended for patients with high- and moderate-risk cardiac conditions.

†This includes restoration of decayed teeth (filling cavities) and replacement of missing teeth.

‡Clinical judgment may indicate antibiotic use in selected circumstances that may create significant bleeding.

TABLE 21-3. Medical Procedures—Recommendations for Endocarditis Prophylaxis

Prophylaxis Recommended

Respiratory tract procedures
  Tonsillectomy or adenoidectomy
  Surgical operations that involve the respiratory mucosa
  Bronchoscopy with a rigid bronchoscope
Gastrointestinal tract procedures*
  Sclerotherapy for esophageal varices
  Esophageal stricture dilatation
  Endoscopic retrogade cholangiography with biliary obstruction
  Biliary tract surgery
  Surgical operations that involve the intestinal mucosa
Genitourinary tract procedures
  Prostatic surgery
  Cystoscopy
  Urethral dilation

Prophylaxis Not Recommended

Respiratory tract procedures
  Endotracheal intubation
  Bronchoscopy with a flexible bronchoscope, with or without biopsy†
  Tympanostomy tube insertion
Gastrointestinal tract procedures
  Transesophageal echocardiography (TEE)†
  Endoscopy with or without gastrointestinal biopsy†
Genitourinary tract procedures
  Vaginal hysterectomy†
  Vaginal delivery†
  Cesarean section
  Urethral catheterization‡
  Uterine dilatation and curettage‡
  Therapeutic abortion‡
  Sterilization procedures‡
  Insertion or removal of intrauterine devices‡
Other procedures
  Cardiac catheterization, including balloon angioplasty
  Implantation of cardiac pacemakers, implanted defibrillators, or coronary stents
  Incision or biopsy of surgically scrubbed skin
  Circumcision

Modified with permission from Dajani AS, Taubert KA, Wilson W, et al: Prevention of bacterial endocarditis—recommendations by the American Heart Association. *JAMA* 277 (22):1797, 1997.
*Prophylaxis is recommended for high-risk patients; optional for medium-risk patients.
†Prophylaxis is optional for high-risk patients.
‡Unless infection is present, in which case prophylaxis is recommended.

TABLE 21-4. Prophylactic Regimens for Dental, Oral, or Upper Respiratory Tract Procedures

Situation	Agent	Regimen
Standard general prophylaxis	Amoxicillin	**Adults:** 2.0 g orally 1 hour before procedure **Children:** 50 mg/kg orally 1 hour before procedure
Unable to take oral medications	Ampicillin	**Adults:** 2.0 g intramuscularly or intravenously 30 minutes before procedure **Children:** 50 mg/kg intramuscularly or intravenously 30 minutes before procedure
Allergic to penicillin	Clindamycin **OR** Azithromycin or clarithromycin	**Adults:** 600 mg orally 1 hour before procedure **Children:** 20 mg/kg orally 1 hour before procedure **Adults:** 500 mg orally 1 hour before procedure **Children:** 15 mg/kg orally 1 hour before procedure

Modified with permission from Dajani AS, Taubert KA, Wilson W, et al: Prevention of bacterial endocarditis—recommendations by the American Heart Association. JAMA 277 (22):1798, 1997.

TABLE 21-5. Prophylactic Regimens for Genitourinary and Gastrointestinal Procedures in Adults

Situation	Agents	Regimen
High-risk patient	Ampicillin plus gentamicin	Ampicillin (2.0 g IM or IV) plus gentamicin (1.5 mg/kg, not to exceed 120 mg) within 30 minutes of procedure Ampicillin (1 g IM or IV) or amoxicillin (1 g orally) 6 hours later
High-risk patient with penicillin allergy	Vancomycin plus gentamicin	Vancomycin (1.0 g IV over 1–2 hours) plus gentamicin (1.5 mg/kg IV or IM, not to exceed 120 mg); complete infusion or injection within 30 minutes of starting procedure
Moderate-risk patient	Amoxicillin or ampicillin	Amoxicillin (2.0 g orally 1 hour before procedure) or ampicillin (2.0 g IM or IV within 30 minutes of procedure)
Moderate-risk patient with penicillin allergy	Vancomycin	Vancomycin (1.0 g IV over 1–2 hours); complete infusion within 30 minutes of starting the procedure

IM = intramuscularly; IV = intravenously.
Modified with permission from Dajani AS, Taubert KA, Wilson W, et al: Prevention of bacterial endocarditis—recommendations by the American Heart Association. JAMA 277 (22):1799, 1997.

venous therapy is recommended (Table 21-5), although practitioners may chose to use oral therapy in moderate-risk patients.

C. Other procedures. Consultation with a cardiologist is recommended when the situation does not conform to the standard guidelines.

References

Dajani AS, Taubert KA, Wilson W, et al: Prevention of bacterial endocarditis — recommendations by the American Heart Association. *JAMA* 277(22):1794–1801, 1997.

Durack DT: Prevention of infective endocarditis. *N Engl J Med* 332(1):38–44, 1995.

22. Lower Extremity Edema

I INTRODUCTION

A. Edema, the excessive accumulation of interstitial fluid in the tissues, results from alterations in one or more of the following parameters:
1. Hydrostatic pressure
2. Oncotic pressure
3. Capillary permeability
4. Lymphatic drainage

B. Lower extremity edema presents as swelling of one or both legs.

II APPROACH TO THE PATIENT

A. Patient history and physical examination. The clinician can use several pieces of information obtained during the history and examination to shorten the extensive differential diagnosis for lower leg edema (Table 22-1).
1. **Duration:** acute or chronic?
2. **Distribution:** unilateral or bilateral?
3. **Associated signs and symptoms:** dyspnea, pain, skin changes, upper extremity swelling?

HOT

Lower extremity edema can be a sign of a life-threatening disease, so a diagnosis should be established promptly.

KEY

B. Laboratory and imaging studies. If the history and physical examination are unrevealing, additional testing may be required. The order of the work-up can be tailored according to any etiologic clues gleaned from the history and physical examination.
1. **Unilateral edema**
   a. Venous duplex ultrasound with Doppler should be obtained.

TABLE 22-1. Causes of Lower Extremity Edema

Cause	Associated History, Signs, and Symptoms
Unilateral, acute onset*	
DVT	Hypercoagulable state; age > 50 years; bed-bound; history of surgery, cancer, or trauma; thigh or calf pain
Cellulitis or abscess	Fever, pain, erythema
Ruptured popliteal cyst	Pain, knee swelling
Trauma	History of recent injury
Compartment syndrome	History of trauma (crush injury) or prolonged pressure on the leg
Ruptured muscle or tendon	Forceful ankle dorsiflexion
Erythema nodosum	Fever, pain, patchy erythema
Unilateral, gradual onset	
Chronic venous insufficiency	Painless, edema worse at day's end but improves with elevation, varicose veins
Lymphedema	Painless, edema worse at day's end, dorsum of toes and feet affected first, dry and scaly skin
External venous compression	Painless, localized enlargement
Soft tissue tumor or vascular tumor	Localized tenderness and enlargement
Congenital venous malformation	Leg length discrepancy from childhood
Reflex sympathetic dystrophy	Taut, shiny skin; extreme sensitivity to touch
Bilateral	
CHF	Dyspnea, orthopnea, PND, elevated jugular venous pressure
Nephrotic syndrome	History of diabetes or lupus
Glomerulonephritis	History of recent fever or sore throat
Hepatic cirrhosis	Jaundice, icterus, ascites, history of alcohol abuse or hepatitis
Hypoproteinemia	History of malnutrition or malabsorption

continued

TABLE 22-1. Causes of Lower Extremity Edema

Cause	Associated History, Signs, and Symptoms
Pretibial myxedema (Graves' disease)	Tachycardia, tremor, weight loss, heat intolerance
Bilateral DVT	Hypercoagulable state; age > 50 years; bed-bound; history of surgery, cancer, or trauma; thigh or calf pain
Bilateral cellulitis	Fever, pain, erythema
Chronic venous insufficiency	Painless, edema worse at day's end but improves with elevation, varicose veins
Lymphedema	Inguinal lymphadenopathy, pelvic symptoms, weight loss
Drug reaction	NSAIDs
	Monoamine oxidase (MAO) inhibitors
	Antihypertensive agents
	β Blockers
	Calcium channel blockers
	Clonidine
	Diazoxide
	Guanethidine
	Hydralazine
	Methyldopa
	Minoxidil
	Reserpine
	Hormones
	Corticosteroids
	Estrogen
	Progesterone
	Testosterone

Modified with permission from Ciocon JO, Fernandez BB, Ciocon DG: Leg edema: clinical clues to the differential diagnosis. *Geriatrics* 48 (5):34–40, 45, 1993. Copyright by Advanstar Communications, Inc. Advanstar Communications, Inc retains all rights to this article.
CHF = congestive heart failure; DVT = deep venous thrombosis; PND = paroxysmal nocturnal dyspnea; NSAIDs = nonsteroidal anti-inflammatory drugs.
*"Acute" = < 72 hours; "gradual" = > 72 hours.

Chapter 22

TABLE 22-2. Evaluation of Bilateral Edema

Studies	Suspected Cause of the Bilateral Edema
Complete blood count (CBC)	Bilateral cellulitis
Urinalysis and renal panel	Glomerulonephritis, nephrotic syndrome
Liver function tests and serum albumin level	Liver disease, malnutrition
Thyroid-stimulating hormone (TSH) level	Thyroid disease
Electrocardiogram (EKG) and chest radiograph, possibly echocardiogram	Congestive heart failure (CHF)
Venous duplex ultrasound with Doppler	Bilateral deep venous thrombosis (DVT), inferior vena cava thrombus
Pelvic ultrasound or pelvic computed tomography (CT) scan	Pelvic malignancy, retroperitoneal fibrosis

    b. A complete blood count (CBC) and a serum creatinine kinase level may also be obtained to evaluate the possibility of infection and compartment syndrome, respectively.

  2. Bilateral edema. Table 22-2 summarizes studies that may be appropriate for the evaluation of bilateral edema.

III TREATMENT

A. Definitive treatment involves addressing the underlying disorder [e.g., anticoagulation for deep venous thrombosis (DVT); antibiotics for cellulitis].

B. Symptomatic treatment

  1. Elevation of the affected limb or limbs is helpful.

  2. Discontinuation of medications. Drugs that may cause or exacerbate the edema should be discontinued, if possible.

  3. Diuretics are helpful for patients with bilateral leg edema associated with congestive heart failure (CHF), renal insufficiency, cirrhosis, or venous insufficiency.

    4. Compression stockings are most useful for patients with edema caused by CHF or venous insufficiency.

IV FOLLOW-UP AND REFERRAL

A. If infection (e.g., cellulitis, abscess) or compartment syndrome is the suspected cause of the edema, the patient should be seen by a surgeon immediately.

B. All patients with leg edema should be advised about the importance of meticulous skin care, proper shoes, and early treatment of minor trauma as a means of preventing serious complications, such as venous stasis ulcers, cellulitis, or osteomyelitis.

References

Ciocon JO, Fernandez BB, Ciocon DG: Leg edema: clinical clues to the differential diagnosis (see comments). *Geriatrics* 48(5):34–40, 45, 1993.

Merli GJ, Spandorfer J: The outpatient with unilateral leg swelling. *Med Clin North Am* 79(2):435–447, 1995.

Powell AA, Armstrong MA: Peripheral edema. *Am Fam Physician* 55(5):1721–1726, 1997.

Sapira J: The extremities. In *The Art and Science of Bedside Diagnosis.* Edited by Sapira J. Baltimore, Lippincott Williams & Wilkins, 1990, p 446.

Weinmann EE, Salzman EW: Deep-vein thrombosis. *N Engl J Med* 331(24):1630–1641, 1994.

PART IV

....

Pulmonology

23. Chronic Cough

I INTRODUCTION

A. Chronic cough, generally defined as a **cough of greater than 3 weeks duration,** is a common problem in the outpatient setting, accounting for **30 million office visits annually** in the United States. Fortunately, in most patients, a treatable cause of chronic cough can be identified.

B. Chronic cough afflicts 10%–20% of nonsmoking adults, and as many as 80% of adults who smoke.

II CAUSES OF CHRONIC COUGH

A. Common causes. Postnasal drip syndrome, gastroesophageal reflux disease (GERD), and asthma account for more than 90% of cases of chronic cough in non-smoking adults. As many as 60% of patients have more than one of these conditions as the underlying cause.

    1. Postnasal drip syndrome secondary to allergic or viral rhinitis or sinusitis is the cause in **20%–50%** of non-smoking patients.

    2. GERD is the cause in **10%–40%** of non-smoking patients. Cough receptors in the distal esophagus may trigger episodes of coughing in response to reflux without actual aspiration into the tracheobronchial tree.

    3. Asthma is the cause in **15%–35%** of non-smoking patients.

    4. Cigarette use [by itself or in association with chronic obstructive pulmonary disease (COPD)] is an extremely common cause of chronic cough.

B. Less common causes include:

    1. Bronchiectasis

    2. Congestive heart failure (CHF)

    3. Angiotensin-converting enzyme (ACE) inhibitor therapy (approximately 10%–15% of patients taking these medications develop a chronic cough, usually within 1 year of starting therapy)

    3. Post-pertussis cough

    4. Malignancy or **chronic infection** (usually accompanied by systemic symptoms; more than 80% of patients with lung cancer who present with a cough also complain of weight loss, hemoptysis, pain, or dyspnea)

5. **Psychogenic cough** (fewer than 2% of patients)

III **APPROACH TO THE PATIENT.** The approach to evaluation and treatment of chronic cough is **largely empiric.** There is no confirmatory diagnostic test for postnasal drip syndrome, and diagnostic tests for GERD and asthma are relatively expensive relative to treatment measures. As a result, a pragmatic and cost-effective approach to chronic cough involves identifying the most likely cause or causes of cough, treating appropriately, and considering more invasive testing only if initial therapy is unsuccessful (Figure 23-1).

A. The **history** and **physical examination** should be directed toward identifying the underlying cause.

HOT

The timing and character of the cough are not helpful in accurately identifying the cause.

KEY

---

1. **Smoking.** All patients who are chronic smokers should be encouraged to stop smoking. Smoking-associated cough may be exacerbated in the first few days after quitting, but generally resolves in 1–2 months.

2. **ACE inhibitor therapy.** Discontinuation of therapy usually resolves the cough in 2–3 weeks. An angiotensin II receptor antagonist (e.g., losartan) or another type of antihypertensive agent should be used instead of the ACE inhibitor. Switching to an alternative ACE inhibitor is generally not helpful in ameliorating the cough.

3. **Postnasal drip syndrome**
   a. In as many as 25% of patients, cough is the only manifestation of postnasal drip, and patients will not report a sensation of secretions dripping down the throat.
   b. The physical examination is insensitive for postnasal drip. A cobblestone appearance of the posterior pharynx may be present in 20% of patients with postnasal drip as a result of lymphoid hyperplasia from chronic irritation.

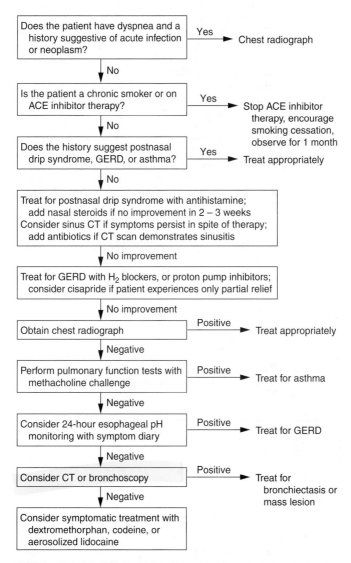

FIGURE 23-1. Algorithm for evaluation and treatment of chronic cough.
ACE = angiotensin-converting enzyme; *CT* = computed tomography;
GERD = gastroesophageal reflux disease.

      4. GERD. As with postnasal drip syndrome, cough may be the only manifestation of reflux.

      5. Asthma. So-called "cough variant" asthma may be seen in patients who do not complain of more classic asthma symptoms, such as wheezing and episodic shortness of breath.

B. Empiric therapy. If no obvious cause for the cough can be identified, then empiric therapy should be initiated based on the most common underlying causes, before extensive diagnostic testing is performed (see Figure 23-1).

C. Invasive testing. In general, invasive testing should be used only when patients fail to respond to empiric therapy.

      1. 24-Hour esophageal pH monitoring is useful for diagnosing **GERD-associated cough** and assessing response to therapy. Patients should be asked to keep a **symptom diary.**

      2. Pulmonary function tests with a **methacholine challenge** are useful for diagnosing **asthma** in patients who fail to respond to empiric therapy for postnasal drip.

        a. A negative result virtually excludes asthma as a cause of cough. Patients with positive results should be treated for asthma.

        b. False-positive results may occur if the test is performed within 8 weeks of an upper respiratory tract infection.

 TREATMENT. In general, response to treatment may take 2–3 weeks, and full resolution of symptoms may require 1–2 months.

HOT

Patients who have only a partial response to treatment may have more than one underlying cause for their cough; these patients may require combination therapy.

KEY

A. Postnasal drip syndrome

      1. Antihistamines

        a. Initial treatment is with an **antihistamine,** such as **pseudoephedrine** (60 mg orally every 4–6 hours) or **phenylpropanolamine/brompheniramine** (25/4 mg orally every 4–6 hours). These agents are available over-the-counter and in sustained-release forms.

    b. If the older antihistamines cause problematic sedation, more selective antihistamines, such as **astemizole** (10 mg orally daily) or **fexofenadine** (60 mg orally daily) may be used during the day.

  2. Nasal steroids, such as **beclomethasone** or **flunisolide** (1–2 sprays per nostril once or twice daily), may be a useful adjunct for patients with seasonal or allergic rhinitis.

  3. Antibiotics are not helpful unless there are clear signs of sinusitis.

B. GERD

  1. Histamine-2 (H$_2$) blockers, such as **cimetidine** (800 mg orally twice daily), **ranitidine** (150 mg orally twice daily), or **famotidine** (20 mg orally twice daily), constitute first-line therapy.

  2. Proton pump inhibitors may be necessary for patients with refractory or severe cases. Agents include **omeprazole** (20–40 mg orally daily) and **lansoprazole** (15–30 mg orally daily).

  3. Cisapride (10 mg twice daily) may be required by some patients to decrease the frequency of reflux, because even nonacidic reflux can trigger the cough.

  4. Surgery may be necessary for patients with a persistent cough and positive results on 24-hour esophageal pH monitoring.

C. Asthma is treated using **inhaled β agonists** (e.g., albuterol metered-dose inhaler, 2–4 puffs four times daily) and/or **inhaled steroids** (e.g., triamcinolone acetonide, 2 puffs three to four times daily).

V FOLLOW-UP AND REFERRAL

A. Follow-up. Patients should be seen every 2–4 weeks until symptoms abate or a diagnosis is made.

B. Referral

  1. A pulmonologist should be consulted if bronchoscopy is being considered for patients with persistent symptoms.

  2. Consultation with a gastroenterologist is useful if GERD is strongly suspected and the patient remains symptomatic despite maximum therapy.

  3. Consultation with an otolaryngologist may be helpful

if a patient with suspected postnasal drip syndrome continues to have symptoms despite aggressive therapy.

References

Mello CJ, Irwin RS, Curley FJ: Predictive value of the character, timing and complications of chronic cough in diagnosing its cause. *Arch Intern Med* 156(9):997–1003, 1996.

Pratter MR, Bartter T, Akers S, et al: An algorithmic approach to chronic cough. *Ann Intern Med* 119(10): 977–983, 1993.

Rosenow EC 3rd: Persistent cough: causes and cures. *Hosp Pract* 31(9):121–127, 1996.

24. Dyspnea

I **INTRODUCTION.** Dyspnea (shortness of breath) refers to discomfort associated with breathing. There are three main subtypes of dyspnea:

A. **Paroxysmal nocturnal dyspnea (PND)** is dyspnea that wakes a person from sleep after she has been sleeping for 1–2 hours. PND is usually a manifestation of increased left atrial pressure caused by congestive heart failure (CHF).

B. **Orthopnea** is dyspnea that begins suddenly when a patient lies down but is immediately relieved when he sits up. Orthopnea implies heart failure or, occasionally, pulmonary disease.

C. **Platypnea** is the opposite of orthopnea—i.e., the dyspnea occurs when the patient sits up but is relieved when he lies down. Platypnea is caused by right-to-left shunting [e.g., hepatopulmonary syndrome, atrial septal defect (ASD)].

II **CAUSES OF DYSPNEA**

A. **Chronic and subacute dyspnea.** The common causes of subacute and chronic dyspnea (the focus of this chapter) are outlined in Table 24-1. The **five most common causes of chronic dyspnea** are:
1. Chronic obstructive pulmonary disease (COPD)
2. Asthma
3. CHF
4. Idiopathic pulmonary fibrosis
5. Ischemic heart disease

B. **Acute dyspnea.** Although this chapter focuses on chronic dyspnea, it is important to be aware of the common causes of acute dyspnea, because many are life-threatening (Table 24-2).

HOT **KEY** Most patients with acute onset of dyspnea should be referred immediately to an emergency department (ED). The only exceptions are those patients with mild asthma or COPD exacerbations. Occasionally, these patients can be evaluated and treated in the clinic.

TABLE 24-1. Common Causes of Subacute and Chronic Dyspnea

General Causes	Specific Disorders
Pulmonary disorders	Asthma
	COPD
	Interstitial lung disease (e.g., idiopathic pulmonary fibrosis)
	Pneumonia (primarily caused by an atypical bacterial pathogen, *Mycobacterium tuberculosis,* fungi, or *Pneumocystis carinii*)
	Chronic pulmonary embolism
Cardiac disorders	CHF
	Myocardial ischemia
	Paroxysmal arrythmias
Physiologic conditions	Pregnancy
Metabolic or	Obesity
endocrine disorders	Thyrotoxicosis
Neuromuscular	ALS
disorders	Guillaine-Barré syndrome
	Myasthenia gravis
	Severe kyphoscoliosis
Hematologic disorders	Anemia
Psychiatric disorders	Anxiety disorder

ALS = amyotrophic lateral sclerosis; CHF = congestive heart failure; COPD = chronic obstructive pulmonary disease.

III APPROACH TO THE PATIENT

HOT

When a patient reports a history of dyspnea, a full evaluation is required, even if the patient is not obviously in respiratory distress.

KEY

TABLE 24-2. Common Causes of Acute Dyspnea

General Causes	Specific Disorders
Pulmonary disorders	Asthma
	COPD
	Pneumonia (usually caused by a typical bacterial pathogen)
	Pulmonary embolism
	Pneumothorax
	Upper airway obstruction
	Aspiration
Cardiac disorders	CHF
	Myocardial infarction
	Myocardial ischemia
	Arrhythmias
	Pericardial tamponade
Metabolic disorders	Sepsis
	Metabolic acidosis
Hematologic disorders	Anemia
Psychiatric disorders	Anxiety disorder
	Panic attack

CHF = congestive heart failure; COPD = chronic obstructive pulmonary disease.

A. **Patient history.** It is crucial to obtain a complete and detailed history. Be sure to investigate the following:
1. The duration of the dyspnea
2. Exacerbating and alleviating factors
3. Associated symptoms (e.g., chest pain, palpitations, weight loss)
4. The patient's past medical history, smoking history, and travel history

B. **Physical examination** must also be thorough. Particular areas of focus include the following:
1. **Vital signs,** including the oxygen saturation
2. **Lungs.** Are wheezing, rales, or rhonchi present?
3. **Heart.** Is the jugular venous pressure elevated? Is the point of maximal impulse (PMI) displaced? Can a third heart sound (S_3) or pathologic murmur be detected?

4. **Neuromuscular system.** Does the patient have obvious weakness or kyphoscoliosis?
5. **Extremities.** Is there any evidence of clubbing, edema, or cyanosis?

HOT

KEY

A useful maneuver to perform in patients who are not acutely dyspneic is to have them walk while monitoring their oxygen saturation. If the patient becomes dyspneic during ambulation, a lung examination should be performed. Listen for new rales or wheezing, which could imply CHF or exercise-induced bronchospasm. A pronounced drop in oxygen saturation on ambulation is a hallmark of interstitial lung disease (e.g., idiopathic pulmonary fibrosis, *Pneumocystis carinii* pneumonia).

C. **Laboratory studies**
1. The following studies should be obtained for most patients with dyspnea:
    a. Blood urea nitrogen (BUN) and creatinine level
    b. Chemistry panel
    c. Complete blood count (CBC)
    d. Chest radiograph
    e. Electrocardiogram (EKG)
    f. Blood gases
2. The following tests should be considered, depending on the suspected cause of the dyspnea.
    a. Pulmonary function tests (PFTs)
    b. Echocardiogram
    c. Exercise stress testing
    d. Chest high-resolution computed tomography (HRCT) scan

 IV **THERAPY** depends on the underlying disorder.

HOT

This is an appropriate time to counsel patients who smoke about health concerns associated with smoking.

KEY

V FOLLOW-UP AND REFERRAL

A. **Follow-up.** Initially, patients should be seen in clinic frequently (i.e., **approximately weekly)** until the cause of the dyspnea is diagnosed. During follow-up visits, smoking cessation counseling should be repeated.

B. **Referral.** When a clear cause cannot be determined, consultation with a **pulmonologist** is often appropriate. Patients with severe COPD, asthma, or interstitial lung disease may also need to see a pulmonologist.

References

Mahler DA, Horowitz MB: Clinical evaluation of exertional dyspnea. *Clin Chest Med* 15(2):259–269, 1994.

Manning HL, Schwartzstein RM: Pathophysiology of dyspnea. *N Engl J Med* 333(23): 1547–1553, 1995.

25. Asthma

I INTRODUCTION

A. Asthma is an **obstructive lung disease** that is most common in children and young adults. Patients generally present with a history of **episodic shortness of breath, chest tightness,** and **wheezing,** often in response to specific stimuli (e.g., exercise, cold air, pollution, allergens).
  1. **Three major components**
     a. **Airway hyperresponsiveness** to various stimuli
     b. **Airway inflammation**
     c. **Airway obstruction** that is reversible
  2. **Two patterns**
     a. **Acute attacks** usually occur within minutes to hours of exposure to an inhaled stimulus (e.g., pollen, dust, fumes) or an ingestion (e.g. aspirin, sulfites).
     b. **Subacute attacks** develop over hours to days and are most often caused by viral respiratory infections.
B. Currently, in the United States, asthma affects **3%–5% of the population,** and the morbidity and mortality attributable to the disease is increasing.

II DIFFERENTIAL DIAGNOSIS

A. **Acute shortness of breath.** The differential diagnosis for acute shortness of breath is broad, but can be simplified by considering five major categories of disease (see Chapter 24, Table 24-2).
B. **Chronic shortness of breath (See Chapter 27, Table 27-1).** Remember, **not all that wheezes is asthma.** Patients with apparent chronic asthma may have another condition that causes wheezing, and a physician who "CARES" will consider these alternate diagnoses.

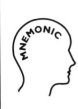

Other Causes of Wheezing ("CARES")

Cardiac asthma (i.e., CHF) or **C**hurg-Strauss syndrome
Allergic bronchopulmonary aspergillosis
Reflux esophagitis
Exposures (irritants, medications) or **E**mbolism (pulmonary)
Sinusitis or **S**trongyloides infection

 III APPROACH TO THE PATIENT

A. **Acute attack.** Patients with a moderate to severe attack of asthma should be evaluated in an emergency setting where cardiopulmonary resuscitation (CPR) is readily available.

  1. **Patient history.** It is always useful to ask the patient how severe the attack is in comparison with others he has had. Be sure to make the following inquiries:

     a. What is the **time course** of the current attack?

     b. Are there any **known triggers?**

     c. What has been the **frequency** and **severity of past attacks** (e.g., was the patient ever intubated or hospitalized)?

     d. What **medications** is the patient using?

     e. What is the **peak flow** and how does it compare to baseline measurements?

  2. **Physical examination.** Findings vary depending on the severity of the attack, but may include:

     a. Tachypnea

     b. Use of the accessory muscles

     c. Intercostal retraction

     d. Wheezing

     e. A prolonged inspiratory-to-expiratory (I:E) ratio

     f. Hyperresonance

     g. Pulsus paradoxus

  3. **Additional studies**

     a. **Pulmonary function tests (PFTs).** Obtain an initial **peak flow** or **forced expiratory volume in 1 second (FEV$_1$)** as an objective measure of disease severity. This baseline measurement will also enable you to evaluate the patient's response to acute treatment.

   b. A **chest radiograph** should be obtained for most patients with moderate to severe attacks.

   c. **Laboratory studies** are generally not necessary, unless another cause of dyspnea is suspected.

B. Chronic asthma

   1. Patient history. Inquire about the following:

      a. History of attacks

      b. Triggers

      c. Nocturnal symptoms (wheezing or shortness of breath at night may indicate a trigger, such as cold temperatures or reflux disease, or suggest that current medications are inadequate)

      d. Medication use

   2. Physical examination. Findings vary, depending on current disease activity. Wheezing, a prolonged I:E ratio, and hyperresonance may be present if the patient is experiencing a mild exacerbation, or if medications are inadequate.

   3. Additional studies

      a. Spirometry and **bronchial provocation testing** are useful for diagnosis and monitoring of disease progression. A positive test is defined by a 20% reduction in the FEV_1 in response to methacholine, histamine, hypertonic saline, or other stimulants.

      b. A **chest radiograph** is generally not required for patients younger than 40 years.

      c. Laboratory studies are rarely useful.

IV TREATMENT

A. Acute treatment. Treatment considerations for a patient with an acute asthma attack can be remembered using the mnemonic, "ASTHMA."

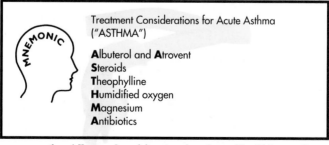

Treatment Considerations for Acute Asthma ("ASTHMA")

Albuterol and **A**trovent
Steroids
Theophylline
Humidified oxygen
Magnesium
Antibiotics

   1. Albuterol and **ipratropium bromide (Atrovent)** are both effective **bronchodilators.**

   a. Albuterol (2–4 puffs from a metered-dose inhaler
       or 0.5 ml of a 0.5% solution in 3 ml of normal
       saline given as a nebulizer) should be the initial
       treatment in most patients.
   b. Ipratropium bromide may be a useful adjunct.
2. **Steroids.** Most patients with an acute attack should
   be treated with a steroid taper (e.g., prednisone, 3
   days each of 60 mg, 40 mg, and 20 mg) to prevent the
   development of a delayed inflammatory response.
3. **Theophylline.** The use of theophylline in acute exacerbations of asthma is controversial but is advocated
   by some authorities.
4. **Humidified oxygen** should be administered to any
   patient with moderate to severe shortness of breath
   until symptoms are controlled.
5. **Magnesium.** The intravenous administration of magnesium may offer improvement for patients with severe attacks.
6. **Antibiotics** are generally not indicated for asthma exacerbations because most attacks are caused by allergens or viral infections.

HOT **KEY** Patients who do not respond rapidly to pharmacologic therapy and those with significant respiratory distress at presentation should be hospitalized for observation. Patients
who are not hospitalized should have close home monitoring with a clear plan for return if symptoms worsen.

B. **Chronic treatment**
   1. **Pharmacologic agents** commonly used for the ongoing
      treatment of asthma are summarized in Table 25-1.
      a. β agonists. Therapy should be initiated with a β
         agonist (e.g., **albuterol**); agents can be added in
         the order they are listed in Table 25-1 if symp-
         toms are not controlled.

HOT **KEY** Patients with mild asthma who require more than 4 doses
per week of a β agonist should begin treatment with inhaled
steroids or a long-acting β agonist.

TABLE 25-1. Medications for the Chronic Treatment of Asthma		
Class of Drug	**Examples**	**Dose**
β Agonists	Albuterol	2 puffs every 4–6 hours as required
Inhaled steroids	Triamcinolone acetonide	2–4 puffs twice daily (200 μg/puff)
Long-acting β agonists	Salmeterol	2 puffs twice daily
Inhibitors of histamine release	Nedocromil	2 puffs four times daily
Methylxanthines	Theophylline	100–300 mg orally twice daily

    b. **Inhaled steroids** (e.g., **triamcinolone acetonide**) may reduce the frequency and severity of exacerbations. The systemic effects associated with steroid use are not believed to occur at doses of approximately 1600 μg/day or less (e.g., 4 puffs twice daily of triamcinolone acetonide).

    c. **Long-acting β agonists** (e.g., **salmeterol**) provide consistent drug levels and should be considered for patients who frequently use short-acting agents (more than 4 doses per week).

HOT

Long-acting β agonists cannot be used for acute attacks because they can accumulate, causing toxicity.

KEY

    d. **Nedocromil,** which is believed to stabilize mast cells, may be useful for prophylaxis prior to animal exposure or exercise.

    e. **Theophylline** may be useful in patients with nocturnal symptoms.

    f. **Leukotriene antagonists** are a newer class of medications for asthma that are designed to reduce the inflammatory response by interfering with leukotriene production or binding to cell receptors. **Zafirlukast** has been shown to improve both symptom scores and objective measures in patients with chronic asthma. The exact role and long-term safety of these agents in the treatment of asthma have not been established.

2. **Inhaler use.** One of the most common causes of inadequate therapy is poor technique when using an inhaler. Patients should be instructed to:
   a. Use a spacer
   b. Shake the canister and exhale completely
   c. Activate the canister and inhale slowly
   d. Hold their breath for 5–10 seconds
3. **Monitoring.** Patients should be given a peak flow meter and advised to call when their baseline peak flow is worsening (signaling the onset of an attack).

V FOLLOW-UP AND REFERRAL

A. Patients who have had an acute attack treated in an urgent care setting should be **re-evaluated in 1–5 days.** Those who experience a near-fatal asthma attack are at very high risk for short-term mortality and should be evaluated by a specialist and seen regularly to monitor symptoms.

B. **Specialized asthma treatment centers** are available and should be considered for the following patients:
   1. Those with newly diagnosed asthma (as a source of patient education and treatment recommendations)
   2. Those with symptoms that do not respond to inhaler therapy
   3. Those who require more than 2 courses of oral steroids per year
   4. Those who have experienced a near-fatal attack of asthma

References

Donahue JG, Weiss ST, Livingston JM, et al: Inhaled steroids and the risk of hospitalization for asthma. *JAMA* 277(11) :887–891, 1997.

Drazen JM, Israel E, Boushey HA, et al: Comparison of regularly scheduled with as-needed use of albuterol in mild asthma. *N Engl J Med* 335(12):841–847, 1996.

Lemanske RF, Busse WW: Asthma. *JAMA* 278(22):1855–1873, 1997.

26. Chronic Obstructive Pulmonary Disease

I. INTRODUCTION

A. Chronic obstructive pulmonary disease (COPD) is characterized by **abnormal expiratory flow** (as evidenced on pulmonary function testing) **that does not change markedly over time.** Underlying causes include chronic bronchitis and emphysema; most patients have a combination of both disorders.

1. **Chronic bronchitis** is defined as the presence of a cough with sputum production for at least 3 months of the year in 2 consecutive years.

2. **Emphysema** is defined pathologically as permanent enlargement of the airspaces distal to the terminal bronchioles and destruction of the walls, but no fibrosis.

B. Most patients with COPD present in the **fifth to sixth decades** of life, have a **history of smoking,** and report some combination of **dyspnea, chronic cough, sputum production,** and **wheezing.**

C. COPD affects more than 15 million Americans and is the **fourth leading cause of death in the United States.**

II. DIFFERENTIAL DIAGNOSIS

A. **Asthma** generally is differentiated from COPD on the basis of reversibility of the airway obstruction, which is suggested by the history and can be confirmed with spirometry.

B. **Bronchiectasis** should be suspected if there is a history of chronic productive cough, frequent pneumonia, and hemoptysis. The chest radiograph often demonstrates characteristic markings of peribronchial fibrosis.

C. **Cystic fibrosis** is an inherited disorder causing chronic productive cough and dyspnea in childhood or early adulthood. A sweat chloride test establishes the diagnosis.

D. **Central airway obstruction** can be caused by any process that narrows the large central airways (e.g., subglottic stenosis, laryngeal carcinoma). Patients may present with progressive dyspnea. The obstruction can be distinguished from COPD on the basis of spirometry.

E. α_1-**Antitrypsin deficiency** is an inherited enzyme deficiency. Because the enzyme is normally protective against lung damage, patients with low levels of the enzyme are at increased risk for development of COPD at an early age.

III APPROACH TO THE PATIENT

A. **Initial diagnosis**

1. **Patient history.** Answers to the following questions should be sought.

a. What is the **timing** and **severity** of the **dyspnea** and **cough?**

b. What is the patient's **smoking history?**

c. What is the patient's **environmental exposure to pollutants** or **second-hand smoke?**

d. Is there a **family history of pulmonary disease?**

2. **Physical examination**

a. Examination of the lungs may reveal **decreased breath sounds,** a **prolonged inspiratory-to-expiratory (I:E) ratio, wheezing,** and **rhonchi.**

b. Patients with moderate to severe disease may exhibit an increased anteroposterior chest diameter (**"barrel chest"), clubbing,** or **central cyanosis.**

3. **Other studies**

a. A **chest radiograph** is indicated for most patients with suspected COPD. Findings may include **hyperinflation, parenchymal bullae,** and an **enlarged pulmonary artery** (suggestive of pulmonary hypertension).

b. **Spirometry** is indicated for most patients with suspected COPD. The diagnosis of COPD is suggested by a **low forced expiratory volume in 1 second (FEV_1)** and a **low FEV_1%.** [i.e., the ratio of the FEV_1 to the forced vital capacity (FVC)].

HOT KEY In a patient who smokes, history, physical, and radiographic findings consistent with COPD and a low FEV_1 or FEV_1% on spirometry establish the diagnosis of COPD. The low spirometry measurements do not improve following the administration of bronchodilators.

---

c. **Laboratory studies**

(1) A **complete blood count (CBC)** may show **polycythemia** as a result of chronic hypoxemia.

(2) **Arterial blood gases (ABGs)** are often useful for determining the **degree of hypoxemia** and **hypercarbia.**

(3) An α_1**-antitrypsin level** is indicated for patients with COPD and no history of smoking, and for those who present with the disease at an early age.

B. **Acute exacerbations** of COPD are common. Most episodes are thought to be caused by **viral infection,** but **bacterial infection** and **inhaled irritants** may also play a role.

HOT
KEY

All patients with COPD should receive a flu vaccination annually and a pneumococcal vaccination every 5–10 years. In addition, they should minimize their exposure to air pollutants, second-hand smoke, and particulate matter.

---

1. Patients present with an **increase in cough, worsening dyspnea,** or a **change in the color or quantity of sputum.**
2. Patients with COPD are at risk for a number of other conditions that may cause acute shortness of breath [e.g., pneumonia, pneumothorax, cardiac ischemia, congestive heart failure (CHF), medication side effect]. Always perform a thorough history and physical and **consider all possible causes of shortness of breath in these patients.**

IV THERAPY

A. **Chronic therapy**
1. **Smoking cessation** has been shown to slow the progression of COPD and is the most important aspect of prevention. Patients with COPD who smoke should be enrolled in a smoking cessation program.
2. **Oxygen therapy.** Long-term oxygen therapy has been shown to improve survival and should be considered in patients with either a resting arterial oxygen tension (Pao_2) of less than 55 mm Hg or a resting Pao_2 of 55–59 mm Hg with clinical evidence of cor pulmonale or secondary erythrocytosis.
3. **Pharmacologic therapy.** Agents should be used in the order in which they are presented in Table 26-1; add the next medication if the patient remains symptomatic.

TABLE 26-1. Agents Used in the Treatment of Chronic Obstructive Pulmonary Disease (COPD)			
Drug Class	Examples	Dose	Side Effects and Cautions
Anticholinergics	Ipratropium metered-dose inhaler	4–6 puffs, four times daily	Minimal side effects
β Agonists	Albuterol metered-dose inhaler	2–4 puffs every 4–6 hours* as needed	May cause tremor, agitation, and tachycardia; use with caution in patients with heart disease
Methylxanthines	Theophylline	100–300 mg twice daily†; monitor serum drug levels for range of 8–12 µg/ml	Multiple drugs interact with theophylline
Corticosteroids	Triamcinolone acetonide	2–10 puffs twice daily	Refer to pulmonologist before initiating oral steroids; consider spirometry before and after initiating oral steroids to monitor effect

*Longer-acting agents are available.
†Once-a-day dosing is available.

B. **Acute exacerbations.** There are three main treatments that should be considered for patients with acute exacerbations of COPD.

1. **Inhalers.** Both inhaled β agonists and ipratropium are effective in improving symptoms and spirometric measurements. When used properly, metered-dose inhalers are as effective as nebulizers.

2. **Corticosteroids.** Although the role of corticosteroids in the treatment of COPD has not been well studied, steroid tapers (e.g., prednisone, 3 days each of 60 mg, 40 mg, and 20 mg) appear to be effective in reducing symptoms. Longer tapers may be appropriate for patients with severe disease.

3. **Antibiotics** (e.g., 1 trimethoprim-sulfamethoxazole double-strength tablet orally twice daily for 10 days) may improve expiratory flow.

HOT

Hospitalization should be considered for all patients with moderate to severe symptoms, hypoxia, or hypercarbia.

KEY

V **FOLLOW-UP AND REFERRAL**

A. **Follow-up.** Stable patients should be seen **every 3–4 months** to monitor symptoms and adjust medications. **Annual spirometry** can be considered to document disease progression, and may help motivate the patient's efforts to stop smoking.

B. **Referral.** Patients with **symptoms that cannot be controlled,** those who require **frequent oral steroids for control,** and those who have α_1-**antitrypsin deficiency** should be referred to a pulmonologist for evaluation.

References

Ferguson GT, Cherniack RM: Management of chronic obstructive pulmonary disease. *N Engl J Med* 328(14):1017–1022, 1993.

Saint S, Bent S, Vittinghoff E, et al: Antibiotics in chronic obstructive pulmonary disease exacerbations: a meta-analysis. *JAMA* 273(12):957–960, 1995.

27. Pulmonary Function Tests

I. INTRODUCTION

A. Background. Pulmonary function tests (PFTs) usually evaluate three areas: **expiratory flow rate** (spirometry), **lung volumes,** and **diffusion capacity** (Table 27-1)

B. Applications. PFTs can be used to:
1. Distinguish obstructive lung disease from restrictive lung disease (Table 27-2)
2. Assess the severity of lung disease
3. Evaluate the patient's response to therapy

II. OBSTRUCTIVE VERSUS RESTRICTIVE LUNG DISEASE

A. Flow rate = lung volume/(resistance)(compliance). The following conclusions can be drawn from examining this equation:
1. The **flow rate** (as **measured by FEV_1**) will decrease under any of the following conditions:
   a. The lung volume decreases (as seen in restrictive disorders)
   b. The resistance increases (as seen in asthma and chronic bronchitis)
   c. The compliance increases (as seen in emphysema)
2. Therefore, the **flow rate will be decreased in both restrictive and obstructive lung diseases,** and looking at the FEV_1 alone will not enable you to distinguish between these two types of disorders.

B. $FEV_1\% = FEV_1/FVC$. In order to distinguish between obstructive and restrictive lung disorders, the lung volume must be removed from the equation. Dividing by the FVC will accomplish this goal.

III. QUICK APPROACH TO THE INTERPRETATION OF PULMONARY FUNCTION TESTS (PFTs). Interpreting

PFTs requires a systematic approach (Figure 27-1).

TABLE 27-1. Abbreviations Associated with Pulmonary Function Tests (PFTs)

Abbreviation	Meaning
Expiratory flow rate	
FEV_1	Forced expiratory volume in 1 second
FVC	Forced vital capacity
$FEV_1\%$	Ratio of the FEV_1 to the FVC
Lung volume	
TLC	Total lung capacity
VC	Vital capacity
RV	Residual volume
Diffusing capacity	
D_{LCO}	Diffusing capacity of the lungs for carbon dioxide

TABLE 27-2. Common Diseases Leading to Abnormal Findings on Pulmonary Function Tests (PFTs)

Obstructive disorders
 Asthma
 Chronic obstructive pulmonary disease (COPD)
 Bronchiectasis
 Cystic fibrosis

Restrictive disorders
 Pleural fibrosis or effusion
 Alveolar edema or inflammation
 Interstitial disorders (e.g., sarcoidosis, idiopathic pulmonary fibrosis, fungal infection)
 Neuromuscular disorders (e.g., myasthenia gravis, myopathy)
 Thoracic or extrathoracic disorders (e.g., kyphoscoliosis, pregnancy, obesity)

HOT

KEY

When interpreting PFTs, it is important to note both the observed values and the percent of predicted values.

HY

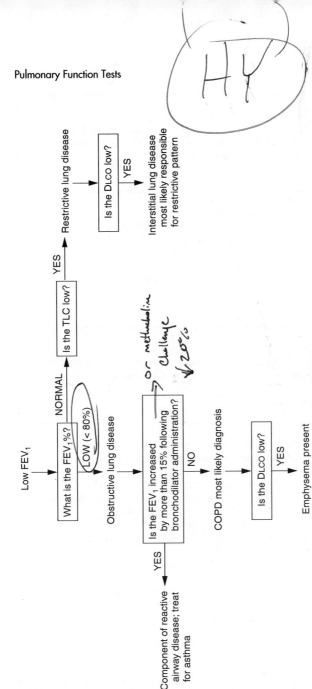

FIGURE 27-1. Approach to interpreting pulmonary function tests (PFTs). DlCO = diffusing capacity of the lungs for carbon dioxide; FEV₁ = forced expiratory volume in 1 second; FEV₁% = ratio of the FEV₁ to the forced vital capacity (FVC); TLC = total lung capacity.

HOT

The range of normal for all values seen on PFTs will vary slightly depending on the PFT laboratory; however, these values can be obtained easily.

KEY

A. First, look at the FEV_1.
B. If the FEV_1 is low, look at the FEV_1%.
   1. **Obstructive disease.** Both the FEV_1 and the FEV_1% will be **decreased.**
   2. **Restrictive disease.** The FEV_1 will be **decreased** but the FEV_1% will be **normal** (or increased). A low TLC supports the diagnosis of a restrictive lung disorder.

HOT

The incidence of postoperative complications tends to increase if the FEV_1 is less than 2.0 L/sec and the FEV_1% is less than 50%.

KEY

C. **If the patient has obstructive lung disease, determine if the obstruction is reversible** by administering bronchodilators and re-evaluating the FEV_1.
   1. **Improvement** of the FEV_1 by more than 15% following bronchodilator administration implies reversible airway obstruction (i.e., **asthma**).
   2. If there is **no improvement,** the patient probably has **chronic obstructive pulmonary disease (COPD).**
D. **Look at the DLCO.** A decreased DLCO is seen whenever there is an inability to transfer gas across the alveolar–capillary interface.
   1. If the patient has **restrictive disease,** a low DLCO implies that **interstitial lung disease** is the cause of the restrictive pattern.
   2. If the patient has **obstructive lung disease,** a low DLCO implies **emphysema.**

References

Enright PL, Lebowitz MD, Cockroft DW: Physiologic measures: pulmonary function tests. Asthma outcome. *Am J Respir Crit Care Med* 149(2 part 2): S9–S18, 1994.

28. Acute Bronchitis

I INTRODUCTION

A. Acute bronchitis is the **acute onset of cough** and **sputum production** in a patient with **no history of chronic pulmonary disease** and **no evidence of pneumonia or sinusitis.**

1. **Sputum production** is the **hallmark** of the disorder.
2. Fever may or may not be present.

B. Acute bronchitis **accounts for more than 10 million annual office visits** in the United States; direct costs are in the hundreds of millions of dollars.

II CAUSES OF ACUTE BRONCHITIS

A. **Viral infections** cause **most cases** of acute bronchitis.

B. **Atypical bacteria** (e.g., *Mycoplasma pneumoniae, Chlamydia pneumoniae, Legionella*) may cause as many as **25% of cases.**

C. **Typical bacteria** (e.g., *Streptococcus pneumoniae, Haemophilus influenzae, Moraxella catarrhalis*) are rarely involved.

D. **Allergic reactions** and **air pollutants** may be responsible for some cases.

III DIFFERENTIAL DIAGNOSIS

A. **Acute, productive cough.** Acute bronchitis must be distinguished from the other common causes of an acute productive cough in otherwise healthy individuals: **pneumonia** and **sinusitis** (in sinusitis, the cough is stimulated by postnasal drip).

B. **Nonproductive cough.** Acute bronchitis must also be distinguished from the many causes of a nonproductive cough in healthy patients, including **upper respiratory tract infections** (e.g., pharyngitis, rhinitis, laryngitis), **asthma,** and **pleural** or **diaphragmatic irritation.**

IV APPROACH TO THE PATIENT

A. **Patient history.** Focus on three questions:

1. **Is the cough productive?** If not, consider upper respiratory tract infections and other causes of nonproductive cough.

2. **Does the patient have a history of pulmonary disease?** A history of asthma, chronic obstructive pulmonary disease (COPD), or another pulmonary disorder suggests the possibility of an exacerbation of the underlying condition.
3. **How severe are the symptoms?**
   a. A productive cough accompanied by fever, shortness of breath, pleuritic pain, or worsening malaise suggests pneumonia.
   b. Sinus pain and purulent nasal discharge in combination with fever suggests sinusitis.

B. **Physical examination.** The examination should be focused to exclude pneumonia and sinusitis.
   1. Pneumonia is suggested by an abnormal lung exam.
   2. Sinusitis is suggested by fever, purulent nasal discharge, and abnormal transillumination.

C. **Imaging studies**
   1. A **chest radiograph** is usually indicated for patients with abnormal findings on lung examination.
   2. A **sinus computed tomography (CT) scan** is occasionally necessary to rule out sinusitis.

D. **Laboratory studies** [e.g., a complete blood count (CBC), sputum Gram stain or culture] are usually not necessary.

 TREATMENT. Symptoms should improve gradually over 1–2 weeks.

HOT

Most authorities do not recommend antibiotics for the treatment of acute bronchitis in healthy adults.

KEY

A. **Albuterol.** Regular use of an albuterol metered-dose inhaler (e.g., 2 puffs very 4–6 hours) may decrease the duration of coughing.
B. **Cough suppressants, throat lozenges,** and **decongestants** may relieve symptoms but have not been shown to alter the course of the illness.

 FOLLOW-UP AND REFERRAL. Otherwise healthy patients do not need to have scheduled follow-up, unless their symptoms do not improve within 2 weeks.

References
Gonzales R, Steiner JF, Sande MA: Antibiotic prescribing for adults with colds, upper respiratory tract infections, and bronchitis by ambulatory care physicians. *JAMA* 278(11):901–904, 1997.
Mainous AG III, Zoorob RJ, Hueston WJ: Current management of acute bronchitis in ambulatory care: the use of antibiotics and bronchodilators. *Arch Fam Med* 5(2):79–83, 1996.

29. Community-Acquired Pneumonia

I. INTRODUCTION

A. Community-acquired pneumonia is a **leading cause of death** and the **number one cause of infectious disease-related mortality in the United States.**

B. **Approximately 80% of patients** with community-acquired pneumonia **are treated entirely as outpatients.**

II. CLINICAL MANIFESTATIONS OF COMMUNITY-ACQUIRED PNEUMONIA.

Community-acquired pneumonia may be classified as "typical" or "atypical" on the basis of the causative organism. Practitioners often attempt to classify community-acquired pneumonia as "typical" or "atypical" on the basis of the patient's signs and symptoms; however, this approach may only partially predict the underlying pathogen.

A. **Typical community-acquired pneumonia**
  1. **Symptoms** commonly include subjective fever, cough, sputum production, pleuritic chest pain, and dyspnea.
  2. **Signs** commonly include fever, tachypnea ($>$ 20 respirations/min), and signs of lobar consolidation (bronchial breath sounds, egophony, dullness to percussion, crackles).

B. **Atypical community-acquired pneumonia** classically is characterized by the **gradual onset of disease,** a **dry cough** (or cough productive of only scant sputum), and **prominent extrapulmonary symptoms** (e.g., headache, myalgia, diarrhea, hepatosplenomegaly, elevated aminotransferase levels).

III. CAUSES OF COMMUNITY-ACQUIRED PNEUMONIA

A. **Typical community-acquired pneumonia** is usually caused by *Streptococcus pneumoniae, Haemophilus influenzae, Staphylococcus aureus,* or Gram-negative bacilli (e.g., *Klebsiella*).

1. **S. pneumoniae** is one of the most common organisms responsible for community-acquired pneumonia. **Respect the "pneumococcus"—it can kill quickly!**

HOT

Usually, pneumococcal pneumonia presents abruptly; however, an indolent presentation is common when pneumococcal disease follows a viral respiratory tract infection.

KEY

---

2. **H. influenzae** is an especially common cause of community-acquired pneumonia in patients with **chronic obstructive pulmonary disease (COPD).**
3. **S. aureus** infection may be seen in patients who have **influenza,** are **immunocompromised,** or live in **nursing homes.**
3. **Aerobic Gram-negative rods.** Infection caused by aerobic Gram-negative rods is more common in **patients older than 60 years** and in **alcoholic patients.**
B. **Atypical community-acquired pneumonia** is usually caused by **Mycoplasma pneumoniae, Chlamydia pneumoniae, Legionella pneumophila,** or **Moraxella catarrhalis.**
   1. **M. pneumoniae** usually causes a **mild pneumonia** in adults. *M. pneumoniae* infection has been associated with even more **prominent extrapulmonary involvement** than other atypical causes of community-acquired pneumonia, including **hemolytic anemia, erythema multiforme, myocarditis, erythema nodosum, bullous myringitis,** and **several neurologic abnormalities.**
   2. **C. pneumoniae** also usually causes a **mild pneumonia.** Although the clinical manifestations are generally similar to those of other causes of atypical pneumonia, **hoarseness with severe pharyngitis** is considered a distinguishing feature of pneumonia caused by *C. pneumoniae.*

HOT

M. pneumoniae and *C. pneumoniae* together account for 25% of all cases of community-acquired pneumonia managed by primary care providers.

KEY

3. *Legionella* species can cause **severe pneumonia. Gram-staining** usually reveals **numerous polymorphonuclear neutrophils (PMNs) but no organisms.**
4. *M. catarrhalis, Mycobacterium tuberculosis, Pneumocystis carinii,* respiratory **viruses** (e.g., influenza virus) and **fungi** can also cause an atypical community-acquired pneumonia.

IV APPROACH TO THE PATIENT

HOT

KEY

In most patients with community-acquired pneumonia, the responsible pathogen is not identified.

A. **Diagnostic tests**
    1. **Chest radiograph.** Posterior-anterior (PA) and lateral views are indicated for most patients with suspected community-acquired pneumonia. In young, otherwise healthy patients who will be treated as outpatients, a chest radiograph may be all that is needed for patient evaluation.
    2. **Laboratory studies.** The following tests may be appropriate for some patients:
        a. **Complete blood count (CBC)**
        b. **Serum electrolyte panel**
        c. **Blood urea nitrogen (BUN)** and **creatinine levels**
        d. **Peripheral blood cultures,** on samples drawn from two separate sites
        e. **Arterial blood gases (ABGs),** especially appropriate if the room air oxygen saturation is < 92%
        f. **Sputum analysis**
            (1) Gram-staining and culture of even a properly expectorated sputum sample may not yield the responsible organism; therefore, it is reasonable to omit this test if it cannot be readily obtained.
            (2) If *M. tuberculosis* or *P. carinii* infection is suspected, sputum analysis using special stains should always be done.
        g. **Thoracentesis.** If a pleural effusion is present and the patient has clinical evidence of empyema

(e.g., hypotension, toxic appearance), thoracentesis should be performed promptly and the pleural fluid should be sent for a cell count and differential, Gram staining and culture, and total protein and lactate dehydrogenase (LDH) levels.

B. Criteria for hospital admission. There are no absolute criteria for hospital admission, but specific factors place the patient at greater risk for a complicated clinical course, mortality, or both. The following mnemonic can help you remember some of the most important criteria for admitting a patient: "ADMIT NOW."

Criteria for Hospital Admission of Patients with Community-Acquired Pneumonia ("ADMIT NOW")

Age > 65 years (depending on individual situation)
Decreased immunity (e.g., cancer, diabetes, AIDS, splenectomy)
Mental status changes
Increased A-a gradient or increased respiratory rate
Two or more lobes involved

No home (i.e., homeless patients)
Organ system failure (increased creatinine, bone marrow suppression, systolic blood pressure ≤ 90 mm Hg, liver failure)
WBC count greater than 30,000/mm^3 or less than 4000/ mm^3

In general, if a patient meets more than one of these criteria, hospitalization is reasonable. Sometimes the most important criterion is the **"eyeball" test** (i.e., how sick a person looks to an experienced physician).

V **TREATMENT.** When a patient does not meet the criteria for hospital admission and has passed the "eyeball" test, **outpatient management** is usually indicated.

A. Empiric therapy
    1. First-line agents. Dosages are given in Table 29-1.
        a. Erythromycin is appropriate initial therapy for most patients younger than 60 years. The newer macrolides (i.e., **clarithromycin, azithromycin**) should be considered if *H. influenzae* is suspected

TABLE 29-1. Dosages for First-Line Agents Used Empirically in the Outpatient Treatment of Community-Acquired Pneumonia

Agent	Dose
Erythromycin	500 mg orally, four times daily for 10–14 days
Clarithromycin	500 mg orally, twice daily for 10–14 days
Azithromycin	500 mg orally on the first day, 250 mg orally daily on days 2–5
Cefuroxime	500 mg orally, twice daily for 10–14 days
Amoxicillin–clavulanic acid	875 mg orally, twice daily for 10–14 days

(e.g., in smokers) or if the patient cannot tolerate erythromycin.

    b. A second-generation cephalosporin (e.g., **cefuroxime**) or a β-lactam combined with a β-lactamase inhibitor (e.g., **amoxicillin-clavulanic acid**) may be considered first-line therapy in patients older than 60 years and in those with comorbid conditions. (Occasionally, a macrolide will be added to the cephalosporin if *Legionella, Mycoplasma,* or *Chlamydia* is of particular concern; however, most patients suspected of having *Legionella* are admitted to the hospital.)

  2. **Second-line agents.** Many of the newer **quinolone drugs** (e.g., **levofloxacin, sparfloxacin**) provide broad-spectrum activity against most of the suspected pathogens. However, because of their expense and the desire to avoid the development of resistance, they remain second-line drugs.

B. Specific therapy. If the causative organism is identified and the patient has not shown expected clinical improvement, antibiotic susceptibility testing should be done to direct further therapy.

VI FOLLOW-UP AND REFERRAL

  A. Follow-up

    1. All patients treated in the ambulatory setting should be instructed to call if their symptoms worsen, dyspnea develops, or they are unable to continue taking medication orally.

2. Most outpatients should experience subjective improvement and decreased fever within 2–4 days of initiating antibiotic therapy.

   a. Office follow-up within 4–7 days to assess response to treatment is reasonable in older patients and in those with comorbid conditions, such as COPD or diabetes.

   b. All patients who smoke or who used to smoke, and any patient with a lingering cough despite resolution of other symptoms should have a follow-up chest radiograph at 4–6 weeks.

HOT

Approximately 3% of patients with bronchogenic carcinoma present initially with pneumonia.

KEY

B. **Referral.** Consultation with a pulmonologist or an infectious disease specialist may be helpful for patients who do not respond to standard therapy or have severe symptoms. In general, however, most patients with community-acquired pneumonia can be adequately managed by primary care physicians.

References

Atlas SJ, Benzer TI, Borowsky LH, et al: Safely increasing the proportion of patients with community-acquired pneumonia treated as outpatients: an interventional trial. *Arch Intern Med* 158(12):1350–1356, 1998.

Bartlett JG, Breiman RF, Mandell LA, et al: Community-acquired pneumonia in adults: guidelines for management. The Infectious Diseases Society of America. *Clin Infect Dis* 26(4):811–838, 1998.

Metlay JP, Kapoor WN, Fine MJ: Does this patient have community-acquired pneumonia? Diagnosing pneumonia by history and physical examination. *JAMA* 278(17):1440–1445, 1997.

30. Solitary Pulmonary Nodule

I INTRODUCTION

A. Solitary pulmonary nodules are **asymptomatic, spherical densities** discovered on chest radiographs or computed tomography (CT) scans.

B. These nodules are **relatively common,** occurring in approximately **one in every five hundred chest radiographs.** They present a problem for the primary care provider, because it is often difficult to determine whether the nodule is malignant or benign.

II DIFFERENTIAL DIAGNOSIS (Table 30-1)

A. Malignant tumors account for approximately 40% of all solitary pulmonary nodules. Most malignant solitary pulmonary nodules are **primary lung tumors.**

B. Benign lesions. Most benign pulmonary nodules are **healed granulomas** caused by tuberculosis or fungal infections (e.g., histoplasmosis, coccidioidomycosis).

III APPROACH TO THE PATIENT. The goal of evaluation is to determine the likelihood of malignancy so that an informed decision can be made about the risks and benefits of surgery.

A. Patient history. Older patients and patients with a **history of smoking** are more likely to have malignant nodules.

B. Imaging studies
  1. **Comparison of recent and old chest films** is a crucial part of the evaluation.
     a. Growth rate. If the nodule is present on an old film and has shown no growth for 500 days or more, then malignancy is unlikely. However, lesions that have shown growth, especially those with a doubling time of less than 500 days, are more likely to be malignant.
     b. Nodule size is also important. Larger nodules are more likely to be malignant (especially those greater than 3 centimeters in diameter).
  2. **CT.** All patients should have a chest CT scan to allow better evaluation of the nodule. CT characteristics that increase the likelihood of malignancy include an

---

TABLE 30-1. Differential Diagnosis of Solitary Pulmonary Nodule

Malignancy
  Primary lung tumor (e.g., bronchogenic carcinoma, carcinoid)
  Metastatic cancer
Benign lesion
  Healed granuloma
  Hamartoma
  Arteriovenous malformation
  Rheumatoid nodule
  Pseudolymphoma
  Hydatid cyst
  Wegener's granulomatosis

---

uncalcified nodule, an **irregular (spiculated) border,** and a **nodular cavity with a thick wall.**

IV TREATMENT

  A. The treatment strategy depends on the likelihood of malignancy and the desires of the patient. Some patients may prefer to have nodules resected that have only a remote possibility of malignancy. Others, such as those with multiple medical problems, may be reluctant to undergo surgery because of the associated risks.

  B. There are no precise "cutoffs" where the probability of malignancy dictates treatment strategy. The following treatment options should be discussed with each patient.

  1. **Observation** entails obtaining serial chest radiographs over an extended period of time to see if the nodule is growing. Nodules that exhibit no growth or have a doubling time greater than 500 days are less likely to be malignant.

   a. The risk of observation is that if the lesion is malignant, the delay in resection may result in a lower chance of curative surgery. Generally, this approach is not recommended unless the probability of malignancy is very low.

   b. Patients who have chosen the observation strategy should be followed in consultation with a pulmonologist.

  2. **Biopsy** can be **transbronchial** (i.e., performed during bronchoscopy) or **transthoracic** (i.e., CT-guided).

   a. A positive diagnosis is helpful for ruling in can-
        cer, but a negative biopsy does not rule out ma-
        lignant disease.
   b. Transthoracic biopsy carries a risk of pneumoth-
        orax; transbronchial biopsy has a low yield but
        carries less risk of pneumothorax.
3. **Thoracotomy with resection** is the treatment of choice
   for malignant lesions as long as the CT scan does not
   reveal extensive, inoperable disease.
   a. The mortality rate associated with thoracotomy
        for malignant lesions depends on the presence of
        comorbid disease, but can be as high as 10%.
   b. Thoracotomy for benign lesions has a very low
        mortality rate.
4. **Video-assisted thoracoscopy,** a new technique for resection of nodules, has a low complication rate and
   should be considered as an alternative to thoracotomy.

 FOLLOW-UP AND REFERRAL. Consultation with a radiologist, a pulmonologist, and a surgeon is always helpful in determining the best strategy.

References
Gurney JW: Determining the likelihood of malignancy in solitary pulmonary nodules
    with Bayesian analysis. Part I. Theory. *Radiology* 186(2):405–413, 1993.

31. Sleep Apnea Syndrome

I INTRODUCTION

A. Recurrent cessation of breathing (i.e., apnea) during sleep leads to a symptom complex marked by daytime hypersomnolence.

   1. **Apnea** is **defined as cessation of airflow at the mouth for at least 10 seconds.** More than five apneic episodes an hour suggests the presence of sleep apnea syndrome.

   2. The **apnea** can be **obstructive, central,** or **mixed.**

     a. **Obstructive apnea** is the most common type; airflow cessation is caused by upper airway obstruction (usually from the tongue, uvula, tonsils, or nasopharynx).

     b. **Central apnea** is rare. In these patients, ventilatory effort is absent during the apneic episode.

     c. **Mixed apnea** is a combination of the obstructive and central types.

B. Sleep apnea syndrome is **common,** affecting approximately 2% and 4% of middle-aged women and men, respectively.

II CLINICAL MANIFESTATIONS OF SLEEP APNEA SYNDROME

A. **Symptoms** may include the following:

   1. **Snoring**

   2. **Daytime hypersomnolence,** which may lead to accidents, poor work performance, depression, or personality changes

   3. **Morning headache**

   4. **Impotence**

   5. **Nocturia** and sometimes **enuresis**

   6. **Pedal edema** or **exercise fatigue** (as a result of right-sided heart failure caused by pulmonary hypertension)

HOT

KEY

Often, a history of snoring is noted only if you ask the patient's spouse.

B. Signs. Physical examination may reveal the following:
   1. **Systemic hypertension**
   2. **Characteristic body habitus** (i.e., obese; large neck; red, florid complexion)
   3. **Evidence of right-sided heart failure** (e.g., **elevated jugular venous pressure, ascites, hepatosplenomegaly),** if pulmonary hypertension has occurred
C. Laboratory abnormalities
   1. A **complete blood count (CBC)** may reveal **polycythemia.**
   2. Waking **arterial blood gases (ABGs)** are **usually normal,** although in some obese patients with sleep apnea syndrome, **hypoxemia** will be apparent. These patients are often considered to have **obesity-hypoventilation (Pickwickian) syndrome.**
   3. The **electrocardiogram (EKG)** may reveal evidence of systemic or pulmonary **hypertension.**

III **DIFFERENTIAL DIAGNOSIS.** Sleep apnea syndrome should be distinguished from:

A. Narcolepsy, which is characterized by sudden sleep attacks during any type of activity, cataplexy, sleep paralysis, and auditory or visual hallucinations either preceding or occurring during the sleep attacks
B. Kleine-Levin syndrome, which is usually seen in young men and consists of sleep attacks a few times a year, with hypersexuality, hyperphagia, and confusion on awakening

IV **APPROACH TO THE PATIENT**

A. Exclude hypothyroidism and **acromegaly** as causes of the apnea. Thyroid-stimulating hormone (TSH) levels should be obtained for all patients to exclude hypothyroidism.
B. Consider sleep studies.
   1. **Indications.** Sleep studies are appropriate for chronic snorers with daytime somnolence and those with observed periods of apnea (even if daytime sleepiness is not a complaint).
   2. **Types.** Sleep studies are generally of two types.
      a. **Nocturnal polysomnography,** the gold standard test, is performed in a specialized sleep center.
      b. **Portable nocturnal oximetry** is less expensive and easier to perform than nocturnal polysomnography, and is useful for ruling out significant sleep apnea.

V TREATMENT

A. **Behavioral modifications** include:
1. **Weight loss**
2. **Avoidance of alcohol** and **sedatives**
3. **Establishment of regular sleeping hours** (in order to avoid sleep deprivation)
4. **Adoption of the lateral position for sleep**

B. **Medical management**
1. **Continuous positive airway pressure (CPAP)** should be guided by polysomnography.
2. **Oral devices** (e.g., tongue-retaining devices, mandible-forward devices) should be considered for those with mild sleep apnea who do not tolerate CPAP.
3. **Protriptyline** (10–20 mg orally each night) may benefit some patients.

C. **Surgical intervention** should only be considered in consultation with a sleep apnea expert. Procedures include:
1. **Uvulopalatopharyngoplasty**
2. **Genioglossal** or **maxillomandibular advancement**
3. **Tracheostomy** (the definitive therapy for obstructive sleep apnea)

VI FOLLOW-UP AND REFERRAL

A. **Follow-up.** Initially, patients should be seen frequently (e.g., every 2–4 weeks) in order to monitor adherence with treatment.

B. **Referral**
1. Consultation with a **nutritionist** may be required to help the patient lose weight.
2. The patient should be referred to a **sleep center** or **pulmonologist specializing in sleep apnea** if the diagnosis remains unclear or formal polysomnography or surgery is being considered.

References

Indications and standards for use of nasal continuous positive airway pressure (CPAP) in sleep apnea syndrome. American Thoracic Society. *Am J Respir Crit Care Med* 150(6 pt 1):1738–1745, 1994.

Strollo PJ, Rogers RM: Current concepts: obstructive sleep apnea. *New Engl J Med* 334(2), 99–104, 1996.

V

Gastroenterology

32. Abdominal Pain

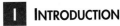 INTRODUCTION

A. The following factors complicate evaluation of abdominal pain:
1. Multiple potential diagnoses
2. Nonspecific signs and symptoms
3. Limited usefulness of radiographic studies
B. Life-threatening conditions can easily "hide" in the abdomen, initially causing few, if any, symptoms. The consequences of wrongly attributing the pain to a benign condition (e.g., gastritis) can be catastrophic.

HOT

Patients older than 65 years with acute abdominal pain frequently have an illness requiring surgery.

KEY

II CAUSES OF ABDOMINAL PAIN

A. **Pain of abdominal origin.** A broad differential diagnosis can be formed by remembering that **infection, obstruction,** or **ischemia** can cause pain in any intra-abdominal organ.
B. **Referred pain.** Disorders of the **thoracic region** (e.g., myocardial ischemia or infarction, pneumonia) and **pelvic region** [e.g., testicular torsion, pelvic inflammatory disease (PID)] can present with abdominal pain.
C. **Systemic and metabolic causes of abdominal pain** can be remembered with the following mnemonic:

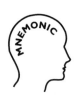

Systemic and Metabolic Causes of Abdominal Pain ("Puking My Very BAD LUNCH")

Porphyria
Mediterranean fever
Vasculitis
Black widow spider bite
Addison's disease or **A**ngioedema
Diabetic ketoacidosis

Lead poisoning
Uremia
Neurogenic (impingement on spinal nerves or roots, diabetes, syphilis)
Calcium (hypercalcemia)
Herpes zoster

III APPROACH TO THE PATIENT

A. **Patient history**

1. **Past medical history.** Knowledge of epidemiologic factors and the patient's past medical history can help narrow the differential diagnosis. For example, a history of intravenous drug abuse may suggest hepatitis; alcohol abuse may suggest pancreatitis or alcoholic hepatitis; and hypertension may suggest myocardial ischemia or abdominal aneurysm.

2. **Time course**

   a. Discern whether the pain is **acute** or **chronic.** Chronic pain is more likely than acute pain to have a benign cause (e.g., irritable bowel syndrome).

   b. The **progression of certain symptom complexes** can also provide important clues. For instance, appendicitis begins with pain (usually periumbilical) that almost always precedes nausea and vomiting; the pain may later move to the right lower quadrant.

3. **Symptoms**

   a. **Pain.** An effort should be made to characterize the pain:

   (1) Quality. Judgements regarding the quality of the pain are often not helpful in narrowing the differential diagnosis.

     (2) Location. Defining the location of the pain may help determine the likely cause (Table 32-1).

TABLE 32-1. Differential Diagnoses for Abdominal Pain as Suggested by Location

Location of Pain	Associated Organs	Common Diseases
Right upper quadrant	Liver, gallbladder	Hepatitis, hepatic tumors or abscesses, cholecystitis, choledocholithiasis, ascending cholangitis, AIDS cholangiopathy
Epigastric region	Stomach, pancreas, duodenum, abdominal aorta	Gastritis, peptic ulcer disease, pancreatitis, abdominal aortic aneurysm, biliary disease, cardiac disease
Left upper quadrant	Spleen	Splenic enlargement, infarct, or abscess
Left or right lower quadrant	Appendix, intestines, ovary, fallopian tubes, testes, kidney, ureters	Appendicitis*, right- or left-sided diverticulitis, ovarian cyst or torsion, ectopic pregnancy, pelvic inflammatory disease, epidydimitis, testicular torsion, nephrolithiasis, pyelonephritis
Periumbilical region	Small intestine, appendix, abdominal aorta	Small bowel obstruction, gastroenteritis, appendicitis, abdominal aortic aneurysm, ischemic bowel†
Suprapubic region	Bladder, uterus, ovaries, fallopian tubes	Urinary tract infection, pelvic inflammatory disease, endometriosis, ovarian cyst, ectopic pregnancy

*Although the pain of appendicitis eventually localizes to the right lower quadrant, it usually begins in the periumbilical region.
†The location of pain from ischemic bowel is variable.

      b. Other symptoms. Always question the patient about cardiac, pulmonary, and pelvic symptoms, as well as associated gastrointestinal symptoms (Table 32-2).

B. Physical examination

    1. Auscultation is usually not helpful because the presence or absence of bowel sounds usually does not narrow the differential diagnosis. For example, bowel sounds are still present in most cases of peritonitis.

    2. Palpation. Always start away from the area of the patient's complaint and move gently toward it.

    3. Rectal and pelvic examinations should always be performed. Pain during rectal or pelvic examination may indicate pelvic pathology, or a disorder involving a lower intra-abdominal structure (e.g., a retrocolic appendix).

C. Laboratory and imaging studies

    1. Basic tests. These tests can help to narrow the differential diagnosis.

        a. Complete blood count (CBC). Look for leukocytosis or anemia. These findings may indicate a serious disorder.

        b. Renal panel. Electrolyte disturbances can be the cause or a result of the illness. Elevated blood urea nitrogen (BUN) and creatinine levels may suggest volume depletion or renal pathology.

        c. Liver function tests screen for liver or biliary pathology.

        d. Amylase level. The addition of a lipase level may increase the sensitivity and specificity of this test for pancreatitis.

TABLE 32-2. Symptoms and Associated Organ Systems

Symptom	Likely Site of Pathology
Dysuria, frequency	Kidney, bladder
Nausea, vomiting, diarrhea	Gastrointestinal tract
Jaundice, pruritus	Liver, gallbladder
Pain that decreases on sitting up	Pancreas
Abrupt onset of midline pain that is out of proportion to the exam	Mesenteric vessels

     e. **Urinalysis** is helpful to rule out diabetic ketoacidosis and renal pathology.

     f. **Urine pregnancy test.** Any woman of childbearing age should have a urine pregnancy test, regardless of how probable pregnancy seems to her.

2. **Ancillary tests** should be ordered on the basis of your initial diagnostic impressions.

     a. A **serum calcium level** can rule out hypercalcemia.

     b. **Serum albumin level.** A low value may increase suspicion for an intra-abdominal malignancy.

     c. A **fecal white blood cell (WBC) count** may be ordered to screen for bowel inflammation in a patient with diarrhea.

     d. **Abdominal radiographs** are useful to evaluate bowel obstruction and kidney stones.

       (1) Layering air-fluid levels are seen in small bowel obstruction.

       (2) Abdominal radiographs have a sensitivity of approximately 50% for detecting kidney stones.

     e. **Thoracic radiographs**

       (1) **Posterior-anterior (PA)** and **lateral views** are indicated for patients with upper abdominal pain (to rule out a lower lobe pneumonia) and when there is suspicion of peritonitis (to rule out free air). Lateral views may demonstrate free air that is not visible on a PA film.

HOT KEY The patient must be maintained upright for at least 5 minutes prior to taking the film to increase the test's sensitivity for detecting air beneath the diaphragm. Left lateral decubitus views can be used to evaluate possible free air in a patient who cannot be maintained upright (e.g., as a result of pain or hypotension).

     f. **Abdominal ultrasound** is often the best study when gallbladder, biliary, or renal disease is suspected.

     g. **Abdominal computed tomography (CT)** is better than ultrasound for evaluating most intra-abdominal structures, except for the biliary tree and perhaps the kidney. **Triple-contrast studies** (i.e., intravenous, oral, and rectal) are usually performed and yield much finer detail. For patients with elevated creatinine, intravenous contrast can sometimes be avoided if the bowel is of primary concern; however, abscesses will often be missed unless intravenous contrast is used.

   h. Paracentesis. If the patient has ascites, you should always do a tap to rule out peritonitis.
   i. Electrocardiogram (EKG). Every patient with abdominal pain (especially upper abdominal pain) and a history of, or risk factors for, cardiac disease should have an EKG to rule out myocardial ischemia.

IV TREATMENT depends on the cause of the abdominal pain. When the cause of the pain is not apparent but the patient appears ill (e.g., fever, diaphoresis, resting tachycardia, abdominal tenderness), observation in the hospital is usually necessary. In these situations, there is no substitute for frequent follow-up examinations and the tincture of time.

V FOLLOW-UP AND REFERRAL

   A. When appendicitis, cholecystitis, peritonitis, or another disorder requiring surgical observation or intervention is suspected, a **surgeon** should be consulted. Early consultation often avoids long delays in diagnosis and unnecessary tests.
   B. Consultation with a **gastroenterologist** may be necessary when a diagnosis cannot be determined, even after performing an extensive and thorough work-up.

References
DeDombal FT: Acute abdominal pain in the elderly. *J Clin Gastroentreol* 19(4):331–335, 1994.
Sanson TG, O'Keefe KP: Evaluation of abdominal pain in the elderly. *Emerg Med Clin North Am* 14(3):615–627, 1996.

33. Diarrhea

I INTRODUCTION

A. Diarrhea is a common presenting complaint in the out-patient setting. It is estimated that the average adult in the United States experiences one to two acute diarrheal illnesses per year.

B. Diarrhea is defined as the passage of **more than 200 grams of stool per 24-hour period.** A more practical definition uses the subjective complaints of **increased frequency** and **increased fluidity** of bowel movements.

C. In order to evaluate and manage a patient with diarrhea, it is critical to determine whether the diarrhea is acute or chronic.

    1. Acute diarrhea is present for less than 3 weeks.

    2. Chronic diarrhea is present for more than 3 weeks.

II CAUSES OF ACUTE DIARRHEA

A. Acute diarrhea can be **inflammatory** (i.e., characterized by the presence of blood or leukocytes in the stool) or **noninflammatory.** Causes are listed in Table 33-1.

B. Chronic diarrhea. There are several major types of chronic diarrhea, which can be remembered using the mnemonic, "SOME MD FUNCTION."

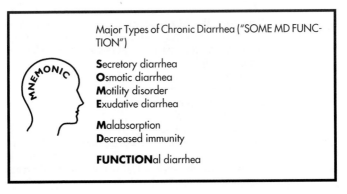

Major Types of Chronic Diarrhea ("SOME MD FUNCTION")

Secretory diarrhea
Osmotic diarrhea
Motility disorder
Exudative diarrhea

Malabsorption
Decreased immunity

FUNCTIONal diarrhea

TABLE 33-1. Causes of Acute Diarrhea

Inflammatory	Noninflammatory
Infection	**Infection**
Campylobacter jejuni	Rotavirus
Shigella species	Norwalk agent
Salmonella species	*Giardia lamblia*
Clostridium difficile	*Cryptosporidium parvum*
Escherichia coli	*Microsporidia* species
Entamoeba histolytica	*Yersinia enterocolitica*
Yersinia enterocolitica	*Vibrio* species
Other	**Food poisoning**
Ischemic colitis	*Staphylococcus aureus*
Radiation enteritis	*Bacillus cereus*
Inflammatory bowel	*Clostriduim botulinum*
disease	*Clostridium perfringens*
	Drugs
	Alcohol
	Magnesium-containing
	antacids
	Laxatives
	Theophylline
	Colchicine
	Antibiotics
	Lactulose
	Other
	Fecal impaction

1. **Secretory diarrhea** occurs following active intestinal secretion of electrolytes and water into the bowel lumen. Secretory diarrhea persists despite fasting. Causes include:
    a. **Thyrotoxicosis**
    b. **Carcinoid syndrome**
    c. **Colon cancer**
    d. **Colonic polyps**
    e. **Drugs** (see Table 33-1)
2. **Osmotic diarrhea** occurs when poorly absorbed materials retain fluid in the gut. The stool osmolality exceeds that of the serum. Causes of osmotic diarrhea include:

    a. Lactase deficiency (i.e., **lactose intolerance**)
    b. Fructose intolerance
    c. Laxatives
    d. Celiac disease
    e. Drugs (see Table 33-1)
    f. Pancreatic insufficiency

3. **Exudative diarrhea** is characterized by the release of protein, blood, and mucus from an inflamed gut wall. The **stools typically contain leukocytes and blood.** Causes of exudative diarrhea include:
    a. Ulcerative colitis
    b. Crohn's disease
    c. Lymphoma
    d. Ischemic colitis
    e. Whipple's disease
    f. Collagenous colitis

4. **Motility disorders** may cause diarrhea or constipation; often, the patient complains of both. Pain may be a prominent feature. Motility problems can be associated with:
    a. Irritable bowel syndrome
    b. Diabetes mellitus
    c. Narcotic use
    d. Systemic sclerosis
    e. Fecal impaction
    f. Surgery (i.e., postgastrectomy syndrome, postvagotomy syndrome)

5. **Malabsorption** occurs in the small bowel and results in large-volume diarrhea that may be associated with evidence of malnutrition or vitamin deficiencies. Causes of malabsorption include:
    a. Short bowel syndrome
    b. Ileal resection
    c. Enteric fistula
    d. Radiation enteritis
    e. Bacterial overgrowth

6. **Decreased immunity.** Some patients with immunodeficiencies, HIV-positive patients in particular, are susceptible to organisms that generally do not cause disease in immunocompetent hosts. Consider the following organisms in an immunocompromised patient with chronic diarrhea:
    a. *Cryptosporidium parvum*
    b. *Microsporidia species*
    c. *Isospora belli*
    d. *Giardia lamblia*

      e. *Strongyloides stercoralis*
      f. *Entamoeba histolytica*
      g. *Mycobacterium avium-intracellulare* **complex**
      h. *Clostridium difficile*
      i. **Cytomegalovirus (CMV)**
7. **Functional diarrhea** has no organic cause and accounts for approximately 50% of cases of chronic diarrhea referred to gastroenterologists. Irritable bowel syndrome is sometimes placed in this category. Often, diarrhea is present for months or years before the patient seeks medical attention.

HOT

KEY

The causes of acute and chronic diarrhea overlap to some degree. In general, infections (including food poisoning) are more commonly a cause of acute diarrhea, whereas medications, systemic disorders, and noninfectious gastrointestinal disorders are more commonly causes of chronic diarrhea.

▐ Approach to the Patient

HOT

KEY

Because there is substantial variability among individuals, it is important to establish the patient's normal bowel pattern as a baseline for evaluation.

  A. **Patient history.** Answers to the following questions should be sought:
     1. Has the diarrhea been **present for less than 3 weeks?**
     2. Is the stool **bloody?**
     3. Is the **volume** large or small?
     4. Has the patient experienced **fever** or **weight loss?**
     5. Is the diarrhea **nocturnal?**
     6. Does the diarrhea **persist despite fasting?**
     7. What is the patient's **medication history?**
     8. Is the diarrhea **associated with a certain food?**
     9. Does the patient have **diabetes mellitus?**
    10. What is the patient's **travel history?**
    11. What are the patient's **HIV risk factors?**
    12. Does the patient have any **extraintestinal symptoms?**

B. Physical examination

1. **Volume status.** Orthostatic hypotension and resting tachycardia indicate volume depletion.

2. **Abdominal examination.** Check for masses or focal tenderness.

3. **Rectal examination.** Evaluate for sphincter tone, masses, fecal impaction, anal pain or fissures, and blood in the stool.

4. **General examination.** Extraintestinal manifestations may provide clues to the underlying cause:

   a. Spondyloarthritis and pyoderma gangrenosum—inflammatory bowel disease

   b. Systemic atherosclerosis—ischemic bowel

   c. Lower extremity edema—malabsorption and protein loss

   d. Dermatitis herpetiformis—celiac disease

C. Laboratory studies are ordered according to the duration of the diarrhea and the patient's clinical manifestations.

HOT   **KEY**

If the patient's history suggests that lactase deficiency or a medication is the cause of the diarrhea, a trial with a lactose-exclusion diet or medication withdrawal is reasonable prior to launching into laboratory work-up.

---

1. **Acute diarrhea**

   a. **Acute diarrhea lasting less than 3 days.** No laboratory work-up is usually necessary unless gross blood is present in the stool or the patient appears systemically ill.

   b. **Acute diarrhea lasting more than 3 days,** or **gross blood in the stool**

      (1) A stool sample should be collected for **methylene blue staining** and **stool guaiac testing** to screen for fecal leukocytes and occult blood, respectively.

      (2) A second stool sample should be sent for **bacterial culture,** to look for *Campylobacter, Shigella, Salmonella, Escherichia coli,* and *Yersinia* species. Depending on the patient's history, it may be appropriate to send a stool sample for *C. difficile* **toxin assay, stool ova and parasites (O&P),** or *Giardia* **antigen assay.**

HOT

KEY

C. difficile is a common and often unrecognized cause of diarrhea; therefore, have a low threshold for sending a *C. difficile* toxin assay.

        (3) If the patient has bloody diarrhea, fever, or volume depletion, a **complete blood count (CBC) and differential, serum electrolyte panel,** and **blood urea nitrogen (BUN) and creatinine level** should be ordered.

  2. **Chronic diarrhea**

    a. **General screening tests.** Initially, a stool sample should be submitted for the following tests:

      (1) **Methylene blue staining** (to evaluate for leukocytes)

      (2) **Stool guaiac** (to evaluate for occult blood)

      (3) **Sudan staining** (to evaluate for fat)

      (4) *C. difficile* **toxin assay**

      (5) *Giardia* **antigen assay**

      (6) **Stool O&P**

    b. **Specific tests** may be appropriate depending on the patient's history and physical examination findings:

      (1) If **laxative abuse** is suspected, test the stool for **phenolphthalein.**

      (2) If **immunodeficiency** is the suspected cause of the diarrhea, the laboratory evaluation should include tests to identify the most likely causative organisms.

      (3) If **malabsorption** is suspected, a **quantitative fecal fat collection** should be performed. A **D-xylose test** or **small bowel biopsy** may be necessary to make a definitive diagnosis.

    c. **Blood studies** should include a **CBC and differential;** a **serum electrolyte panel;** and **BUN, creatinine, albumin,** and **thyroid-stimulating hormone (TSH) levels.**

IV TREATMENT

  A. Most patients in the outpatient setting can be treated with **diet** or **medication adjustments, oral rehydration,** and **antidiarrheal agents** (Table 33-2).

TABLE 33-2. Antidiarrheal Agents

Generic Name	Brand Name	Dosage
Loperamide	Imodium	2 tablets orally initially, followed by 1 tablet after each loose stool (to a maximum of 8 tablets per day)
Diphenoxylate	Lomotil	2 tablets orally 4 times daily
Bismuth subsalicylate	Pepto-Bismol	2 tablets or 30 ml initially; repeat every 30–60 minutes as needed
Kaolin	Kaopectate	30 ml or 1.5–2 tablets (1200–1500 mg) orally after each loose stool
Tincture of opium	. . .	15–30 ml orally after each loose stool, up to 4 times daily

HOT
KEY

Antidiarrheal agents are usually safe to use in patients with mild to moderate diarrhea. However, they should not be used in those with bloody diarrhea or severe systemic illness. If the patient's symptoms worsen despite therapy, use of antidiarrheal agents should be discontinued.

B. Antibiotic therapy
 1. **Empiric therapy.** Patients who are systemically ill or who have blood or pus in their stool may require empiric antibiotic therapy. Typically, **trimethoprim-sulfamethoxazole** or **ciprofloxacin** is used (ciprofloxacin is preferred where *Campylobacter jejuni* infection is common). For patients with an increased risk of *C. difficile* infection (e.g., those who have recently had antibiotic therapy) or parasitic infection (e.g., travelers to endemic regions), **metronidazole** is frequently added to the regimen.
 2. **Specific therapy.** Once a specific pathogen is identified, one of the regimens described in Table 33-3 can be used.

HOT
KEY

Antibiotic therapy may not shorten symptom duration when the causative agent is *Campylobacter*, nontyphoidal *Salmonella*, *Yersinia*, or *E. coli*.

V FOLLOW-UP AND REFERRAL
 A. Referral to a gastroenterologist for evaulation and possible endoscopy is appropriate when:
  1. A thorough evaluation has been performed and the cause of the diarrhea still cannot be identified
  2. Neoplasia or malabsorption is the suspected cause
  3. Toxic megacolon or ischemic bowel is the suspected cause
 B. Patients with inflammatory bowel disease may benefit from referral to a gastroenterologist for ongoing management.

TABLE 33-3. Selected Antibiotic Regimens for the Specific Treatment of Infectious Diarrhea

Pathogen	Antimicrobial Agent	Dosage	Duration
Shigella species	Trimethoprim–sulfamethoxazole	160 mg/800 mg orally twice daily	5 days
	Ciprofloxacin	500 mg orally twice daily	3–5 days
Salmonella typhi	Trimethoprim–sulfamethoxazole	160 mg/800 mg orally twice daily	5 days
	Ciprofloxacin	500 mg orally twice daily	3–5 days
Campylobacter jejuni	Ciprofloxacin	500 mg orally twice daily	5 days
	Azithromycin	500 mg orally once daily	3 days
Clostridium difficile	Metronidazole	250 mg orally three times daily	7–14 days
	Vancomycin	125 mg orally four times daily	7–14 days
Entamoeba histolytica	Metronidazole	750 mg orally three times daily	10 days, followed by
	Iodoquinol	650 mg orally three times daily	20 days
Giardia lamblia	Metronidazole	250 mg orally three times daily	5 days
	Tinidazole	2 g orally	Single dose
Yersinia enterocolitica	Ciprofloxacin	500 mg orally twice daily	3–5 days
	Norfloxacin	400 mg orally twice daily	3–5 days
Vibrio cholerae	Ciprofloxacin	1000 mg orally	Single dose
	Norfloxacin	400 mg orally twice daily	3 days
	Doxycycline	300 mg orally	Single dose

References

Donowitz M, Kokke FT, Saidi R: Evaluation of patients with chronic diarrhea. *N Engl J Med* 332(11):725–729, 1995.

Talal AH, Murray JA: Acute and chronic diarrhea: how to keep laboratory testing to a minimum. *Postgrad Med* 96(3):30–46, 1994.

Wilcox CM, Schwartz DA, Cotsonis G, et al: Chronic unexplained diarrhea in human immunodeficiency virus infection: determination of the best diagnostic approach. *Gastroenterology* 110(1):30–37, 1996.

34. Constipation

I INTRODUCTION

A. Constipation is the most common gastrointestinal complaint in the United States. Approximately 30% of people older than 60 years use laxatives routinely.

B. Constipation is diagnosed when a patient reports fewer than three bowel movements per week or the presence of severe straining with defecation.

II CAUSES OF CONSTIPATION.
The causes of constipation can be easily remembered with the mnemonic, "DUODENUM." In most patients, a definitive cause cannot be determined.

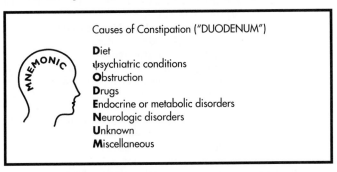

Causes of Constipation ("DUODENUM")

Diet
ψsychiatric conditions
Obstruction
Drugs
Endocrine or metabolic disorders
Neurologic disorders
Unknown
Miscellaneous

A. **Diet.** Constipation can be related to a **low-fiber diet** or **low water intake.**

B. **Psychiatric conditions,** such as **depression, somatization disorders,** and **obsessive-compulsive disorders,** may be associated with constipation.

C. **Obstruction**
1. **Neoplasia.** Colon cancer must always be considered in an adult patient with changes in bowel habits. In addition, other types of malignant masses in the abdomen can compress the sigmoid colon or rectum, leading to constipation.
2. **Strictures** may result from diverticuli, ischemic bowel, or radiation therapy.
3. **Surgical adhesions** or **rectoceles** can also cause mechanical obstruction.

D. **Drugs** that can cause constipation include opiates, tricyclic antidepressants, neuroleptics, antihistamines, calcium channel blockers, iron supplements, and antacids.

E. Endocrine and metabolic disorders that can be associated with constipation include diabetes mellitus, hypothyroidism, hypercalcemia, hypokalemia, hypomagnesemia, and uremia.

F. Neurologic disorders associated with constipation include spinal cord compression, Parkinson's disease, multiple sclerosis, and cerebrovascular disease.

G. Miscellaneous causes of constipation include irritable bowel syndrome, amyloidosis, scleroderma, and immobility.

III APPROACH TO THE PATIENT

A. Exclude colon cancer in adults.

   1. Patient history. Be sure to assess the patient's **risk factors** for colon cancer.

      a. Have the patient's **bowel habits changed** recently after a long period of "normality"?

      b. Has the patient **lost weight?**

      c. Has the patient observed **blood** in the stools, or stools that have **changed in shape or form?**

      d. Does the patient have a **family history** of colon cancer?

   2. Physical examination. Perform abdominal and rectal examinations to detect possible masses.

   3. Colonoscopy should be considered for adult patients with new-onset constipation.

B. Evaluate the patient for other causes of constipation.

   1. Patient history

      a. Does the patient have any **symptoms suggestive of hypothyroidism, diabetes,** or **uremia?**

      b. Does the patient have a history of any **rectoanal pathology,** such as strictures or fissures?

      c. Has the patient ever had **abdominal surgery?**

      d. What **medications,** including laxatives and over-the-counter drugs, is the patient currently taking?

      e. What is the patient's **dietary** and **exercise history?**

   2. Laboratory studies. Depending on the patient's history, it may be appropriate to order certain laboratory studies, such as:

      a. Thyroid-stimulating hormone (TSH) level

      b. Glucose level

    c. Serum electrolyte panel, including calcium and magnesium levels

    d. Blood urea nitrogen (BUN) and creatinine levels

  3. Imaging studies. Abdominal plain films (flat and upright) should be obtained in patients with abdominal pain or distention.

IV TREATMENT takes a step-wise approach.

A. Perform fecal disimpaction in patients with impacted stool in the rectal vault.

B. Discontinue constipation-causing medications, if possible.

C. Recommend lifestyle changes. The patient should be advised to **increase exercise, water intake** (to at least 1.5–2 liters daily), and **fiber intake** (preferably to at least 10–20 grams daily). Sources of fiber include:

  1. Wheat bran or **high-bran cereals**

  2. Psyllium (Metamucil), 2–3 tablespoons per day, mixed with water

  3. Methylcellulose (Citrucel) or **calcium polycarbophil (Fibercon),** which are often associated with less intestinal gas, but are significantly more expensive than psyllium

D. Consider laxatives if the patient continues to experience constipation despite implementing dietary changes and increasing the amount of exercise.

HOT

Side effects of prolonged laxative therapy include laxative-dependent stooling, incontinence, and abdominal cramping.

KEY

---

  1. Oral laxatives (in order of increasing potency)

    a. Docusate sodium (Colace), 100 mg once or twice daily

    b. Milk of magnesia, 15–30 ml twice daily

    c. Sorbitol, 15–30 ml once or twice daily

    d. Lactulose, 15–60 ml daily

    e. Magnesium citrate, 15–30 ml daily

  2. Rectal suppositories [e.g., **bisacodyl (Dulcolax),** 1 suppository 3 times per week] can be used as an alternative or an adjunct to oral laxatives.

3. **Enemas**
    a. **Tap water enema,** 500 ml daily
    b. **Mineral oil enema,** 100–250 ml daily

HOT

KEY

If the patient has been constipated for more than 5–7 days, it is preferable to initiate therapy with an enema because oral laxatives may be ineffective and result in worsening abdominal distention.

V FOLLOW-UP AND REFERRAL

A. **Follow-up.** Patients with constipation often must implement significant lifestyle changes in order to achieve lasting relief. The importance of careful patient education and continual reinforcement cannot be overemphasized.

B. **Referral.** The primary indication for referral to a gastroenterologist is to rule out colon cancer. Those with chronic constipation unresponsive to conservative measures may also benefit from consultation.

References

Camilleri M, Thompson WG, Fleshman JW, et al: Clinical management of intractable constipation. *Ann Intern Med* 121(7):520–528, 1994.

Romero Y, Evans JM, Fleming KC, et al: Constipation and fecal incontinence in the elderly population. *Mayo Clin Proc* 71 (1):81–92, 1996.

35. Heartburn and Gastroesophageal Reflux Disease

I. INTRODUCTION

A. **Heartburn** (i.e., a retrosternal burning sensation), believed to be caused by the abnormal reflux of acid from the stomach into the esophagus, **is a symptom of** the process known as **gastroesophageal reflux disease (GERD).** GERD has three underlying mechanisms:
   1. Recurrent, abnormal relaxation of the lower esophageal sphincter, which allows reflux of gastric acid into the esophagus
   2. Impaired clearance of the acid from the esophagus (inadequate peristalsis and swallowing of saliva)
   3. Susceptibility of the esophageal mucosa to the acid

B. Heartburn is experienced daily by approximately 5%–10% of American adults, and at least once a month by approximately 40% of the adult population.

II. COMPLICATIONS OF GASTROESOPHAGEAL REFLUX DISEASE

A. **Esophageal complications**
   1. **Esophagitis** results from prolonged exposure of the esophageal mucosa to gastric acid. The severity of the pain does not correlate well with the severity of the esophagitis.
   2. **Esophageal ulcer** (i.e., erosion of the mucosa) can result from persistent esophagitis. Patients usually have more severe pain than that experienced with esophagitis and may present with bleeding or anemia.
   3. **Esophageal stricture,** which may result from chronic inflammation or ulceration, causes luminal narrowing and often presents as dysphagia or odynophagia.
   4. **Barrett's syndrome** results when columnar epithelium replaces the normal squamous epithelium in the distal esophagus after prolonged exposure to gastric acid. Barrett's syndrome is a strong risk factor for esophageal adenocarcinoma.

B. **Extraesophageal complications**
   1. **Asthma.** Symptoms of asthma may be worsened or even caused by GERD. Bronchoconstriction is

thought to be caused by either aspiration of small amounts of gastric acid or stimulation of a vagal reflex arc by esophageal acid.

2. **Otolarnygologic complications.** Persistent acid reflux can irritate any structure in the pharynx or larynx, possibly leading to chronic cough, hoarseness, laryngitis, difficulty clearing the throat, and dental decay.

III APPROACH TO THE PATIENT

HOT

KEY

All patients with retrosternal pain should be evaluated for other causes of chest pain, especially those with risk factors for coronary artery disease (CAD; see Chapter 17).

A. **Patient history**
   1. Patients with GERD typically complain of **heartburn** (which is relieved by antacids and exacerbated by eating, lying down, or bending over) and a **feeling of regurgitation.** These symptoms are fairly (approximately 90%) specific for GERD.
   2. Patients may present with symptoms resulting from complications of GERD, including **esophageal pain** or **bleeding, dysphagia** or **odynophagia, worsening asthma, chronic coughing, hoarseness, laryngitis, difficulty clearing the throat,** and **dental decay.**

HOT

KEY

A history of exercise-induced symptoms, or of new symptoms in a patient with risk factors for heart disease, should prompt an evaluation for CAD.

B. **Physical examination** should focus on identifying **signs of conditions that can exacerbate GERD** (e.g., Raynaud's disease as a sign of scleroderma; palmar erythema or spider angioma as a sign of chronic alcohol use). Use the mnemonic "ACIDS" to remember the conditions that can exacerbate GERD:

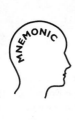

Conditions That Can Exacerbate GERD ("ACIDS")

Acid hypersecretion (e.g., Zollinger-Ellison disease) or **A**lcohol abuse
Connective tissue disease (e.g., scleroderma)
Infections of the esophagus (e.g., cytomegalovirus, herpes, candidiasis)
Diabetic gastroparesis or **D**rug therapy (e.g., calcium channel blockers, β agonists, α blockers, theophylline, narcotics, progestins)
Smoking

C. **Other studies**
1. **Endoscopy.** Patients with a history suggestive of complications (e.g., dysphagia, odynophagia, early satiety, weight loss, anemia, asthma exacerbations, oropharyngeal pathology) should be referred to a gastroenterologist promptly for endoscopy.
2. **Esophageal biopsy** may be indicated, depending on the endoscopy findings. Patients with **esophageal ulcer** or **stricture** should have esophageal biopsies to rule out dysplastic changes and adenocarcinoma.

IV TREATMENT

A. **Mild GERD** is treated with diet and lifestyle changes. Antacids or over-the-counter histamine-2 (H_2) antagonists can be used on an as-needed basis.
1. **Diet.** Patients should be advised to avoid coffee, alcohol, chocolate, high-fat meals, and acidic or spicy foods. In addition, they should eat smaller, more frequent meals and avoid lying supine within 3 hours after eating.
2. **Lifestyle changes.** Weight loss and smoking cessation are indicated for obese patients and those who smoke, respectively. Tight-fitting garments should be avoided. Elevating the head of the bed may help alleviate symptoms at night.
3. **Antisecretory therapy** (Table 35-1). If the patient's symptoms do not improve with conservative methods, an 8- to 12-week trial with an H_2 **antagonist** is indicated. Some physicians may prefer to start with a **proton-pump inhibitor.** Failure of pharmacologic therapy should prompt referral to a gastroenterologist.
B. **Moderate to severe GERD.** Some physicians attempt an

TABLE 35-1. Pharmacologic Therapy for Gastrointestinal Reflux Disease (GERD)

Generic Name	Brand Name	Dose Range
Histamine-2 (H$_2$) antagonists*		
Cimetidine	Tagamet	400–800 mg twice daily
Ranitidine	Zantac	150–300 mg twice daily
Nizatidine	Axid	150–300 mg twice daily
Famotidine	Pepcid	20–40 mg twice daily
Proton-pump inhibitors†		
Omeprazole	Prilosec	20–40 mg daily
Lansoprazole	Prevacid	15–30 mg daily
Prokinetic agents‡		
Cisapride	Propulsid	10 mg four times daily (before meals and at bedtime)

*H$_2$ antagonists are reasonable first choices for patients with mild symptoms. No agent has proven superiority. For patients with more severe symptoms, use higher doses.
†Proton-pump inhibitors are more effective than H$_2$ antagonists for treatment of esophagitis and prevention of relapse.
‡Prokinetic agents increase lower esophageal sphincter tone and speed gastric emptying. May be a useful adjunct in patients with refractory symptoms.

8-to 12-week trial with a **proton-pump inhibitor** followed by withdrawal of the medication and reassessment. Consultation with a gastroenterologist for early endoscopy is also an appropriate option.

C. Complications of GERD

    1. Esophagitis

        a. Antisecretory therapy. An 8- to 12-week course of therapy with a **proton-pump inhibitor** is the treatment of choice. Many patients experience a relapse after initial therapy; therefore, long-term proton-pump inhibitor therapy is usually indicated.

            (1) Although an H$_2$ antagonist may be used instead, proton-pump inhibitors are more effective for preventing relapse.

            (2) The safety of long-term treatment with

proton-pump inhibitors has not been fully established.

b. **Surgery** (e.g., laparoscopic Nissen fundoplication) may be an option for patients with symptoms refractory to medical therapy.

2. **Esophageal ulcer** is treated with a **proton-pump inhibitor** for at least 12 weeks, and then **repeat endoscopy** is performed to document ulcer healing. Long-term pharmacologic treatment is often necessary.

3. **Esophageal stricture**
    a. Most patients have dramatic improvement with **serial dilatation** of the stricture, which can be repeated periodically.
    b. Long-term **proton-pump inhibitor therapy** can help prevent recurrence of strictures.
    c. **Surgery** may be considered for patients with severe symptoms or frequent recurrence.

4. **Barrett's syndrome**
    a. Long-term **proton-pump inhibitor therapy** is usually indicated.
    b. **Surgery** is the treatment of choice when severe dysplasia is found on biopsy.

5. **Asthma.** It is difficult to know which patients with asthma will benefit from treatment of GERD.
    a. Patients with symptoms of both diseases can be given a trial of **proton-pump inhibitors.**
    b. **Surgery** may be more effective than medical therapy for relieving asthmatic symptoms in these patients.

6. **Otolaryngologic complications.** A trial of **proton-pump inhibitors** is indicated when symptoms are believed to be caused by GERD.

V FOLLOW-UP AND REFERRAL

A. **Follow-up**
    1. Patients with mild GERD should be followed monthly until symptoms are controlled. Patients with more severe symptoms require closer follow-up.
    2. All patients with documented esophageal disease should be followed in consultation with a gastroenterologist. In patients with Barrett's syndrome, periodic surveillance with endoscopic biopsies is required because the syndrome carries a significant risk for progression to esophageal cancer.

   B. Referral to a gastroenterologist is useful when GERD is
        the suspected cause of asthmatic or otolaryngological
        disease.

References
Kahrilas PJ: Gastroesophageal reflux disease. *JAMA* 276 (12):983–988, 1996.
Weinberg DS, Kadish SL: The diagnosis and management of gastroesophageal reflux
    disease. *Med Clin North Am* 80(2):411–429, 1996.

36. Dyspepsia

I INTRODUCTION

A. Dyspepsia is an imprecise term that refers to **chronic** or **recurrent epigastric** or **upper abdominal pain,** often accompanied by bloating, nausea, or postprandial fullness (i.e., "indigestion").

B. Approximately 25% of Americans complain of dyspepsia, one of the leading causes of office visits to primary care providers.

II CAUSES OF DYSPEPSIA. The differential diagnosis list for dyspepsia is long, encompassing pathology in all of the abdominal organs (Table 36-1). Fortunately, the list of common causes is short.

A. **Peptic ulcer disease** is diagnosed in **10%–20% of patients** with dyspepsia. Duodenal and gastric ulcers are approximately equal in incidence.

   1. *Helicobacter pylori* **infection** is responsible for approximately 95% of duodenal ulcers and 70% of gastric ulcers.

   2. **Nonsteroidal anti-inflammatory drug (NSAID) use** is responsible for most ulcers not caused by *H. pylori* infection.

B. **GERD.** As many as **20% of patients** with dyspepsia have GERD. Most patients with GERD have symptoms of "heartburn" or a sensation of acid reflux. However, some patients with GERD have a more vague sensation of pain without heartburn.

C. **Non-ulcer dyspepsia** is a term used to describe dyspepsia that is not associated with any abnormalities of the gastric mucosa on endoscopy. More than **50% of patients** with dyspepsia have non-ulcer dyspepsia, and the exact cause of the pain is unclear.

D. **Medication side effect.** A number of commonly prescribed medications, such as NSAIDs, theophylline, and iron, may induce dyspepsia.

III APPROACH TO THE PATIENT

A. **Patient history.** Because many of the causes of dyspepsia have similar symptoms, the history may not provide much useful diagnostic information.

Table 36-1. Selected Causes of Dyspepsia

Common Causes
  Peptic ulcer disease
  Gastroesophageal reflux disease (GERD)
  Non-ulcer dyspepsia
  Medication side effect (e.g., NSAIDs, theophylline, iron)
Less common causes
  Gastric cancer
  Gastroparesis
  Crohn's disease involving the stomach
  Biliary tract disease (e.g., cholelithiasis, hepatobiliary
    neoplasm)
  Pancreatic disease (e.g., chronic pancreatitis, pancreatic
    cancer)
  Malabsorption
  Parasitic infection (e.g., *Giardia, Strongyloides*)
  Chronic intestinal ischemia
  Systemic conditions (e.g., thyroid disease, diabetes,
    hyperparathyroidism, pregnancy, collagen vascular disease)

NSAIDs = nonsteroidal anti-inflammatory drugs.

    1. Always ask about NSAID use.
    2. In general, patients who have nocturnal pain or pain that is relieved by food or antacids are more likely to have peptic ulcer disease.
  B. Physical examination. All patients should have a thorough physical examination, including a stool guaiac test. The abdomen should be palpated for masses, organomegaly, and ascites.
  C. Laboratory studies
    1. Standard work-up. A complete blood count (CBC), serum electrolyte panel, calcium and glucose levels, and liver function tests are usually ordered for all patients with unexplained abdominal pain.
    2. *H. pylori* testing. Because *H. pylori* is responsible for most cases of peptic ulcer disease, it is reasonable to test patients with dyspepsia for *H. pylori* so that antibiotic therapy can be initiated in those who test positive. This strategy results in the treatment of many *H. pylori*-positive patients who do not actually have peptic ulcer disease because the infection results in ulcer formation in only 10%–15% of infected patients.

     a. Noninvasive testing methods include **serology** and the **urease breath test.** Both have a sensitivity and specificity of approximately 90%.

     b. For patients who undergo endoscopy, **biopsy specimens** can be tested for *H. pylori* using a **urease test, histologic stains,** or **culture.**

D. Imaging studies

    1. Upper endoscopy should be performed in patients with severe symptoms or any of the following DANGER signs:

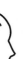

Indications for Upper Endoscopy ("DANGER")

Drop in weight
Anemia or **A**bdominal mass
New onset of pain and age > 40 years
Guaiac-positive stool
Endemic risk (patient from area with endemic gastric cancer, such as Japan)
Response to treatment inadequate

---

    2. An **upper gastrointestinal series** is less accurate than endoscopy and does not allow biopsy of suspicious lesions. This study is generally used only when patients cannot tolerate endoscopy.

    3. Abdominal ultrasound is useful if biliary or pancreatic disease is suspected.

    4. Computed tomography (CT) and **magnetic resonance imaging (MRI)** are rarely indicated; they may be useful when an intra-abdominal malignancy is suspected.

IV **TREATMENT**

HOT

Advise patients who are taking NSAIDs to discontinue the medication.

KEY

A. **Peptic ulcer disease**
  1. **Antisecretory therapy**. Patients who do not have any of the "danger" signs listed in III D can be treated initially with a 6- to 8-week trial of **histamine-2 (H$_2$) antagonists or proton-pump inhibitors** (Table 36-2). These agents block the secretion of acid by parietal cells in the stomach, neutralizing the pH and allowing for ulcer healing. Patients whose symptoms do not improve within 10 days and those whose symptoms recur after 8 weeks of therapy should be referred for endoscopy.
  2. **Anti-*H. pylori* therapy.** Patients who test positive for *H. pylori* infection should receive therapy to eradicate the organism in addition to antisecretory therapy. Two of the most effective regimens are given in Table 36–3 (both are approximately 90% effective).

HOT

KEY
Patients with a documented duodenal ulcer should receive anti-*H. pylori* therapy regardless of the results of *H. pylori* testing (due to the high prevalence of the infection in these patients).

B. **GERD**. Therapy is described in Chapter 35 IV.
C. **Non-ulcer dyspepsia**
  1. Patients may benefit from a trial of an H$_2$ antagonist or a prokinetic agent [e.g., cisapride, 10–20 mg orally four times daily (before meals and at bedtime)]. In addition, patients should be advised to avoid alcohol, tobacco, and caffeine.
  2. Treatment for *H. pylori* is not currently recommended for patients with non-ulcer dyspepsia.
D. **NSAID-induced ulcer.** Most NSAID-induced ulcers will heal with withdrawal of the NSAID and 4–8 weeks of antisecretory therapy.
  1. If the patient must continue NSAID use, **omeprazole** may be more effective than an H$_2$ antagonist to speed ulcer healing. For patients with ulcers who require long-term NSAID treatment, **misoprostol** (100–200 mg four times daily) may prevent new ulcer formation and should be considered. H$_2$ antagonists do not prevent NSAID-induced ulcers.

Table 36.2. Antisecretory Therapy for Peptic Ulcer Disease

Generic Name	Brand Name	Dose
Histamine-2 (H₂) antagonists		
Cimetidine	Tagamet	400 mg twice daily (or 800 mg at bedtime)
Ranitidine	Zantac	150 mg twice daily (or 300 mg at bedtime)
Nizatidine	Axid	150 mg twice daily (or 300 mg at bedtime)
Famotidine	Pepcid	20 mg twice daily (or 40 mg at bedtime)
Proton-pump inhibitors		
Omeprazole	Prilosec	20 mg every morning
Lansoprazole	Prevacid	30 mg every morning

Table 36-3. Selected Regimens for the Eradication of *Helicobacter pylori*

	Regimen
Option 1	**FOR 1 WEEK:** **Bismuth subsalicylate:** 2 tablets (525 mg) four times daily **Metronidazole:** 250 mg four times daily* **Tetracycline:** 500 mg four times daily **Omeprazole:** 20 mg twice daily before meals
Option 2	**FOR 1 WEEK:** **Metronidazole:** 500 mg twice daily with meals† **Clarithromycin:** 500 mg twice daily with meals **Omeprazole:** 20 mg twice daily before meals

*Amoxicillin, 500 mg four times daily, may be substituted for metronidazole.
†Amoxicillin, 1 g given twice daily, may be substituted for metronidazole.

   2. Patients with suspected NSAID-induced ulcers who are *H. pylori*-positive should be treated for the infection.

V FOLLOW-UP AND REFERRAL

A. Follow-up

   1. Patients started on a trial of H_2 antagonists should be advised to call if their symptoms have not improved within 10 days; otherwise, they should return for a follow-up visit in 6–8 weeks.
   2. In patients with a documented gastric ulcer, the possibility of gastric cancer presenting as a gastric ulcer needs to be considered. Consultation with a gastroenterologist is required, and repeat endoscopy is often performed to document healing of the ulcer.

B. Referral to a gastroenterologist is warranted if any of the danger signs are present or if the patient has severe or persistent symptoms.

References
NIH Consensus Development Panel on *Helicobacter pylori* in Peptic Ulcer Disease: *Helicobacter pylori* in peptic ulcer disease. *JAMA* 272(1):65–69, 1994.
Soll AH: Medical treatment of peptic ulcer disease. *JAMA* 275(8):622–629, 1996.

37. Involuntary Weight Loss

I **INTRODUCTION.** Weight loss is a common outpatient complaint with important prognostic significance. Weight loss of 5%–10% of the body mass index (BMI) is a predictor of increased mortality for patients older than 60 years.

$$BMI = weight(kg)/height(m^2)$$

II **CAUSES OF WEIGHT LOSS.** There are many causes of involuntary weight loss. The most common are presented here.

A. Cancer. Gastrointestinal cancers (e.g., colon, pancreatic, gastric) are the primary cause of neoplasia-associated weight loss. Lung cancer, prostate cancer, lymphoma, and myeloma are other common causes.

B. Gastrointestinal disorders. Think about the entire gastrointestinal tract, from the mouth to the anus. Loss of teeth, oral ulcers, mechanical or functional esophageal obstruction, peptic ulcer disease, pancreatic insufficiency, cholelithiasis, liver disease, and diseases of the small bowel or colon (infectious, inflammatory, ischemic, and malabsorptive) should be considered.

C. Psychiatric disorders that can be associated with weight loss include depression, dementia, anxiety, anorexia nervosa, and bipolar disorder.

D. Other causes of involuntary weight loss include:
1. **Congestive heart failure (CHF)**
2. **Chronic obstructive pulmonary disease (COPD)**
3. **Alcohol abuse** and **illicit drug use**
4. **Therapeutic drug use**
5. **Chronic infections,** such as AIDS, tuberculosis, abscess, endocarditis, and osteomyelitis
6. **Endocrine disorders,** such as hyperthyroidism, diabetes, hypercalcemia, and adrenal insufficiency
7. **Metabolic disorders,** such as uremia and cirrhosis
8. **Collagen vascular disorders,** such as systemic lupus erythematosus (SLE) and rheumatoid arthritis

III **APPROACH TO THE PATIENT**

A. Patient history. Patients will usually volunteer that they think they have lost weight. Often, they will have associated complaints, such as pain, weakness, or gastrointestinal symptoms. Your job is to identify those who really have lost weight and figure out why.

HOT

KEY

As many as 50% of patients who claim to have lost weight have not actually lost any weight.

1. **Patient records.** Obtaining the patient's weight should be a routine part of every patient visit, making it possible to document weight loss by using the weights recorded in the patient's chart as a basis for comparison with his current weight.
   a. Like sphygmomanometers, scales can vary greatly in accuracy, so it is best to use hospital scales and to follow trends instead of individual readings.
   b. Weight loss can be corroborated by noting a change in clothing size (e.g., pants, belts, shirt collar). Family members may also be able to give an objective opinion.
2. **Questions** should be designed to identify symptoms of and risk factors for the common causes of involuntary weight loss. Do not forget to screen patients for evidence of depression (depressed mood and anhedonia) and dementia (use the mini-mental state examination; see Chapter 65, Table 65-1).

B. **Physical examination.** A complete examination should be performed.
   1. The major **lymph node groups** (i.e., the cervical, supraclavicular, axillary, and inguinal nodes) should be palpated.
   2. A careful **abdominal examination** should be performed.
   3. A **prostate examination** should be performed in men and a **pelvic examination** is required for women.

C. **Laboratory and imaging studies.** When the cause of the weight loss remains unclear despite a detailed history and physical examination, the following tests are usually obtained.
   1. **Laboratory tests**
      a. Complete blood count (CBC)

   b. Serum electrolyte panel
   c. Glucose and calcium levels
   d. Liver panel
   e. Thyroid-stimulating hormone (TSH) level
   f. Erythrocyte sedimentation rate (ESR)
   g. Urinalysis
   h. Prostate-specific antigen (PSA), in men

HOT

Obtain an HIV test in any patient with weight loss and risk factors for HIV disease.

KEY

---

   2. Imaging studies
   a. A **chest radiograph** should be obtained.
   b. **Mammography** is indicated for women older than 50 years and should also be considered for younger women with weight loss.
   c. **Colonoscopy** is usually recommended for patients older than 50 years and should be considered for younger patients with weight loss.
   d. **Upper endoscopy** may be performed if symptoms suggest an upper gastrointestinal tract disorder or colonoscopy is unremarkable.
   e. An **abdominal computed tomography (CT) scan** may be obtained if symptoms, signs, or laboratory test results suggest an abdominal disorder or if no other cause has been identified.

IV TREATMENT

A. Definitive treatment entails treating the underlying cause.
B. Symptomatic treatment
   1. Consider the use of **megestrol acetate** (800 mg orally daily) or **dronabinol** (5–10 mg orally twice daily) to stimulate the appetite and quell nausea in patients with cancer- or AIDS-related cachexia. The utility of these drugs in the treatment of other causes of involuntary weight loss is unproven.
   2. **Testosterone, growth hormone,** or **thalidomide** may be useful for those with AIDS-associated weight loss.

FOLLOW-UP AND REFERRAL

   A. Patients with documented involuntary weight loss that has eluded diagnosis after 1 month should be referred to a gastroenterologist for endoscopy.

   B. Psychiatric consultation should be considered for patients with persistent weight loss that remains unexplained despite a complete evaluation.

References
Reife CM: Involuntary weight loss. *Med Clin North Am* 79(2):299–313, 1995.

38. Abnormal Liver Function Tests

I INTRODUCTION

A. Liver function tests may be ordered because a patient presents with suggestive symptoms (e.g., jaundice, abdominal pain) or as part of a screening laboratory examination. In the outpatient setting, as many as one third of all screening liver function tests are abnormal. Of these, only about 1% represent clinically significant yet unsuspected liver disease. Clinicians must decide what these biochemical abnormalities mean and how far to pursue them.

B. A liver profile most often includes **total bilirubin, alkaline phosphatase (AP), aspartate aminotransferase (AST),** and **alanine aminotransferase (ALT) levels,** as well as a **prothrombin time (PT).**

1. Obtaining the **conjugated** and **unconjugated bilirubin levels** may help clarify the cause of an elevated total bilirubin level.

2. Similarly, a **γ-glutamyl transferase (GGT) level** may help define the cause of an elevated AP level.

II APPROACH TO THE PATIENT

A. **Consider the possibility that the abnormality could represent an extrahepatic disorder.** Table 38-1 summarizes some of the common extrahepatic disorders that could lead to abnormal liver function test results.

B. **Categorize the abnormality as either cholestatic or hepatocellular.**

1. The **cholestatic pattern** is characterized by markedly **increased AP** and **bilirubin levels.** Aminotransferase levels may be elevated, but not as markedly as the AP and bilirubin levels.

HOT **KEY**   If the AP level is increased but the bilirubin level is not, it is important to determine whether the abnormality is from the liver or the bone. A GGT level can be obtained to make this distinction. Because GGT is not found in bone, an elevated AP level in the presence of an elevated GGT level confirms a hepatic source.

TABLE 38-1. Extrahepatic Causes of Abnormal Liver Function Tests

Abnormality	Potential Extrahepatic Cause
Elevated AST	Myocardial infarction, muscle disorder
Elevated AP	Bone disease, pregnancy, hyperthyroidism
Elevated bilirubin	Hemolysis, sepsis
Increased PT	Malaborption, anticoagulant or antibiotic use, vitamin K deficiency
Decreased albumin	Malnutrition, protein-losing enteropathy, nephrotic syndrome, congestive heart failure (CHF)

AP = alkaline phosphatase; AST = aspartate aminotransferase; PT = prothrombin time.

2. The **hepatocellular pattern** is characterized primarily by **increased AST** and **ALT levels.** The bilirubin level and the PT can also be increased in patients with chronic hepatocellular disease; in later stages, the serum albumin level may decrease.

   a. AST is a sensitive but not a specific marker of hepatocyte necrosis.

   b. ALT is found primarily in the liver and is thus a better indicator of hepatocellular injury.

HOT KEY

Sometimes it can be difficult to distinguish a cholestatic pattern from a hepatocellular pattern (because elevated transaminase levels can occur in both). By determining the relative elevation of the AP, AST, and ALT levels (i.e., how many times normal the levels are), you can determine which pattern is more likely. Elevations in the AP level that are out of proportion to the AST and ALT levels imply a cholestatic pattern, whereas AST and ALT levels that are out of proportion to the AP level imply a hepatocellular pattern.

C. **Narrow the differential diagnosis.**

   1. **Cholestatic pattern.** Figure 38-1 presents an algorithm for narrowing the differential diagnosis in pa-

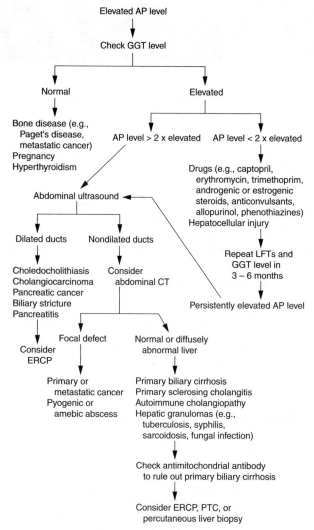

FIGURE 38-1. Approach to the patient with liver function test results suggestive of cholestasis. *AP* = alkaline phosphatase; *CT* = computed tomography; *ERCP* = endoscopic retrograde cholangiopancreatography; *GGT* = γ-glutamyl transferase; *LFTs* = liver function tests; *PTC* = percutaneous transhepatic cholangiogram. (Modified with permission from Moseley RH: Evaluation of abnormal liver function tests. *Med Clin North Am* 80(5):887–906, 1996.)

tients with liver function test results suggestive of cholestasis.

HOT KEY

Infiltrative liver disease often presents with a markedly elevated AP level that is out of proportion to the elevated bilirubin level.

2. **Hepatocellular pattern.** Elevated transaminases are the most common liver function test abnormality. Figure 38-2 presents an algorithm for narrowing the differential diagnosis in patients with liver function test results suggestive of a hepatocellular disorder.

   a. The **most common causes** of elevated transaminases in the United States include the following.

     (1) **Alcohol-induced hepatitis** is associated with high morbidity and mortality rates. Patients usually have an AST level of less than 500 U/L and an AST:ALT ratio that is greater than or equal to 2.

     (2) **Drug-induced hepatitis.** Common offenders include acetaminophen, nonsteroidal anti-inflammatory drugs (NSAIDs), vitamin A, sulfonamides, isoniazid, tetracyclines, 3-hydroxy-3-methylglutaryl coenzyme A (HMG-CoA) reductase inhibitors, valproic acid, and propylthiouracil.

     (3) **Viral hepatitis.** Patients with chronic hepatitis B or C are often asymptomatic. Infection leads to end-stage liver disease in approximately 20% of infected patients and may be associated with the development of hepatocellular carcinoma.

     (4) **Nonalcoholic steatohepatitis (NASH)** is a clinical and biochemical diagnosis made after excluding significant alcohol consumption and other identifiable liver diseases. It is associated with obesity, possibly diabetes, and hypertriglyceridemia. The natural history is poorly understood but suggests that as many as 15% of patients with NASH will progress to end-stage liver disease.

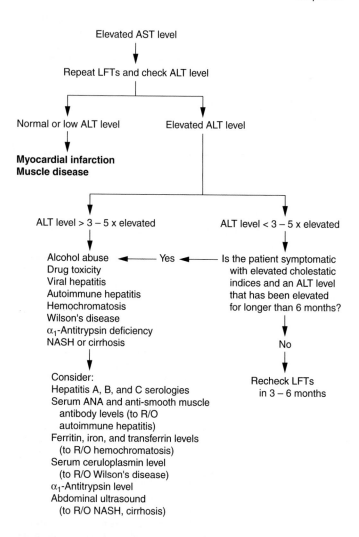

FIGURE 38-2. Approach to the patient with liver function test results suggestive of a hepatocellular disorder. *ALT* = alanine aminotransferase; *ANA* = antinuclear antibody; *AST* = aspartate aminotransferase; *LFTs* = liver function tests; *NASH* = nonalcoholic steatohepatitis; *R/O* = rule out. (Modified with permission from Kamath PS: Clinical approach to the patient with abnormal liver test results. *Mayo Clin Proc* 71(11):1089–1095, 1996.)

        (a) NASH presents with mild to moderate AST elevations. Characteristically, the AST:ALT ratio is less than 1.

        (b) Ultrasound often reveals the hyperechoic texture of fatty infiltration.

        (c) Although a liver biopsy confirms the presence of steatosis with parenchymal inflammation, the role of biopsy in diagnosis is controversial because there are no specific therapies for NASH.

    b. Rarer but potentially treatable causes include the following.

      (1) Hemochromatosis (clinical iron overload) is an autosomal recessive multisystemic disease that predominantly affects Caucasian men. Early recognition and therapy with phlebotomy is crucial in preventing complications.

HOT KEY The College of American Pathologists now recommends widespread screening for hemochromatosis by evaluating the serum ferritin level and the transferrin saturation. A transferrin saturation greater than 60% in men or 50% in women is suggestive of iron overload.

---

      (2) Wilson's disease results from copper overload in the liver and is most common in patients younger than 30 years. A low serum ceruloplasmin level suggests the diagnosis.

      (3) Autoimmune hepatitis is found primarily in young women. Positive results on antinuclear antibody (ANA) or anti-smooth muscle antibody testing suggest the diagnosis.

      (4) α_1-Antitrypsin deficiency. Patients may also have emphysema. A serum α_1-antitrypsin level can be obtained to evaluate possible deficiency.

III FOLLOW-UP AND REFERRAL

A. Cholestasis. Patients with biliary dilatation should be referred to a gastroenterologist.

    1. Extrahepatic biliary dilatation

      a. Patients should see a **gastroenterologist** to undergo **endoscopic retrograde cholangiopancre-**

atography (ERCP). ERCP can be helpful both diagnostically and therapeutically: it permits visualization of the entire biliary tree and facilitates sphincterotomy to decompress a distally obstructed biliary tract.

    b. Referral to a **general surgeon** may also be appropriate for these patients.

  2. Intrahepatic biliary obstruction. ERCP or **percutaneous transhepatic cholangiography (PTC)** should be performed to confirm the suspicion of intrahepatic biliary obstruction. A **percutaneous liver biopsy** may be needed to further clarify the diagnosis.

B. Hepatocellular Disorders

  1. Referral to a gastroenterologist for percutaneous liver biopsy may be indicated for the following patients:

    a. Chronic carriers of either the hepatitis B or C virus

    b. Patients with elevated transferrin saturations

    c. Patients with low serum ceruloplasmin levels

    d. Patients with persistent evaluation of AST or ALT of unclear etiology.

  2. Patients diagnosed with autoimmune hepatitis or α_1-antitrypsin deficiency should be referred to a gastroenterologist for treatment and follow-up.

  3. Patient with cirrhosis should be referred to a gastroenterologist for further evaluation and consideration for liver transplantation.

References

Kamath PS: Clinical approach to the patient with abnormal liver test results. *Mayo Clin Proc* 71(11):1089–1095, 1996.

Moseley RH: Evaluation of abnormal liver function tests. *Med Clin North Am* 80(5):887–906, 1996.

PART VI

Nephrology and Urology

39. Hematuria

I INTRODUCTION

A. Hematuria is defined by the presence of **3 or more red blood cells (RBCs) per high-power field** in a centrifuged urine sample. Hematuria may be **gross** (i.e., characterized by the presence of visible blood or blood clots in the urine) or **microscopic.**

B. The most important reason for understanding hematuria is the fact that **hematuria is a presenting sign of certain potentially curable malignancies.**

C. Hematuria **rarely requires emergent attention:** hemodynamic instability due to urinary blood loss is unusual. However, significant degrees of anemia are not uncommon, and bladder outlet obstruction from clots frequently occurs with gross hematuria, necessitating immediate catheterization and urologic evaluation.

II DIFFERENTIAL DIAGNOSIS

A. **Pseudohematuria.** It is important to ensure that hematuria is truly present. "Pseudohematuria" refers to discolored urine that is mistaken (usually by the patient) for bloody urine. Causes of pseudohematuria include:

1. Certain foods (e.g., beets)
2. Certain drugs (e.g., phenazopyridine, rifampin, methyldopa)
3. Hyperbilirubinemia
4. Highly concentrated urine
5. Myoglobinuria (as a result of rhabdomyolysis)
6. Hemoglobinuria (as a result of hemolysis)

HOT

If a patient has a urinary dipstick positive for heme but no RBCs are seen on microscopic examination, consider the diagnosis of rhabdomyolysis.

KEY

B. Hematuria. The differential diagnoses for gross and microscopic hematuria are the same, although urologic cancer is much more frequently found in patients with gross hematuria. On most standard urine dipsticks, the presence of heme causes a color change from yellow to green. Think, "GREEN PIS" to remember the causes of hematuria:

Causes of Hematuria ("GREEN PIS")

Glomerulonephritis
Renal cyst or trauma
Exercise
Embolism or infarction
Neoplasm

Prostate hypertrophy
Infection
Stones

1. **Glomerulonephritis** of any cause (e.g., IgA nephropathy, poststreptococcal glomerulonephritis, vasculitis) can cause hematuria.
2. **Renal cysts** or **trauma.** Hemorrhage into cysts (usually seen in the setting of polycystic kidney disease) or blunt trauma to the kidneys can lead to hematuria.
3. **Exercise-induced hematuria** usually occurs within 24–48 hours of vigorous exercise and is thought to be associated with transient glomerular changes. The hematuria may be microscopic or gross.
4. **Embolism** or **infarction.** Renal infarction may occur as a result of emboli (e.g., cardiac thrombus, endocarditis, aortic atherosclerosis) or as a result of some other form of arteriolar pathology [e.g., sickle cell disease (SCD), vasculitis, malignant hypertension, hemolytic-uremic syndrome/thrombotic thrombocytopenic purpura (HUS/TTP)].
5. **Neoplasm. Transitional cell carcinoma** (usually of the bladder, but also possibly of the ureter or renal pelvis), **renal cell carcinoma,** and **prostate carcinoma** are important to consider in patients with hematuria.
6. **Prostate hypertrophy.** Benign prostatic hypertrophy (BPH) is a common finding in elderly men and may, on occasion, cause hematuria.
7. **Infection** of any part of the urinary or seminal tract can lead to hematuria. Common infections include

urethritis [seen in association with certain sexually transmitted diseases (STDs)], cystitis, prostatitis, epididymitis, pyelonephritis, tuberculosis, and schistosomiasis.

8. **Stones** anywhere in the urogenital tract can lead to hematuria. Ureteral calculi are usually associated with pain.

III APPROACH TO THE PATIENT

A. **Verify the presence of hematuria using urinalysis.**
B. **Try to determine the cause** by obtaining a careful history, performing a physical examination, and ordering selected laboratory tests.
   1. **Patient history.** Be sure to ask:
      a. Does the patient have any **risk factors for malignancy?** Risk factors include a prior history of urologic cancer or smoking, age greater than 50 years, and male sex.
      b. Does the patient have **pain with urination or flank or groin pain?** Pain suggests the presence of infection or stones.
      c. What is the patient's **medication history** and **travel history?** Is there a history of **vigorous exercise, sexual activity,** or **trauma** (including iatrogenic trauma)?
   2. **Physical examination** should include palpation of the flank and abdomen for tenderness, genital inspection, and a digital rectal examination.
   3. **Standard laboratory studies**
      a. **Urinalysis**
         (1) **Proteinuria** (2+ or greater) on the urine dipstick suggests glomerular pathology if seen in the setting of microscopic hematuria. With gross hematuria, proteinuria is a less reliable marker, due to the presence of protein in blood.
         (2) **Pyuria.** White blood cells (WBCs) in the urine suggest infection but may also be seen with any form of nephritis, especially tubulointerstitial nephritis. As with protein, small numbers of WBCs may be a "normal" finding with gross hematuria. WBC casts suggest a renal source.
         (3) **RBC casts** are nearly pathognomonic for glomerulonephritis. Dysmorphic or crenated

RBCs suggest glomerular disease but are not reliably seen without using phase-contrast microscopy.

   b. **Blood urea nitrogen (BUN)** and **creatinine levels** should be assessed in nearly all patients.

   c. A **complete blood count (CBC), prothrombin time (PT),** and **partial thromboplastin time (PTT)** are indicated for patients with gross hematuria.

C. **Initiate a diagnostic work-up if the cause of the hematuria is not evident from the history, physical examination, and initial laboratory studies.** Patients meeting any one of the criteria given in Table 39-1 should undergo further evaluation to determine the cause of the hematuria.

   1. **Intravenous pyelography (IVP)** has traditionally been considered the preferred first test in the work-up of hematuria, especially when ureteral pathology (e.g., calculi) is suspected.

      a. **Advantages.** IVP is the best test for showing pathology in the renal collecting system and ureters.

      b. **Disadvantages.** IVP may miss some renal malignancies. In addition, IVP requires intravenous contrast, which may be contraindicated if the patient has renal insufficiency.

   2. **Ultrasound and radiographic examination of the kidneys, ureters, and bladder (ultrasound/KUB).** Re-

---

TABLE 39-1. Criteria for Diagnostic Work-Up of Hematuria

1. Suspicion of malignancy
2. Two of three urinalyses showing 3 or more RBCs/HPF
3. One urinalysis showing more than 100 RBCs/HPF
4. Any single episode of gross hematuria and both of the following:
   a. No clear reason for benign, transient hematuria (e.g., vigorous exercise, minor trauma, bladder catheterization, sexual activity) **and**
   b. No obvious diagnostic clues (e.g., dysuria or pyuria suggesting UTI)

RBCs/HPF = red blood cells per high-power field; UTI = urinary tract infection.

cent studies have suggested that ultrasound/KUB may be safer, more accurate, and less costly than IVP. Ultrasound is generally better than IVP for identifying renal tumors, but not as good at imaging the collecting system and ureters.

3. **Cystoscopy.** In most centers, cystoscopy is performed if either IVP or ultrasound/KUB is negative or suggests a bladder lesion. Cystoscopy is the preferred first test if there is active, gross hematuria, because it may reveal a bleeding bladder lesion or determine from which side an upper tract lesion is bleeding.

4. **Urine cytology** may detect bladder carcinoma when all other tests are negative (as may be the case in patients with *in situ* carcinoma), but the sensitivity is only 67% overall. Urine cytology is mostly used in following patients who have had negative work-ups. The test must be performed on the first morning specimen to guarantee that the urine has had prolonged exposure to the bladder wall.

5. **Other tests** (e.g., serologic studies, hemoglobin electrophoresis, blood and urine cultures, renal or prostate biopsy, angiography) may be indicated, depending on the patient's history and physical examination findings.

IV FOLLOW-UP AND REFERRAL

A. **Active, gross hematuria.** A urologist should be consulted promptly.

B. **Negative initial work-up.** In patients with negative evaluations initially (including negative results on urine cytology), standard follow-up includes urinalysis with urine cytology every 6 months, and IVP (or ultrasound/KUB) every year for up to 3 years if the hematuria persists. The yield of such follow-up for detecting malignancy is about 2% in patients with microscopic hematuria and 20% in those with gross hematuria.

References

Ahmed Z, Lee J: Asymptomatic urinary abnormalities: hematuria and proteinuria. *Med Clin North Am* 81(3):641–652, 1997.

McCarthy JJ: Outpatient evaluation of hematuria: locating the source of bleeding. *Postgrad Med* 101(2):125–128, 131, 1997.

40. Proteinuria and Nephrotic Syndrome

I INTRODUCTION

A. **Proteinuria** is considered significant when more than 150 mg of protein are excreted over a 24-hour period. Proteinuria is classified as either **nonrenal ("benign")** or **renal.**
 1. **Nonrenal (benign) proteinuria** is proteinuria in the absence of known renal disease and in the presence of an otherwise normal urinary sediment. These patients usually do not develop progressive renal insufficiency.
 2. **Renal proteinuria** is caused by a renal disorder. A small but significant percentage of these patients develop progressive renal insufficiency.
B. **Nephrotic syndrome.** The hallmark of nephrotic syndrome is **insidious proteinuria.** Patients also have **hypoalbuminemia, hyperlipidemia,** and **peripheral edema.** These patients may look "PALE" because they are excreting so much protein.

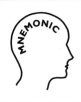

Characteristics of the Nephrotic Syndrome ("PALE")

Proteinuria (> 3.5 grams/24 hours)
Albumin (low)
Lipids (elevated)
Edema

II CAUSES OF PROTEINURIA

A. **Nonrenal (benign) proteinuria.** Use the mnemonic "PROTEIN" to remember the causes of nonrenal proteinuria.

Causes of Nonrenal Proteinuria ("PROTEIN")

Pulmonary edema or congestive heart failure (CHF)
Relative lordotic position
Orthostatic proteinuria (i.e., proteinuria when sitting
upright but not in the supine position)
Temperature increase (i.e., fever)
Exercise (following vigorous exercise)
Injury to the head or cerebrovascular accident (CVA)
Idiopathic (diagnosis of exclusion)
Norepinephrine excess (emotional stress)

HOT

Benign proteinuria can exacerbate renal proteinuria; thus,
it is important to note complete resolution of the proteinuria
(not just a decrease in the amount) before ascribing it to a
benign cause.

KEY

B. **Renal proteinuria.** Several renal disorders are associated
   with proteinuria.
   1. **Nephrotic syndrome.** Causes of nephrotic syndrome
      include the following.
      a. **Renal disease.** Nephrotic syndrome is caused by
         primary renal disease in two-thirds of patients. Pri-
         mary glomerular diseases associated with nephro-
         tic syndrome in adults include:
         (1) Membranous nephropathy
         (2) Minimal change disease
         (3) Focal glomerulosclerosis
         (4) Membranoproliferative glomerulonephritis
         (5) Rapidly progressive glomerulonephritis
      b. **Systemic disease.** In the remainder of patients,
         nephrotic syndrome occurs secondary to a sys-
         temic disease. Although there is a long list of pos-
         sible secondary causes, they can be remembered
         easily using the mnemonic, "THIS LAD HAS
         nephrotic syndrome."

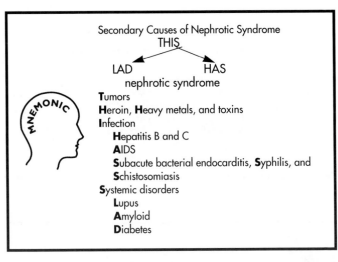

Secondary Causes of Nephrotic Syndrome

THIS

LAD ← → HAS

nephrotic syndrome

Tumors
Heroin, **H**eavy metals, and toxins
Infection
  Hepatitis B and C
  AIDS
  Subacute bacterial endocarditis, **S**yphilis, and
  Schistosomiasis
Systemic disorders
  Lupus
  Amyloid
  Diabetes

(1) Tumors. Many cancers can cause nephrotic syndrome. In elderly patients with unexplained nephrotic syndrome, an underlying malignancy is a real concern. Both **hematologic malignancies** (e.g., lymphoma, leukemia) and **solid tumors** can cause nephrotic syndrome.

(2) Heroin, heavy metals, and **toxins.** "Street" heroin, organic gold, mercury, antitoxins, and contrast media can cause nephrotic syndrome.

(3) Infections. There are many infections that can cause nephrotic syndrome; the most important ones are **hepatitis B** and **C, AIDS, subacute bacterial endocarditis, syphilis,** and **schistosomiasis.**

(4) Systemic disorders. Major causes of nephrotic syndrome include **systemic lupus erythematosus (SLE), amyloid,** and **diabetes.**

HOT

The disorders that can cause nephrotic syndrome can also lead to non-nephrotic range proteinuria.

KEY

2. **Other causes** of renal proteinuria include **nephritic syndrome,** acute and chronic **renal failure, urinary tract infection (UTI), hypertension, nephrolithiasis,** and **tubular defects.**

III APPROACH TO THE PATIENT. Proteinuria is usually detected when a urinalysis is done for other reasons. When confronted with a patient with proteinuria on urinalysis, take the following approach:

A. First, **confirm the presence of proteinuria** on two more dipstick urine samples.

B. If the proteinuria is still present, **consider both nonrenal and renal causes.**

1. If the patient has one of the conditions associated with benign proteinuria (e.g., fever, pulmonary edema), **consider repeating the urinalysis** after the condition has resolved. However, remember that a benign cause is usually a diagnosis of exclusion (i.e., the diagnosis is only made after renal causes have been excluded).

2. In younger patients (especially men), consider evaluating the patient for **orthostatic proteinuria** before undertaking an extensive evaluation. Three urine samples are required:

a. Instruct the patient to void in the evening and then immediately lie supine in bed.

b. On awakening the next morning, the patient should collect the second urine sample while still supine.

c. The patient should collect a third sample after he has been ambulatory for several hours. If the patient has orthostatic proteinuria, **proteinuria** will be **present in the first** and **third specimens** and **absent in the second.**

3. If a nonrenal cause cannot be identified and the proteinuria is persistent, obtain a **24-hour urine collection to quantify the proteinuria.** If the 24-hour urine collection reveals an abnormal amount of protein (i.e., more than 150 mg), then the following studies should be performed:

a. **Initial studies**

(1) **Complete urinalysis,** with close attention to the urinary sediment. If the patient has evidence of a UTI, treatment with antibiotics may precede further evaluation.

(2) **Electrolyte panel,** including blood urea nitrogen (BUN), creatinine, and glucose values.

    b. Specific studies. In patients with **suspected nephrotic syndrome,** one or more of the following tests may be indicated in addition to urinalysis and a serum electrolyte panel.

      (1) Antinuclear antibody (ANA) assays

      (2) Hepatitis serologies

      (3) Rapid plasma reagin (RPR) or **Venereal Disease Research Laboratory (VDRL) test** (to rule out syphilis)

      (4) HIV test

      (5) Blood cultures (to rule out endocarditis)

      (6) Fat pad or **rectal biopsy** (to look for amyloidosis)

    c. Renal biopsy should be reserved for those with a suspected underlying renal cause, and only after consultation with a nephrologist. In patients with chronic hypertension or diabetes, biopsy is often not necessary unless there are indications that a superimposed cause for the proteinuria may be present.

IV **TREATMENT** of proteinuria focuses on the underlying disorder.

  A. Nonrenal (benign) proteinuria. Reassurance is usually all that is needed.

  B. Renal proteinuria

    1. Treatment of specific renal lesions (e.g., glomerulonephritis) should be done in consultation with a nephrologist.

    2. General management strategies for the nephrotic syndrome include:

      a. A diet low in sodium and saturated fat

      b. Adequate protein intake (approximately 1 g/kg/day)

      c. Diuretics for edema and hypertension

      d. Fluid restriction (if hyponatremia is present)

V **FOLLOW-UP AND REFERRAL**

  A. If the proteinuria can be attributed to a benign cause, no follow-up is needed.

  B. If the proteinuria is persistent and not attributable to a benign cause, the patient should be referred to a nephrologist for evaluation and possible renal biopsy.

References

Ahmed Z, Lee J: Asymptomatic urinary abnormalities: hematuria and proteinuria. *Med Clin North Am* 81(3):641–652, 1997.

Larson TS: Evaluation of proteinuria. *Mayo Clin Proc* 69(12):1154–1158, 1994.

41. Dysuria

I INTRODUCTION

A. Dysuria (i.e., **pain** or **burning with urination)** is a common complaint in the outpatient setting.

B. Dysuria suggests inflammation or irritation of the urethra or bladder neck and is usually associated with **other irritative symptoms: frequency, urgency, nocturia,** and occasionally, **hematuria.** The duration and severity of the symptoms vary, and do not always correlate with the degree of pathology.

II DIFFERENTIAL DIAGNOSIS

A. Women

1. **Urinary tract infections (UTIs)** are much more common in women than in men. Predisposing factors include failure to void after intercourse, diaphragm use, and postmenopausal status.

   a. **Etiology.** Eighty percent of UTIs in women are caused by *Escherichia coli;* the rest are caused by other Gram-negative rods, *Staphylococcus saprophyticus, Mycobacterium tuberculosis,* adenovirus, and fungi.

   b. **Clinical manifestations.** Patients complain of the acute onset of dysuria with associated frequency and urgency. Examination may reveal suprapubic or costovertebral angle tenderness (or both).

2. **Vaginal infections** (e.g., **candidiasis, trichomoniasis).** Patients usually complain of a vaginal discharge; they may also mention external genital discomfort or pruritus. Examination usually reveals a discharge and erythema of the external genitalia.

3. **Sexually transmitted urethritis.** Infection is caused by *Chlamydia trachomatis, Neisseria gonorrhoeae,* or herpes simplex virus (HSV).

4. **Urethral syndrome without clear etiology.** In 5% of patients, no cause is found for the irritative symptoms. A history of postcoital voiding dysfunction and dyspareunia is suggestive of the idiopathic urethral syndrome.

5. **Interstitial cystitis** most often affects middle-aged women.

       a. Etiology. Symptoms are caused by inflammation of the bladder wall, but the cause is unknown. Cystoscopic examination reveals characteristic findings on the bladder wall.

       b. Clinical manifestations. Symptoms are chronic. A history of nocturia is almost universal; sometimes hematuria and dyspareunia are present as well. Examination may reveal suprapubic tenderness.

B. Men

  1. UTIs are much less common in men than in women. In men, the most common causative organisms are *E. coli, Enterococcus, Proteus,* and *Klebsiella.*

  2. Bladder stones and **tumors** are more common in men than in women and may present with pain or hematuria.

  3. Prostatic disorders

       a. Prostatitis may be acute bacterial, chronic bacterial, or chronic nonbacterial.

         (1) Etiology

           (a) Acute bacterial: *Pseudomonas, E. coli, Enterococcus*

           (b) Chronic bacterial: Gram-negative rods

           (c) Chronic nonbacterial: *Chlamydia, Ureaplasma, Trichomonas*

         (2) Clinical manifestations include obstructive symptoms (i.e., hesitancy, decreased flow) and pain with ejaculation. Patients with acute bacterial prostatitis may have signs of systemic toxicity. Examination reveals a normal or tender boggy prostate.

       b. Prostatodynia is a diagnosis of exclusion.

HOT KEY

Performing a urinalysis before and after prostatic massage can help determine which prostate disorder may be responsible for the dysuria. Chronic bacterial prostatitis results in a positive urine culture. Chronic nonbacterial prostatitis is associated with increased leukocytes after prostatic massage, but the culture is negative. In patients with prostatodynia, the culture is negative and there is no increase in leukocytes after massage.

---

  4. Urethritis may be gonococcal (35% of cases) or nongonococcal.

    a. Etiology

      (1) Gonococcal urethritis is caused by *N. gonorrhoeae.*

      (2) Nongonococcal urethritis is caused by *Chlamydia* or *Ureaplasma.*

    b. Clinical manifestations. Patients usually have a history of a penile discharge, which can be extracted by milking the urethra. A history of multiple sex partners or a new sex partner increases the likelihood of urethritis.

  5. Epididymitis is the most common intrascrotal infection in men.

    a. Etiology

      (1) In **young men,** *C. trachomatis* and *N. gonorrhoeae* are the most common causes.

      (2) In **older men, coliform bacteria** and *Pseudomonas* are more often responsible.

    b. Clinical manifestations include pain in the scrotum and an enlarged or tender epididymis on examination.

III **APPROACH TO THE PATIENT.** Algorithms for the approach to the patient for women and men are given in Figures 41-1 and 41-2, respectively.

IV **TREATMENT.** Selected therapies for the treatment of common causes of dysuria in women and men are summarized in Tables 41-1 and 41-2, respectively.

V **FOLLOW-UP AND REFERRAL**

A. Women

  1. UTI

    a. Symptoms should be eliminated or markedly reduced within 72 hours of initiating antimicrobial treatment.

      (1) If symptoms persist, urine should be cultured (or recultured). If bacteriuria is still present, consider the possibility of noncompliance, an underlying structural anomaly, a resistant organism, or poor renal function that is limiting the amount of antibiotic that is excreted in the urine.

      (2) In women with persistent or recurrent UTIs (i.e., more than 3 episodes per year), a workup should be done to rule out an underlying

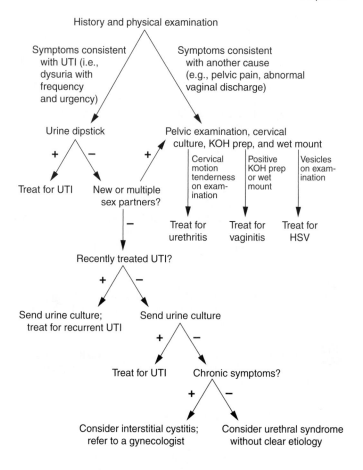

FIGURE 41-1. Approach to a woman with dysuria. *HSV* = herpes simplex virus; *KOH prep* = potassium hydroxide preparation; *UTI* = urinary tract infection.

structural abnormality. If pathology is found, the patient should be referred to a urologist.

b. Measures patients can take to prevent future infections include avoiding diaphragm use and urinating after intercourse. Women with the urethral

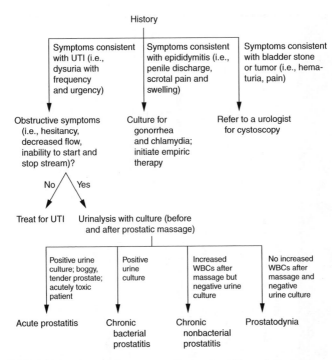

FIGURE 41-2. Approach to a man with dysuria. *UTI* = urinary tract infection; *WBCs* = white blood cells.

syndrome without clear etiology should take similar precautions.

2. **Vaginitis.** These patients do not need follow-up, provided there is an adequate response to therapy.

3. **Sexually transmitted urethritis.** These patients should be counseled about using barrier protection. Follow-up tests for HIV and syphilis are usually performed.

4. **Interstitial cystitis.** Patients should be referred to a urologist or urogynecologist who has experience in managing this condition. Patients may obtain support through national support groups.

B. **Men**

1. **UTI.** In men, any UTI warrants an investigation to rule out an underlying structural abnormality.

2. **Urethritis** or **epididymitis.** These patients should be

TABLE 41-1. Selected Therapies for the Common Causes of Dysuria in Women

Diagnosis	Therapy
Uncomplicated UTI	**Trimethoprim-sulfamethoxazole,** double strength (twice daily for 3 days)* **Phenazopyridine** (200 mg three times daily for 2 days) to relieve symptoms
Recurrent UTI or pyelonephritis	Use culture to guide treatment, which should be given for 7–14 days[†] Therapy may be initiated with **ciprofloxacin** (500 mg PO twice daily)
Urethritis	*Neisseria gonorrhoeae:* **ceftriaxone** (125 mg IM, one dose) or **norfloxacin** (800 mg PO, one dose)[‡] *Chlamydia trachomatis:* **doxycycline** (100 mg PO, twice daily for 7 days) or **azithromycin** (1 g PO, one dose)[‡]
Vaginitis	*Candida albicans:* **fluconazole** (100 mg PO, one dose) or **terconazole** suppositories (for resistant infections) *Trichomonas vaginalis* or *Gardnerella vaginalis:* **metronidazole** (2 g PO, one dose)
HSV infection	**Acyclovir** (200 mg PO, five times daily for 7 days) or **valacyclovir** (500 mg PO twice daily for five days) (less frequent dosing, more expensive than acyclovir)
Interstitial cystitis	**Refer to gynecologist**
Urethral syndrome of unclear etiology	**Sitz baths** and **phenazopyridine** (200 mg orally, three times daily for 5–10 days)

HSV = herpes simplex virus; IM = intramuscularly; PO = orally; UTI = urinary tract infection.

*One-day therapy is not effective. Three-day therapy has the same cure rate (90%–95%) as seven-day therapy. Alternative agents include quinolones, tetracycline, and nitrofurantoin.

[†]The current recommendation for the treatment of pyelonephritis is ciprofloxacin for 14 days; admit the patient for intravenous antibiotics if signs of systemic toxicity develop.

[‡]Patients treated for *N. gonorrhoeae* should receive empiric therapy for *C. trachomatis* and vice versa.

TABLE 41-2. Selected Therapies for the Common Causes of Dysuria in Men

Diagnosis	Therapy
UTI	Use culture to guide treatment, which should be given for 7–14 days Therapy may be initiated with **ciprofloxacin** (500 mg twice daily)
Acute bacterial prostatitis	**Trimethoprim-sulfamethoxazole**, double strength (twice daily until culture results are available); therapy (based on culture results) given for 30 days; admit for IV antibiotics if toxicity is present
Chronic bacterial prostatitis	**Ciprofloxacin** (500 mg PO twice daily for 4–16 weeks)*
Chronic nonbacterial prostatitis	**Doxycycline** (100 mg PO, twice daily for 7 days) or **azithromycin** (1 g PO, one dose)
Young man with urethritis or epididymitis	*Neisseria gonorrhoeae:* **ceftriaxone** (125 mg IM, one dose) or **norfloxacin** (800 mg PO, one dose)† *Chlamydia trachomatis:* **doxycycline** (100 mg PO, twice daily for 7 days) or **azithromycin** (1 g PO, one dose)†
Older man with epididymitis	Use culture to guide treatment, which should be given for 7–10 days Therapy may be initiated with **ciprofloxacin** (500 mg PO twice daily)
Prostatodynia	May respond to α **blockers**
Bladder stone or tumor	**Refer to urologist** for cystoscopy

HSV = herpes simplex virus; IM = intramuscularly; IV = intravenously; PO = orally; UTI = urinary tract infection.
*Cure rates for chronic bacterial prostatitis are reported to be less than 50%. If a patient with chronic bacterial prostatitis does not show improvement in 14 days, additional therapy may not be beneficial.
†Patients treated for *N. gonorrhoeae* should receive empiric therapy for *C. trachomatis* and vice versa.

counseled about using barrier protection. Follow-up
tests for HIV and syphilis are usually performed.

3. **Prostatitis.** Patients with acute bacterial prostatitis
    should be seen expeditiously by a urologist. Patients
    with chronic prostatitis that does not respond to ther-
    apy or prostatodynia may also benefit from consulta-
    tion with a urologist.

4. **Bladder stone** or **tumor.** Patients with suspected
    bladder pathology need to be seen by a urologist.

References

Hamilton-Miller JM: The urethral syndrome and its management. *J Antimicrob Chemother* 33(suppl A:63–73), 1994.

Hooton TM, Stamm WE: Diagnosis and treatment of uncomplicated urinary tract infection. *Infect Dis Clin North Am* 11(3):551–581, 1997.

42. Scrotal Mass

I ■ DIFFERENTIAL DIAGNOSIS. Scrotal masses can be classified as either painful or painless (Table 42-1).

A. **Painful masses.** The main considerations in a patient with an acutely swollen and painful testicle are **epididymitis** and **testicular torsion.** Other causes of painful scrotal masses include **orchitis, Fournier's gangrene,** and **trauma.**

   1. **Epididymitis** is approximately ten times more common than testicular torsion.

      a. In **heterosexual men younger than 35 years,** the infection is usually sexually transmitted and caused by *Chlamydia trachomatis* or *Neisseria gonorrhoeae.*

      b. In **homosexual men** and **men older than 35 years,** the infection is usually caused by **Enterobacteriaceae.**

   2. **Testicular torsion** primarily occurs in teenagers and young adults and is rare after the age of 40 years. The acute pain and swelling result from rotation of the testicle around the vascular pedicle of the spermatic cord, which leads to venous occlusion, edema, and eventual ischemia.

   3. **Orchitis** occurs in association with mumps and develops 7–10 days after parotitis. Involvement is usually unilateral with swelling, pain, and tenderness.

   4. **Fournier's gangrene** is a necrotizing fasciitis of the male external genitalia caused by mixed bacteria. It is more common in older patients and those with serious comorbid disease (e.g., diabetes, chronic renal failure, alcoholism).

B. **Painless masses.** Most painless lesions are discovered by the patient incidentally or cause a feeling of fullness or a dull ache.

   1. **Tumor.** Testicular tumors are usually malignant germ cell tumors (seminoma and nonseminoma). The peak incidence is in men between the ages of 20 and 40 years.

   2. **Hydrocele** is an accumulation of fluid between the two layers of the tunica vaginalis, a potential space created by the descent of the testicle within the "wrapping" of the peritoneum. Hydrocele usually occurs in men older than 40 years.

TABLE 42-1. Differential Diagnosis of a Scrotal Mass

Painful Scrotal Mass	Painless Scrotal Mass
Infection (e.g., epididymitis, orchitis, Fournier's gangrene)	Tumor
Torsion	Hydrocele, spermatocele, varicocele
Trauma	Inguinal hernia
Referred pain (e.g., kidney stone, appendicitis, abdominal aortic aneurysm, prostatitis, retroperitoneal cancer)	Sperm granuloma
	Tuberculous mass

3. **Spermatocele** is a sperm-filled cyst on the superior pole of the testis caused by blockage of an efferent ductule.
4. **Varicocele** is a dilatation of the veins in the pampiniform plexus, which is located above the testis in the spermatic cord. This lesion is more common in young men and on the left side.
5. **Inguinal hernia** presents with the sudden onset of a large inguinal mass following the herniation of an abdominal organ (usually the small bowel) through the inguinal canal and into the testes.
6. **Sperm granulomas** occur in patients with a history of vasectomy and present as tender nodules at the site of surgery.
7. **Tuberculous mass.** *Mycobacterium tuberculosis* can cause infections in the testicle, epididymis, or seminal vesicle. Infection may present as a firm mass or a draining sinus.

II APPROACH TO THE PATIENT
A. Painful mass
  1. **Patient history**
     a. **Epididymitis** presents within hours to days as pain in the scrotum that may radiate along the spermatic cord to the flank. Fever, swelling of the epididymis, urethral discharge, and irritative voiding

symptoms (e.g., dysuria, frequency, urgency) are common.

    b. **Testicular torsion.** Patients often have nausea but rarely have fever or irritative voiding symptoms. There is often a history of previous episodes of pain that resolved spontaneously. A history of trauma does not exclude the possibility of torsion.

2. **Physical examination** should include careful inspection and palpation of the scrotum.

    a. **Epididymitis.** The epididymis, which is swollen and painful, is located posterior to the testicle. In advanced cases, the swelling may involve the entire testicle.

HOT

KEY

Unlike testicular torsion, the pain of epididymitis may improve with testicular elevation (Prehn's sign).

    b. **Testicular torsion** results in a painful, swollen testicle that may be elevated in the scrotum (known as a "high lie").

    c. **Fournier's gangrene** presents with painful swelling of the scrotum, perineum, or penis. Evidence of necrosis may be noted.

HOT

KEY

Referred pain from the retroperitoneum (as in ureterolithiasis, abdominal aortic aneurysm, or retrocecal appendix) or prostate (as in prostatitis) should be suspected if the testicular examination is normal. Referred pain is caused by irritation of one of the nerves supplying the scrotum (e.g., the iliofemoral or genitofemoral nerves).

3. **Laboratory studies**

    a. **Urinalysis** and **urine culture.** Pyuria suggests the diagnosis of epididymitis.

    b. **Urethral culture** should be performed if a sexually transmitted disease (STD) is suspected.

B. **Painless mass**

1. **Patient history.** Certain aspects of the history may provide clues to the diagnosis:

    a. A sudden onset suggests an inguinal hernia; the other processes develop slowly.

    b. Patients who have undergone vasectomy are at risk for sperm granuloma.

    c. Fluid or discharge from a sinus may suggest a tuberculous mass.

2. Physical examination

    a. The mass should be palpated to determine if it is within the testicle or external to it. Masses external to the testicle and masses that transilluminate are more likely to be benign. All intratesticular masses are cancer until proven otherwise.

    b. A varicocele often increases in size when the patient performs a Valsalva maneuver and decreases in size when the patient lies down. When palpated, a varicocele may feel like a "bag of worms."

HOT

KEY

A right-sided or a rapidly enlarging left-sided varicocele should lead to an evaluation for a retroperitoneal tumor with venous obstruction.

---

3. Imaging studies. An **ultrasound** and **urologic consultation** should be obtained for all patients with intratesticular masses. Most extratesticular masses should also be evaluated with ultrasound because many of these lesions can occur in association with cancer (e.g., a hydrocele may be caused by a testicular tumor).

III TREATMENT

A. Painful mass

    1. Epididymitis. Antibiotic therapy should be directed at the likely cause.

        a. For heterosexual patients younger than 35 years, treat for *C. trachomatis* and *N. gonorrhoeae* (see Chapter 81).

        b. For homosexual men or men older than 35 years, treat for Enterobacteriaceae with ciprofloxacin (500 mg orally twice daily for 10–14 days) or ofloxacin (200 mg orally twice daily for 10–14 days).

    2. Testicular torsion is a **surgical emergency.** Surgical consultation should be immediate when testicular torsion is suspected because salvage of the testicle is much more likely when the condition is corrected within 6 hours.

3. **Fournier's gangrene** is also a **surgical emergency,** requiring immediate debridement.

4. **Trauma** can be managed with oral analgesics unless rupture of the testicle is suspected, in which case surgery is required.

B. Painless masses

1. **Testicular cancer** is treated with excision; radiation and chemotherapy are sometimes required.

2. **Tuberculous masses** are treated with antibiotics and may require debridement.

3. **Hydroceles** can be aspirated with a needle, but the fluid often reaccumulates.

HOT

KEY

Needle aspiration of a hydrocele should be performed only after cancer has been excluded because malignant cells can seed the needle tract.

---

4. **Other painless swellings** can be left alone once cancer has been excluded. For conditions that remain uncomfortable or cosmetically unappealing, surgery can be considered.

IV FOLLOW-UP AND REFERRAL

A. Patients with epididymitis must always be reevaluated after treatment to ensure that there are no remaining masses on physical examination, because as many as 50% of patients with testicular cancer initially present with epididymitis.

B. All patients with intratesticular masses or an extratesticular mass suspicious for malignancy should be referred to a urologist.

References

McGee SR: Referred scrotal pain: case reports and review. *J Gen Intern Med* 8(12):694–701, 1993.

43. Impotence

I. INTRODUCTION

A. Impotence is the **consistent inability to maintain an erection sufficient to enable sexual intercourse.** Male erection primarily relies on **sufficient libido,** an **intact nerve supply** to the penis (both autonomic and somatic), and proper **arterial** and **venous function.**

B. Approximately 10 million men in the United States are affected by impotence. The incidence increases with age; over **25% of men older than 65 years** suffer from the condition.

C. Often, men will not be forthcoming with this complaint; thus, it is important to **inquire about this problem during routine health screenings.** Men who experience occasional episodes of impotence should be reassured that this is very common.

II. CAUSES OF IMPOTENCE.
Impotence is either **organic** (i.e., neurogenic, vascular, hormonal, or pharmacologic in origin) or **psychogenic.** Table 43-1 lists the most common causes of impotence.

HOT

Most cases of impotence are organic rather than psychogenic.

KEY

III. APPROACH TO THE PATIENT

A. **Patient history.** Ask about:
1. The presence of any disorder that commonly leads to impotence (e.g., hypertension, atherosclerosis, diabetes, central or peripheral nerve disorders)
2. The use of both prescription and illicit drugs that commonly lead to impotence
3. Any surgeries involving the pelvic area or the vasculature of the pelvis or lower extremities
4. The time course of the impotence

5. The presence or absence of occasional erections during sleep or early morning

TABLE 43-1. Causes of Impotence

Classification of Disease	Specific Examples	Approximate Incidence
Neurogenic	Diabetic neuropathy, peripheral neuropathy, spinal cord injury, surgical damage to pelvic nerves	30%
Vascular	Arteriosclerosis-related, hypertension-related, smoking-related	20%
Pharmacologic	Clonidine, β blockers, spironolactone, alcohol, cimetidine, narcotics, sedatives, tricyclic antidepressants, calcium channel blockers	15%
Pyschogenic	Sexual difficulties, generalized anxiety, depression, performance anxiety	10%
Hormonal	Hypgonadism, hyperprolactinemia, adrenal insufficiency, thyroid disease	5%
Multifactorial	Combination of any of the above	20%

HOT

KEY

Gradual loss of erections or the absence of normal erections at any time usually signals an organic cause.

B. Physical examination

1. Note the presence or absence of secondary sexual characteristics.
2. Perform a neurologic examination (consider evaluating the cremasteric reflex, the anal wink, and rectal tone).
3. Evaluate the peripheral pulses of the lower extremities.
4. Note testicular size and consistency.

C. Laboratory studies should include a **fasting glucose** or

---

HOT

In most patents with impotence, the physical exam is relatively normal.

KEY

---

hemoglobin A_{1c} **level** (to screen for diabetes) and a **testosterone level.**

1. If the testosterone level is decreased, follicle-stimulating hormone (FSH), luteinizing hormone (LH), and prolactin levels should be determined.
2. Additional tests [e.g., a thyroid-stimulating hormone (TSH) level] should be ordered according to clinical suspicion.

IV TREATMENT

A. Definitive therapy depends on the cause. Unfortunately, it is often difficult to ascertain the exact cause in many patients.

1. **Psychogenic impotence.** Consultation with a psychiatrist and **psychosexual therapy** are often helpful.
2. **Hypogonadism with documented androgen deficiency.** Patients can be treated with **intramuscular testosterone injections** (200 mg every 3–4 weeks), or testosterone patches (4–6 mg patch applied to hairless skin once daily)

HOT

Before prescribing exogenous testosterone to any man, always screen for prostate cancer by obtaining a prostate-specific antigen (PSA) level and performing a digital rectal examination.

KEY

3. **Vascular dysfunction.** Patients with vascular disorders who fail more conventional therapy may be eligible for **vascular reconstruction.**

B. **Symptomatic therapy**

1. **Vacuum constriction devices** are useful for most patients and are often considered first-line therapy. A cylinder creates a vacuum that draws the penis into an erect state; the erection is maintained by placing a rubber constriction device at the base of the penis. (This rubber constriction device must be removed after intercourse and should not be worn for an extended period.)

2. **Sildenafil citrate (Viagra)** is the first oral medication to be approved by the Food and Drug Administration (FDA) for the treatment of erectile dysfunction. One 50-mg tablet is taken 1 hour prior to sexual intercourse. Men older than 65 years and those with hepatic or renal dysfunction should begin with a dose of 25 mg.

HOT

Men who are receiving nitrate therapy (including nitrate patches) should not take sildenafil.

KEY

---

3. **Injection therapy** entails the direct injection of vasoactive prostaglandins into the penis and may be considered after consultation with a urologist. Intraurethral prostaglandin suppositories are also available.

4. **Penile prostheses** may be inflatable, rigid, malleable, or hinged. A urologist should be consulted.

V FOLLOW-UP AND REFERRAL

A. Referral to a psychiatrist is appropriate for those with psychogenic impotence.

B. Referral to a urologist or an impotence clinic is usually indicated when the patient:

1. Has a normal testosterone level, the impotence is not psychogenic in origin, and therapy with a vacuum constriction device fails

2. Desires injection or surgical therapy

References

O'Keefe M, Hunt DK: Assessment and treatment of impotence. *Med Clin North Am* 79(2):415–434, 1995.

Sildenafil: an oral drug for impotence. *Med Lett Drugs Ther* 40(1026):51–52, 1998.

44. Benign Prostatic Hyperplasia

I **INTRODUCTION.** Benign prostatic hyperplasia (BPH) is a heterogenous disorder characterized by proliferation of the epithelial and stromal elements of the prostate.

II **CLINICAL MANIFESTATIONS.** Patients classically present with some combination of obstructive and irritative symptoms.

  A. **Obstructive symptoms,** caused by mechanical blockade of the prostatic urethra, include a decreased force of urinary stream, an intermittent stream, hesitancy, and a feeling of incomplete emptying.
  B. **Irritative symptoms,** which are thought to be caused by incomplete emptying and bladder hypersensitivity, include daytime frequency, urgency, nocturia, and dysuria.

III **DIFFERENTIAL DIAGNOSIS.** Many medical conditions mimic the symptoms of BPH (Table 44-1).

IV **APPROACH TO THE PATIENT.** The most important aspect of evaluating a patient with suspected BPH is to rule out other disease (see Table 44-1).

  A. **Patient history**
    1. Does the patient have a **past medical history** or symptoms suggestive of **diabetes, congestive heart failure (CHF), alcoholism,** or **neurologic disease?**
    2. What is the patient's **past urologic history?** Has the patient ever had strictures, a sexually transmitted disease (STD), a urinary tract infection (UTI), or required instrumentation?
    3. What is the patient's **medication history?** Decongestants (α agonists), anticholinergic agents, diuretics, and lithium can cause sudden worsening of the symptoms of BPH.
  B. **Physical examination**
    1. Palpate the abdomen. A palpable bladder suggests severe obstruction.
    2. Examine the prostate for size, tenderness (suggestive of prostatitis), and nodularity (suggestive of prostate cancer).

TABLE 44-1. Differential Diagnosis of Benign Prostatic Hyperplasia (BPH)	
Differential Diagnosis	**Symptoms or Signs Similar to Those of BPH**
Systemic Disorders	
Congestive heart failure (CHF)	Nocturia
Diabetes	Frequency and nocturia
Alcoholism	Frequency and nocturia
Neurologic disease	Incontinence, frequency, incomplete emptying
Medication side effects	Frequency and obstructive symptoms
Genitourinary Disorders	
Infection	Frequency, urgency, nocturia, dysuria
Prostatitis	
STDs	
UTIs	
Renal, bladder, or prostate cancer	Dysuria
Strictures	Incomplete emptying, irritative symptoms

STDs = sexually transmitted diseases; UTIs = urinary tract infections.

3. Assess rectal tone to evaluate for neurologic disease.
4. Focus the rest of the examination on signs suggestive of CHF, diabetes, or alcoholism.

C. **Laboratory studies**
1. A **urinalysis** and **urine culture** should be ordered to rule out infection, hematuria, and glycosuria. If hematuria or glycosuria is detected, the work-up should continue as described in the chapters on hematuria and diabetes (Chapters 39 and 75, respectively).
2. **Serum creatinine level.** If the serum creatinine level is elevated, upper tract imaging (e.g., ultrasound) to rule out obstruction is indicated.
3. **Serum prostate-specific antigen (PSA)** may be ordered to screen for prostate cancer.

D. **Other studies**
1. A **post-void residual (PVR) study** is generally or-

dered when severe obstruction is suspected. If the PVR is greater than approximately 200 ml, the obstruction may be severe, and urology referral is warranted.

2. The **maximum urine flow rate** is often used as a marker of severity. For total voided volumes of 150 ml or more, a maximum flow rate of less than 10 ml/sec is considered low, whereas a rate of more than 15 ml/sec is considered normal.

 TREATMENT. There are three major treatment options: watchful waiting, medical therapy, and surgery.

A. **Watchful waiting** is generally appropriate for patients with mild symptoms. Approximately 50% of patients report improvement without treatment.

B. **Medical therapy**

1. **α Antagonists** decrease the tone of the smooth muscle in the prostate and are usually the first-line treatment for BPH. **Terazosin** is commonly used (initiate therapy with 1 mg orally at bedtime and advance weekly; maximum dose is 20 mg). Patients should be warned that postural hypotension may be a side effect of therapy with these agents, especially with the first few doses.

2. **5α-Reductase inhibitors** should be considered for patients with an enlarged prostate who do not respond to therapy with terazosin. **Finasteride** (5 mg daily) is the only currently available agent.

C. **Surgery** should be considered for patients with severe symptoms and for those who remain symptomatic despite medical therapy. **Transurethral resection of the prostate; transurethral incision;** and **laser, microwave, balloon,** and **stenting procedures** are all effective. No option has proven superiority; the choice of procedure depends on local practice and patient preference.

VI FOLLOW-UP AND REFERRAL

A. Patients with mild symptoms who choose watchful waiting or finasteride treatment can be followed at 3- to 6-month intervals.

B. Treatment with an α antagonist necessitates that the patient be seen 1–3 times over 1–2 months to assess treatment effect and medication side effects.

C. Patients who have signs of impending obstruction (e.g., a palpable bladder, large post-void residual, or severe symptoms) and those who are considering surgical treatment should be referred to a urologist.

References

Lepor H, Williford WO, Barry MJ, et al: The efficacy of terazosin, finasteride, or both in benign prostatic hyperplasia. Veteran Affairs Cooperative Studies Benign Prostatic Hyperplasia Study Group. *New Engl J Med* 335(8):533–539, 1996.

Oesterling JE: Benign prostatic hyperplasia: medically and minimally invasive treatment options. *New Engl J Med* 332(2):99–109, 1995.

VII

Gynecology

45. Amenorrhea

I INTRODUCTION

A. **Primary amenorrhea** is the absence of menses in a patient 16 years or older. An evaluation is started at age 14 if a patient has no signs of secondary sexual characteristics.

B. **Secondary amenorrhea** is the absence of menstrual periods for three consecutive cycles or for 6 months in a woman who had experienced menarche.

II CAUSES OF AMENORRHEA

A. **Primary amenorrhea**

1. **Congenital abnormalities** of the uterus, cervix, or vagina can cause primary amenorrhea.

2. **Pseudohermaphroditism**

   a. **Female pseudohermaphroditism** is the presence of ovarian tissue in a patient with some male morphologic features. **Congenital adrenal hyperplasia** is a common example. In this condition, adrenal hormone (e.g., 21-hydroxylase, 11β-hydroxylase) deficiencies decrease adrenal hydrocortisone production. In response, more adrenocorticotropic hormone (ACTH) is released, causing adrenal hyperplasia and excess androgen production.

   b. **Male pseudohermaphroditism** is the presence of testicular tissue in a patient with female morphologic features. **Testosterone resistance** and **testosterone deficiency** are examples.

3. **Hypothalamic** or **pituitary abnormalities**

   a. Kallmann's syndrome occurs when a deficiency of luteinizing hormone-releasing hormone (LHRH) leads to low luteinizing hormone (LH) and follicle-stimulating hormone (FSH) levels, resulting in primary amenorrhea.

   b. Other causes of abnormal pulsatile LHRH or gonadotropin release (e.g., hypothalamic or pituitary tumors, hypothyroidism, excessive dieting or exercise, stress) can cause primary or secondary amenorrhea.

4. **Ovarian failure**
   a. Primary ovarian failure can be caused by abnormal gonadal development or ovarian dysgenesis. Examples include Turner's syndrome (45,XO karyotype) and chromosomal mosaicism (e.g., 45X/46X,X). A Y chromosome can be present, and is associated with an increased risk for gonadal neoplasm.
   b. Other causes of ovarian failure, which can lead to primary or secondary amenorrhea, include autoimmune destruction and idiopathic ovarian failure.

B. **Secondary amenorrhea**

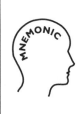

7 Major Causes of Secondary Amenorrhea ("3 + 2 + 1 + 1")

3 Endocrine (hypothalamic or pituitary dysfunction, hyperprolactinemia, thyroid disorder)
2 Ovarian (polycystic ovary syndrome, premature ovarian failure)
1 Uterine (Asherman's syndrome)
1 Obstetric (pregnancy)

1. **Endocrine causes**
   a. **Hypothalamic or pituitary dysfunction**
      (1) Hypothalamic dysfunction, with loss of the normal LHRH pulsatile release, can be caused by stress, heavy exercise, or extreme weight loss (e.g., anorexia nervosa). Hypothalamic masses are rare.
      (2) A pituitary tumor or Sheehan's syndrome (i.e., pituitary necrosis that typically results from postpartum hemorrhage and hypotension) can lead to secondary amenorrhea.
   b. **Hyperprolactinemia** of any cause leads to both pituitary and ovarian dysfunction by disrupting the pulsatile release of FSH and LH. Medications (e.g., tricyclic antidepressants, phenothiazines) or a pituitary tumor can cause hyperprolactinemia.
   c. **Thyroid disorders.** Hypothyroidism (and less commonly, hyperthyroidism) can lead to secondary amenorrhea.

2. **Ovarian causes**
   a. **Polycystic ovary syndrome.** Common features include irregular or absent menses, obesity, hirsutism, infertility, and an LH:FSH ratio greater than 2.
   b. **Premature ovarian failure** is ovarian failure prior to age 40 years accompanied by elevated gonadotropin levels. Autoimmunity, chemotherapy, and radiation are common causes. In women younger than 30 years, a karyotype is necessary to exclude the presence of a Y chromosome (which increases the risk for gonadal neoplasm).
3. **Uterine cause. Asherman's syndrome** (i.e., intrauterine adhesions, usually caused by infection after delivery and curettage) can cause outflow tract obstruction, leading to secondary amenorrhea.
4. **Pregnancy** should be ruled out in all women of reproductive age.

III ▐ APPROACH TO THE PATIENT

A. **Primary amenorrhea.** Perform a physical examination to **evaluate secondary sexual development** and assign the patient to one of the three following groups:
   1. **Normal female secondary sexual characteristics.** The presence of normal female secondary sexual characteristics suggests that the patient has normal levels of estrogen, progesterone, and androgens. A **congenital abnormality of the uterus, cervix,** or **vagina** is the most likely cause.
      a. **Patient history.** Absence of the uterus is usually asymptomatic, whereas an abnormality of the vagina or cervix impairing uterine outflow typically presents with **cyclic crampy pain.**
      b. **Pelvic** and **bimanual examinations** should be performed to assess for congenital abnormalities. If the examination is normal, proceed with work-up of secondary amenorrhea.
   2. **Ambiguous external genitalia (male and female characteristics).** This finding indicates excess androgen exposure *in utero.*
      a. The most common cause of excess androgen exposure *in utero* is **congenital adrenal hyperplasia.** This diagnosis is confirmed by finding elevated **serum dehydroepiandrosterone sulfate (DHEAS)** and **17-OH progesterone levels.**

      b. A less likely cause of ambiguous genitalia is **male** or **female hermaphroditism.** Diagnosis is made by **karyotype.**

   3. **Absent female secondary sexual characteristics.** This finding indicates no prior systemic exposure to estrogen. A serum FSH level distinguishes hypothalamic from ovarian pathology.

      a. A **low** or **normal FSH level** (i.e., < 25 IU/L) indicates a **hypothalamic** or **pituitary abnormality.**

      b. An **elevated FSH level** (i.e., > 25 IU/L) suggests **ovarian failure.** A karyotype analysis should be obtained.

        (1) An **XY karyotype** carries an increased risk of gonadal neoplasm and is treated with gonadectomy and hormone replacement therapy (HRT).

        (2) An **XX karyotype** indicates ovarian insensitivity, premature ovarian failure, or adrenal enzyme deficiency with adrenal hyperplasia.

B. **Secondary amenorrhea**

HOT

KEY

Pregnancy is the most common cause of secondary amenorrhea. A pregnancy test should be performed before undertaking an exhaustive work-up.

   1. **Patient history.** Begin by establishing the pattern of the patient's menses, then think about the seven causes of secondary amenorrhea and use them to guide your questions.

      a. **Pregnancy.** Is the patient sexually active? Does she use contraception, and if so, what form?

      b. **Hypothalamic** or **pituitary dysfunction.** Is there a history of stress, weight loss, or strenuous exercise?

      c. **Hyperprolactinemia.** Has the patient noted galactorrhea? What is the patient's medication history?

      d. **Thyroid disorder.** Does the patient complain of cold intolerance, fatigue, depression, or weight gain? All of these are symptoms of hypothyroidism.

      e. **Polycystic ovarian syndrome.** Is the amenorrhea chronic? Is there a history of obesity or hirsutism?

    f. **Premature ovarian failure.** Has the patient experienced "hot flashes" or atrophic vaginitis?

    g. **Asherman's syndrome.** Does the patient have a history of endometritis, pregnancy, or abortion?

2. Physical examination

    a. Galactorrhea, hirsutism, or thyromegaly may be found on physical examination.

    b. The presence of secondary sexual characteristics (indicating estrogen and progesterone production) should be noted.

    c. A pelvic examination should be performed to assess vaginal patency and uterine or ovarian pathology.

3. Laboratory studies. An algorithm for evaluating secondary amenorrhea is shown in Figure 45–1

HOT **KEY**

Amenorrhea persisting for more than 6 months following the cessation of oral contraceptive use should not be attributed to the oral contraceptives. A work-up for secondary amenorrhea is appropriate for these patients.

 TREATMENT depends on the underlying disorder.

A. Primary amenorrhea

    1. Congenital abnormalities of the uterus, cervix, or **vagina.** Some congenital abnormalities can be treated surgically.

    2. Congenital adrenal hyperplasia is treated with low-dose dexamethasone to suppress production of androgen precursors.

    3. Ovarian failure. Patients with the XY karyotype should have their ovaries removed to reduce the risk of ovarian cancer. All patients with ovarian failure should receive HRT.

B. Secondary amenorrhea

    1. Hypothalamic or **pituitary dysfunction**

    a. Prolactin-secreting tumors can be treated with bromocriptine to suppress prolactin secretion. Other pituitary tumors and prolactinomas that are unresponsive to medical therapy can be resected, either via a transphenoidal approach or, rarely, craniotomy.

    b. Patients with pituitary failure due to neoplasia,

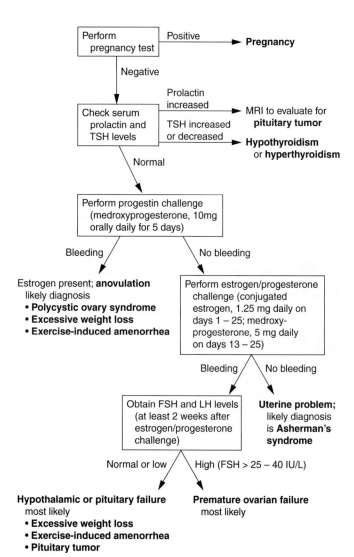

Figure 45-1. Approach to the patient with secondary amenorrhea. *FSH* = follicle-stimulating hormone; *LH* = luteinizing hormone; *MRI* = magnetic resonance imaging; *TSH* = thyroid-stimulating hormone.

Sheehan's syndrome, or other causes require replacement therapy with steroids (i.e., hydrocortisone, 15 mg every morning and 10 mg every evening), thyroid hormone, and estrogen/progesterone.

2. **Polycystic ovarian syndrome.** All patients with polycystic ovarian syndrome benefit from weight loss, which decreases peripheral estrogen formation. In addition, they should receive one of the following three hormonal therapies:
   a. **Oral contraceptives** decrease ovarian androgen production and induce withdrawal bleeding to prevent endometrial hyperplasia.
   b. **Clomiphene** increases FSH production in women who desire fertility.
   c. **Terminal progesterone** induces withdrawal bleeding.

3. **Premature ovarian failure** is treated with ovariectomy (if the patient has an XY karyotype) and HRT.

4. **Asherman's syndrome** is treated with dilatation and curettage (D&C) or lysis of endometrial adhesions, followed by short-term placement of a pediatric Foley catheter or an intrauterine device (IUD) to maintain the endometrial cavity. Estrogens are given to maintain the endometrial lining.

References

Kiningham RB, Apgar BS, Schwenk TL: Evaluation of amenorrhea. *Am Fam Physician* 53(4):1185–1194, 1996.

Warren MP: Clinical review 77: evaluation of secondary amenorrhea. *J Clin Endocrinol Metab* 81(2):437–442, 1996.

46. Abnormal Uterine Bleeding

I. INTRODUCTION

A. A **normal menstrual cycle** lasts 21–35 days, of which 2–7 days involve bleeding. The total blood loss during a normal menstrual cycle is 25–80 milliliters. Any menstrual bleeding outside of these parameters is considered abnormal and should be evaluated.

B. Common terms used to describe **abnormal patterns of menstrual bleeding** are defined in Table 46-1. The terminology can be confusing; it is always appropriate to simply describe the abnormality in terms of the cycle length, days of bleeding, or amount of bleeding.

II. DIFFERENTIAL DIAGNOSIS. Abnormal uterine bleeding can be **pregnancy-related, ovulatory,** or **anovulatory** (Table 46-2).

A. **Pregnancy-related bleeding** occurs in patients who are pregnant or were recently pregnant.

B. **Ovulatory bleeding** is abnormal bleeding in patients who are ovulating normally. Because ovulation requires a functioning endocrine axis, the hypothalamus, pituitary gland, and ovaries are usually normal in these patients. The endometrium cycles normally, with a proliferative (estrogen-dependent) and a secretory (progesterone-dependent) phase. Ovulatory bleeding is usually attributable to either an **anatomic abnormality** of the uterus, cervix, or vagina or a **bleeding disorder** (see Chapter 73).

C. **Anovulatory bleeding** occurs in patients who are not ovulating normally, which usually indicates an abnormality in one of the organs of the endocrine axis. When ovulation does not occur, estrogen is often present for long periods of time without progesterone, leading to the "unopposed estrogen effect." Unopposed estrogen causes the endometrium to continue in the proliferative phase, resulting in periodic shedding of tissue. Bleeding patterns vary, but are often characterized by irregular intervals and irregular amounts.

1. **Hypothalamic-pituitary dysfunction.** Thyroid disease, hyperprolactinemia, excess androgens or cortisol, and stress (emotional, weight loss-related, or exercise-related) can disturb hypothalamic rhythmicity and result in anovulation.

TABLE 46-1. Patterns of Abnormal Uterine Bleeding

Menorrhagia: Prolonged, heavy uterine bleeding occurring at regular intervals

Metrorrhagia: Variable amount of uterine bleeding occuring at frequent, irregular intervals

Menometrorrhagia: Prolonged, heavy uterine bleeding occuring at irregular intervals

Polymenorrhea: Uterine bleeding occuring at regular intervals of less than 21 days

Oligomenorrhea: Uterine bleeding occuring at intervals varying from 35 days to 6 months

Amenorrhea: Absence of uterine bleeding for at least 6 months

Intermenstrual bleeding: Variable amount of uterine bleeding occuring between regular menstrual periods

Dysfunctional uterine bleeding: Abnormal uterine bleeding in which the source is the endometrium; occurs in the absence of anatomic lesions and is most often caused by chronic anovulation

    2. Ovarian dysfunction. Ovarian tumors, polycystic ovary syndrome, or ovarian failure (menopause or premature ovarian failure) may cause anovulatory uterine bleeding.

HOT

KEY

Physiologic anovulatory bleeding accompanies normal aging and occurs in perimenarchal and perimenopausal patients. It is common for adolescent girls to experience anovulation and heavy bleeding for 1–2 years after the onset of menses. Similarly, perimenopausal women have anovulatory cycles that can cause abnormal patterns of bleeding for several years.

III **APPROACH TO THE PATIENT.** Figure 46-1 presents a stepwise approach for evaluating a patient with abnormal uterine bleeding.

  A. Obtain the patient history and perform a general physical examination.
    1. What is the patient's current pattern of menstrual bleeding? Her previous pattern?

TABLE 46-2. Common Causes of Abnormal Uterine Bleeding

Pregnancy-related bleeding
  Ectopic pregnancy
  Threatened or spontaneous abortion
  Retained products of gestation
  Gestational trophoblastic disease
Ovulatory bleeding
  Uterine anomaly
    Uterine carcinoma
    Uterine fibroids
    Uterine polyps
    Adenomyosis
    Foreign body [e.g., intrauterine device (IUD)]
    Sarcoma
  Cervical anomaly
    Cervical carcinoma
    Cervical polyps
    Cervicitis
    Condyloma
    Pelvic inflammatory disease (PID)
    Erosion
    Cervical trauma
  Vaginal anomaly
    Vaginal carcinoma
    Vaginal infection (e.g., vaginitis, herpes)
    Vaginal foreign body
    Vaginal trauma
    Adenosis
  Bleeding disorder
Anovulatory Bleeding
  Hypothalamic-pituitary dysfunction
    Physiologic anovulatory bleeding (perimarchal and
      perimenopausal)
    Thyroid disease
    Hyperprolactinemia
    Stress
    Cushing's syndrome (cortisol excess)
    Adrenal or ovarian tumor (androgen excess)
  Ovarian dysfunction
    Ovarian failure
    Ovarian tumor
    Polycystic ovary disease

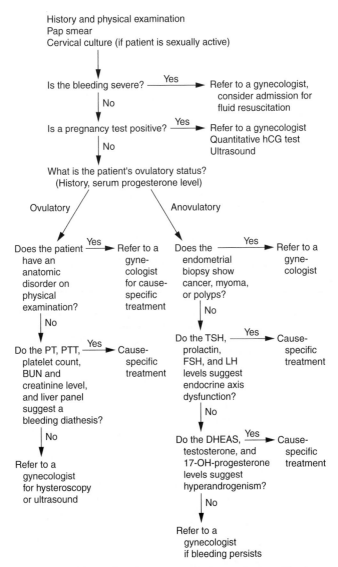

FIGURE 46-1. Approach to the patient with abnormal uterine bleeding. *BUN* = blood urea nitrogen; *DHEAS* = dehydroepiandrosterone sulfate; *FSH* = follicle-stimulating hormone; *LH* = luteinizing hormone; *PT* = prothrombin time; *PTT* = partial thromboplastin time; *TSH* = thyroid-stimulating hormone.

2. Does the patient have any associated symptoms?

HOT KEY

Premenstrual symptoms (e.g., breast tenderness, mood swings, bloating, cramping) accompany ovulation and suggest ovulatory bleeding. Patients with anovulatory cycles often lack premenstrual symptoms.

3. What is the patient's obstetric history, surgical history, past medical history, and medication history?

HOT KEY

Patients who have evidence of severe bleeding on physical examination (e.g., orthostatic vital signs, pallor, brisk bleeding) should be fluid resuscitated, admitted to the hospital, and evaluated emergently by a gynecologist.

B. Attempt to identify an anatomic cause for the bleeding.
   1. Perform a **pelvic examination,** and obtain a **Pap smear.**
   2. Patients who are sexually active should have **cervical cultures** to rule out pelvic inflammatory disease (PID).
C. Narrow the differential diagnosis
   1. Rule out pregnancy-related bleeding by performing a **pregnancy test.** All women of reproductive age with abnormal uterine bleeding should have a pregnancy test. If positive, the patient should be referred to a gynecologist. These patients require a quantitative human chorionic gonadotropin (hCG) level and possibly ultrasonographic evaluation to rule out ectopic pregnancy.
   2. Determine the patient's ovulatory status. The **history** is often suggestive of ovulatory status, obviating the need for laboratory testing. However, if the ovulatory status is in question, a **serum progesterone level** can be obtained 1 week before the next expected menses (during the secretory phase). A level greater than 5 ng/ml indicates that ovulation has occurred.
D. Order additional laboratory and imaging tests as appropriate.
   1. Ovulatory bleeding. These patients should be evaluated for abnormalities of the vagina, cervix, and uterus,

and for bleeding disorders. If a diagnosis is not made after a thorough history, physical examination, and laboratory work-up, referral to a gynecologist is indicated for imaging of the uterus (hysteroscopy or ultrasound).

2. Anovulatory bleeding

   a. Endometrial biopsy. All patients with anovulation of more than 1 year's duration should be considered for endometrial biopsy because unopposed estrogen is a strong risk factor for the development of endometrial cancer.

      (1) The biopsy may reveal cancer, polyps, or myomas. Referral to a gynecologist is indicated for these patients.

      (2) Patients with high estrogen levels usually have a thick endometrium, while those with low estrogen levels have a thin endometrium. A thin endometrium suggests an abnormal endocrine axis.

   b. Evaluate for endocrine axis dysfunction. If the endometrial biopsy does not reveal cancer, polyps, or myoma, patients with chronic anovulation should be evaluated for abnormalities of the endocrine axis organs. The following tests should be ordered:

      (1) Thyroid-stimulating hormone (TSH) level, to evaluate for hypo- and hyperthyroidism

      (2) Prolactin level, to evaluate for hyperprolactinemia

      (3) Follicle-stimulating hormone (FSH) and **luteinizing hormone (LH) levels**

         (a) An FSH level greater than 40 IU/L suggests ovarian failure.

         (b) An LH:FSH ratio of more than 2:1 is compatible with polycystic ovary disease.

   c. Evaluation for hyperandrogenism. A **dehydroepiandrosterone sulfate (DHEAS) level, testosterone level,** and **17-OH progesterone level** should be obtained for patients with a negative endocrine axis evaluation or with signs of hyperandrogenism (e.g., hirsutism, virilization).

      (1) Patients with the rapid onset of hyperandrogenism, elevated testosterone levels, or elevated DHEAS levels may have adrenal or ovarian androgen-producing tumors, and gynecology referral is warranted.

      (2) Elevated DHEAS or 17-OH progesterone levels may indicate an adrenal enzyme deficiency.

IV TREATMENT

A. Ovulatory bleeding. Treatment entails surgical correction of the anatomic abnormality or treatment for the bleeding disorder.

B. Anovulatory bleeding. Definitive treatment depends on the underlying disorder.

    1. Observation is appropriate for perimenarchal patients who have mild bleeding that corrects itself within several months.

    2. Oral contraceptive therapy

        a. Mild to **moderate bleeding** can usually be controlled with combination oral contraceptive pills (i.e., each pill contains both estrogen and progesterone), such as Lo/Ovral, Ortho-Cept, or Desogen. The patient should take 1 tablet daily.

        b. Moderate to **severe bleeding** in a perimenarchal patient can be treated with a 21-day package of combination oral contraceptive pills, each containing 30 μg of estrogen (e.g., Lo/Ovral). The patient should take one pill three times daily for 7 days, and then stop taking the pills for 7 days. Following withdrawal bleeding (often heavy), she can begin another package of pills, this time taking one tablet daily. After 3–6 months, normal cycling usually resumes and the patient can stop therapy with oral contraceptives if she so desires.

        c. Oral contraceptive pills are an effective method of regulating menstrual cycling in patients with chronic anovulation. Possibly advantageous side effects of therapy with oral contraceptives include contraception and reduced hyperandrogenism.

    3. Progesterone therapy

        a. Monthly progesterone therapy may be used for women with chronic anovulation who have contraindications to or do not want to take oral contraceptives. Patients should take 10 mg of medroxyprogesterone acetate daily for 12 days, during the same time each month. This method does not provide contraception.

        b. Monthly progesterone therapy is appropriate for perimenopausal women who present with anovulatory bleeding. When withdrawal bleeding stops (usually after 3–12 months of therapy), the patient has completed menopause (ovarian failure) and should consider hormone replacement therapy (HRT).

HOT

KEY

An endometrial biopsy (to rule out cancer, polyps, or myoma) should be performed prior to initiating progesterone therapy in a perimenopausal woman.

    d. A one-time 12-day course of progesterone may be used for patients without chronic anovulation who have heavy bleeding associated with one anovulatory cycle (once pregnancy has been excluded).

V FOLLOW-UP AND REFERRAL

    A. Follow-up. Patients should be seen every 1–2 weeks until a diagnosis is established and bleeding is satisfactorily controlled.

    B. Referral to a gynecologist is indicated at several points during the work-up of abnormal uterine bleeding (see Figure 46–1), and whenever uncertainty about a diagnosis or management exists.

References

Bayer SR, DeCherney AH: Clinical manifestations and treatment of dysfunctional uterine bleeding. *JAMA* 269(14):1823–1828, 1993.

Jennings JC: Abnormal uterine bleeding. *Med Clin North Am* 79(6):1357–1376, 1995.

47. Pelvic Pain and Dysmenorrhea

I INTRODUCTION

A. **Pelvic pain** accounts for as many as one third of office visits to gynecologists, and it is a common problem seen by primary care providers.

B. **Dysmenorrhea** (i.e., painful menstruation) is experienced by approximately 50% of women and is severe or disabling in 10%.

II DIFFERENTIAL DIAGNOSIS

A. **Acute pelvic pain.** Patients with acute pelvic pain may present with unilateral or bilateral pain, fever, orthostatic vital signs, an elevated white blood cell (WBC) count, or vaginal bleeding or discharge. Causes of acute pelvic pain can be classified as ovarian, tubal, or extrapelvic (i.e., referred pain).

1. **Ovarian causes** include **ovarian torsion** and **ruptured ovarian cyst.**

2. **Tubal causes** include **ectopic pregnancy** and **pelvic inflammatory disease (PID).**

3. **Extrapelvic causes** include **appendicitis, bowel ischemia, kidney stones,** and **urinary tract infection (UTI).**

HOT **KEY** Many of the causes of acute pelvic pain require emergent intervention to prevent serious complications: ectopic pregnancy can result in massive blood loss, PID can result in sepsis and infertility, and ovarian torsion can result in loss of the ovary.

B. **Subacute or chronic pelvic pain** can be categorized as primary dysmenorrhea, secondary dysmenorrhea, or nonmenstrual.

1. **Primary dysmenorrhea** (i.e., **menstrual pain in the absence of underlying organic disease)** is thought to be caused by the production of prostaglandins during menstruation. The prostaglandins cause dysrhythmic muscle contractions, leading to reduced uterine blood flow and endometrial ischemia.

     a. Patients generally begin to experience pain several months after menarche.

     b. The pain begins with the onset of menstrual flow, lasts 2–3 days, and is usually described as a crampy, lower abdominal pain that radiates to the back or inner thigh. Headache, fatigue, and nausea may accompany the pain.

2. **Secondary dysmenorrhea** is menstrual pain that has an **organic cause.** Secondary dysmenorrhea should be suspected in women who begin to have menstrual pain after several years of menstruating without pain. Causes of secondary dysmenorrhea include the following.

     a. **Endometriosis** is the presence of functioning endometrial tissue outside of the uterus (e.g., in the peritoneum, bowel wall, bladder, or ovaries). During the menstrual cycle, hormones can influence this extra-uterine tissue, causing it to undergo changes that cause pain.

     b. **Adenomyosis** is the presence of functioning endometrial tissue in the muscular layers of the uterus. As in endometriosis, hormonal influence may cause growth of this tissue, resulting in pain at the time of menstruation.

     c. **Leiomyomata (uterine fibroids)** are smooth muscle tumors of the uterus that may cause pain with growth.

     d. **Ovarian cysts** may cause pain when they grow rapidly or if they undergo intermittent torsion.

     e. **Congenital abnormalities** can obstruct the normal menstrual flow, leading to fluid accumulation and pressure behind the site of obstruction.

3. **Non-menstrual pelvic pain.** Non-menstrual causes of pelvic pain produce constant or irregular patterns of pain unrelated to the menstrual cycle.

     a. **Gynecologic causes** include **pregnancy, PID,** and **intrauterine device (IUD) use.** Although pregnant women often feel uncomfortable, mildly nauseous, or tired, any new pain requires prompt consultation with a gynecologist.

     b. **Urologic causes** include **UTI** and **kidney stones.**

     c. **Gastrointestinal causes** include **inflammatory bowel disease, irritable bowel syndrome,** and **constipation.**

     d. **Musculoskeletal disorders,** such as abdominal wall or low back muscle strain, can be associated with pelvic pain.

        e. Chronic pelvic pain is pain that lasts longer than 6 months with no clear organic pathology.

HOT

KEY

While it is useful to classify chronic pelvic pain as either cyclic (primary and secondary dysmenorrhea) or non-cyclic (non-menstrual pain), the pattern of pain may vary among individuals with any of the conditions associated with chronic pelvic pain.

III APPROACH TO THE PATIENT

A. Acute pelvic pain

1. **Patient history and physical examination.** A thorough history and physical examination are essential. The approach taken for a patient with acute pelvic pain is similar to that taken for a patient with acute abdominal pain (see Chapter 32 III A-B).

2. **Laboratory studies**

   a. Pregnancy test. If the **urine human chorionic gonadotropin (hCG) pregnancy test** is negative, a **serum hCG level** should be obtained to rule out ectopic pregnancy. (The urine hCG test may remain negative for as long as 6 weeks after conception.)

   b. A **urinalysis, complete blood count (CBC)** and **differential,** and **erythrocyte sedimentation rate (ESR)** are indicated for all patients. The ESR is usually elevated in patients with PID.

3. **Imaging studies. Ultrasound or a computed tomography (CT) scan** of the pelvis is indicated for patients with suspected ectopic pregnancy, appendicitis, or abscess, or when the source of the pain remains unclear.

B. Chronic pelvic pain (Figure 47-1). All patients with chronic pelvic pain should have a thorough **history** and **physical examination,** including a pelvic exam. In addition, all sexually active patients should have a **pregnancy test** and **cervical cultures** for *Neisseria gonorrhoeae* and *Chlamydia trachomatis* (to evaluate for PID). The patient can then be assigned to one of the three diagnostic categories on the basis of this preliminary information.

1. **Primary dysmenorrhea.** If the history, physical examination, cervical cultures, and pregnancy test do not suggest another cause of dysmenorrhea, it is ap-

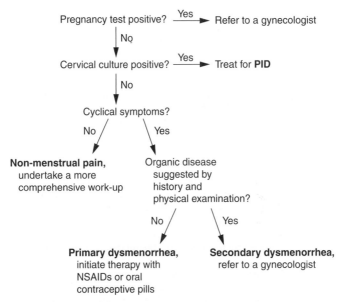

FIGURE 47-1. Approach to the patient with chronic pelvic pain. *NSAIDs* = nonsteroidal anti-inflammatory drugs; *PID* = pelvic inflammatory disease.

propriate to initiate therapy for primary dysmenorrhea.

2. **Secondary dysmenorrhea.** Physical examination findings may help define the cause.
   a. **Endometriosis.** Patients may have focal tenderness on examination and nodularity to palpation of the uterosacral ligaments. The diagnosis can only be established with laparoscopy.
   b. **Congenital abnormalities** may be visualized during speculum examination.
   c. **Leiomyomata** and **ovarian cysts** can often be palpated during bimanual examination.
3. **Non-menstrual pelvic pain**
   a. **Gastrointestinal disorders.** The patient may have a history of constipation (or alternating constipation and diarrhea), nausea, melena, rectal bleeding, or stress-induced symptoms. A more extensive gastrointestinal evaluation is indicated for these patients.

      b. **UTI.** Patients should have a urinalysis and urine culture to rule out UTI.

      c. **PID** is suggested by a history of PID, cervical discharge or cervical motion tenderness on examination, or systemic signs of infection.

      d. **Musculoskeletal pain.** A musculoskeletal source of the pain may be evident on examination (i.e., the lower abdominal or pelvic floor muscles may reveal isolated tenderness).

IV TREATMENT

A. **PID** may be treated on an outpatient basis if the patient is not pregnant or febrile, has no signs of abscess or peritonitis, and is able to tolerate and comply with oral antibiotic therapy. Antibiotic regimens must cover *C. trachomatis* and *N. gonorrhoeae;* one typical regimen is **ceftriaxone,** 250 mg administered intramuscularly once, followed by **doxycycline,** 100 mg orally twice daily for 14 days.

B. **Primary dysmenorrhea**

    1. **Nonsteroidal anti-inflammatory drugs (NSAIDs)** are the initial treatment of choice. One common regimen is oral **naproxen,** 500 mg taken as needed (up to a maximum dose of 1000 mg daily) for the first 2–3 days of menstruation.

    2. **Oral contraceptive pills.** Patients who do not respond to therapy with NSAIDs or who desire contraception can be treated with oral contraceptive pills, which are extremely effective at reducing symptoms.

C. **Secondary dysmenorrhea.** Medical treatment (usually with oral contraceptive pills) is often used to manage many of the conditions that can cause secondary dysmenorrhea, but surgical options are available and may be more appropriate for patients desiring pregnancy (some of the conditions can affect fertility). Patients should be referred to a gynecologist for therapy.

D. **Non-menstrual pelvic pain.** Treatment is cause-specific.

    1. **PID** and **UTI** are treated with appropriate antibiotics.

    2. An **IUD** suspected of causing irritation can be removed.

    3. **Constipation** and **irritable bowel syndrome** may respond to fiber supplementation.

    4. **Chronic pelvic pain,** which is a diagnosis of exclusion, is an incompletely understood syndrome that is best managed with gynecology consultation. Patients may respond to a variety of medical, surgical, and psychosocial treatments.

V FOLLOW-UP AND REFERRAL

A. **Pregnant patients** with acute pelvic pain and patients with suspected **ovarian torsion** require **immediate gynecologic consultation.**

B. Patients with **gastrointestinal symptoms** or **evidence of peritonitis** on physical examination (e.g., rebound, rigidity, guarding) may require imaging [e.g., ultrasound, computed tomography (CT)] and **immediate surgical consultation.**

References

Lipscomb GH, Ling FW: Chronic pelvic pain. *Med Clin North Am* 79(6):1411–1425, 1995.

48. Abnormal Vaginal Discharge

I INTRODUCTION

A. Most often, abnormal vaginal discharge is attributable to **vaginitis** (i.e., inflammation of the vaginal wall), which is almost always caused by one of three common infections: **bacterial vaginosis, candidiasis,** or **trichomoniasis.**

B. Normal vaginal secretions are generally clear or white, odorless, and viscous. An **abnormal discharge** is usually **yellow, gray,** or **green** and **increased in volume,** and is usually accompanied by **itching, vulvar irritation, dyspareunia, dysuria,** or **vaginal odor.**

II DIFFERENTIAL DIAGNOSIS. Abnormal vaginal discharge can be caused by any process that increases or alters secretions from the **vagina, cervix,** or **uterus** (Table 48–1) .

A. **Vaginitis**

1. Infectious vaginitis is the most common cause of abnormal vaginal discharge.

   a. **Bacterial vaginosis,** the most common cause of vaginitis, results from a **disturbance in the normal vaginal flora.** An overgrowth of anaerobes and Gram-negative bacteria (e.g., *Gardnerella vaginalis, Bacteroides* species, *Peptostreptococcus* species, *Mycoplasma hominis*) leads to an increase in the vaginal pH. Patients may be asymptomatic, or they may complain of **itching,** a **"fishy" odor,** or a **whitish discharge.**

   b. *Candida vulvovaginitis,* the second most common cause of vaginitis, is caused by *Candida albicans,* a fungus.

      (1) Patients usually present with a **white, curdlike discharge; vulvar** or **vaginal erythema;** and **itching.**

      (2) **Risk factors** for symptomatic infection include **pregnancy, oral contraceptive use, diabetes, antibiotic** or **corticosteroid use,** and **tight-fitting clothing.**

   c. *Trichomonas* **vaginitis** is caused by the flagellated protozoan, *Trichomonas vaginalis.*

      (1) Patients may be asymptomatic, or they may

TABLE 48-1. Differential Diagnosis of Abnormal Vaginal Discharge

Infectious vaginitis
    Bacterial vaginosis
    Candida vulvovaginitis
    Trichomonas vaginitis
Allergic vaginitis
Atrophic vaginitis
Cervicitis and pelvic inflammatory disease (PID)
    Neisseria gonorrhoeae
    Chlamydia trachomatis
Herpes simplex virus (HSV) infection
Human papillomavirus (HPV) infection (condyloma acuminatum)
Cervical cancer
Endometrial disease (cancer, polyps, foreign body)

---

present with a **copious yellow** or **green frothy discharge, vaginal erythema** and **itching, dysuria, dyspareunia,** or a **"strawberry cervix"** (i.e., reddening and petechial hemorrhage of the cervix, a rare finding).

    (2) Although the infection is **most often sexually transmitted,** it may be acquired from clothing or water.

  2. Allergic vaginitis. Topical creams, such as spermicides, can induce an allergic vaginitis.

  3. Atrophic vaginitis, a common cause of discharge in older women, occurs when lack of estrogen stimulation leads to atrophy and friability of the vagina.

B. Cervicitis and **pelvic inflammatory disease (PID),** which are caused by *Neisseria gonorrhoeae* or *Chlamydia trachomatis* infection, may be associated with increased cervical secretions, leading to a vaginal discharge. Cervicitis and PID are usually associated with **cervical motion** or **adnexal tenderness** and a **purulent cervical discharge.**

C. Herpes simplex virus (HSV) and **human papillomavirus (HPV) infections** can be associated with vaginal discharge. Both have characteristic lesions that are usually visible during a speculum examination.

D. Cervical cancer and **endometrial disease** are rare but important causes of vaginal discharge.

III **APPROACH TO THE PATIENT.** The goal is to determine whether the discharge is attributable to vaginitis, or to a less common, but potentially more dangerous, condition.

- **A. Patient history.** A thorough history is essential. Areas to focus on include the following:
    1. **Nature of the discharge** (i.e., the amount, color, duration, and odor)
    2. **Associated symptoms** (e.g., itching, dysuria, dyspareunia, abdominal pain, fever)
    3. **Gynecologic history** (i.e., sexual history, menstrual history, prior episodes of discharge)
    4. **Medication history**
    5. **Medical history** (i.e., chronic diseases)
- **B. Physical examination**
    1. A **speculum examination** should be performed to examine the cervix for discharge, polyps, or lesions suggestive of herpes, condyloma acuminatum, or cervical dysplasia. Cervicitis is present if a swab inserted into the cervical canal shows a yellow or green exudate.
    2. A **bimanual examination** that reveals adnexal, uterine, or cervical motion tenderness suggests PID as the cause of the discharge.
- **C. Laboratory studies**
    1. A swab of the secretions should be taken from the vagina and placed on two separate microscope slides.
        a. **Potassium hydroxide (KOH) preparation ("whiff" test).** A drop of KOH should be added to one slide. A fishy odor in response to the KOH suggests bacterial vaginosis.
        b. **Wet preparation.** Normal saline should be added to the other slide, and the pH of the discharge should be measured. A pH greater than 4.5 suggests bacterial vaginosis.
    2. **Microscopic examination.** Both slides should be examined microscopically. A microscopic slide that meets the diagnostic criteria given in Table 48-2 is helpful for ruling in the disease, but a slide that does not reveal a suspected pathogen does not rule out the disease.
    3. **Culture** is much more sensitive than microscopic examination for detecting *Candida* and *Trichomonas* infections.

TABLE 48-2. Diagnostic Criteria for Common Causes of Infectious Vaginitis

Diagnosis	Diagnostic Criteria
Bacterial vaginosis	Amsel criteria* 1. pH > 4.5 2. Clue cells on wet preparation 3. Positive "whiff" test 4. Thin, white, homogenous discharge
Candida vulvovaginitis	Hyphae or budding spores on KOH preparation OR Positive culture
Trichomonas vaginitis	Motile trichomonads on wet preparation OR Positive culture

KOH = potassium hydroxide.
*Three of the four criteria must be met.

HOT

KEY

Because the three most common causes of infectious vaginitis have similar signs and symptoms, it is important to follow the diagnostic criteria given in Table 48-2 in order to avoid diagnostic error and incorrect treatment.

IV TREATMENT

A. **Infectious vaginitis** is treated with **antibiotics.** Several common regimens for each of the three types of infectious vaginitis are given in Table 48-3 .

HOT

KEY

Before initiating treatment, always determine if the patient is pregnant, because some of the medications are contraindicated in pregnancy.

TABLE 48-3. Selected Therapeutic Regimens for Infectious Vaginitis

Condition	Drug	Form	Dosage
Bacterial vaginosis*	Metronidazole[†]	Oral	500 mg twice daily for 7 days
			OR
			2 g given as one dose
	Clindamycin	0.75% Gel	5 g intravaginally twice daily for 5 days
		Oral	300 mg twice daily for 7 days
		2% Cream	5 g intravaginally at bedtime for 7 days
Candida vulvovaginitis[‡]	Clotrimazole	500-mg vaginal tablet	1 tablet once
		200-mg vaginal tablet	1 tablet at bedtime for 3 days
		100-mg vaginal tablet	1 tablet at bedtime for 7 days
	Miconazole	200-mg vaginal tablet	1 tablet at bedtime for 3 days
		100-mg vaginal tablet	1 tablet at bedtime for 7 days
	Butonconazole	2% cream	5 g intravaginally at bedtime for 3 days
	Terconazole	0.8% cream	5 g intravaginally at bedtime for 3 days
	Fluconazole[§]	Oral	150 mg given as one dose
Trichomonas vaginitis**	Metronidazole[†]	Oral	2 g given as one dose
			OR
			500 mg given twice daily for 7 days
	Clindamycin	0.75% Gel	5 g intravaginally twice daily for 7 days
		2% cream	5 g intravaginally twice daily for 7 days

*Need for treatment in pregnant patients is controversial.
[†]Metronidazole is contraindicated in the first trimester of pregnancy and should not be taken with alcohol.
[‡]Patients in the first trimester of pregnancy should not undergo treatment for Candida vulvovaginitis.
[§]Fluconazole should not be used during pregnancy.
**Treat the patient and her partner.

B. **Atrophic vaginitis** can be treated with **topical estrogen cream** (2–4 g intravaginally daily for 2 weeks) or with **hormone replacement therapy (HRT),** if contraindications do not exist.

C. **PID.** The treatment of PID is discussed in Chapter 47 IV A.

D. **Cervicitis, HSV infection,** and **HPV infection.** Treatment is discussed in Chapter 81.

V FOLLOW-UP AND REFERRAL

A. **Follow-up.** Patients who respond appropriately to therapy do not require scheduled follow-up.

B. **Referral**
   1. When the diagnosis cannot be established or the abnormal discharge persists despite therapy, referral to a gynecologist is indicated.
   2. Patients with suspected cervical cancer or endometrial disease require prompt referral to a gynecologist.

References

Reed BD, Eyler A: Vaginal infections: diagnosis and management. *Am Fam Physician* 47(8):1805–1816, 1993.

Reife CM: Office gynecology for the primary care physician, part I: vaginitis, the Papanicolaou smear, contraception, and postmenopausal estrogen replacement. *Med Clin North Am* 80(2):299–319, 1996.

49. Urinary Incontinence

I. INTRODUCTION

A. **Urinary incontinence** is **involuntary urine voiding** that presents a **social** or **hygienic problem for the patient** because of the **frequency** with which the incontinence occurs or the **amount of urine** lost with each episode.

B. **Incidence and epidemiology.** The prevalence of urinary incontinence is difficult to assess because many patients are hesitant to discuss the subject with their physicians.

1. It is estimated that **8–12 million people** in the United States are affected.

2. Urinary incontinence is **more common with aging:** 15%–30% of elderly people in the community and at least 50% of patients in nursing homes are affected.

HOT KEY

Always ask elderly patients if they have urinary incontinence.

C. **Physiology of voiding**

1. **Bladder wall.** The **detrusor muscle** forms the bladder wall and consists of three layers of smooth muscle.

   a. **Parasympathetic stimulation** causes the detrusor muscle to contract. **Voiding** is initiated via a reflex arc from the brain stem nucleus, and can be inhibited by higher cortical control.

   b. **Sympathetic** (β-adrenergic) stimulation stretches the bladder dome and relaxes the detrusor muscle.

2. **Bladder neck** and **proximal urethra. Sympathetic (α-adrenergic)** stimulation causes the bladder neck to contract, maintaining normal continence.

3. **Pelvic floor muscles.** The skeletal muscle of the pelvic floor is under **voluntary control** via the **pudendal nerve.** Contraction of the pelvic floor muscles prevents

emptying of the bladder when the intra-abdominal pressure increases.

II DIFFERENTIAL DIAGNOSIS

A. **Acute urinary incontinence**. The causes of acute urinary incontinence can be remembered with the mnemonic, "DAMN DRIPS."

Causes of Acute Urinary Incontinence ("DAMN DRIPS")

Delirium
Atrophic urethritis or vaginitis
Medications— e.g., sedative-hypnotics, diuretics, anticholinergics, α-adrenergic agonists or antagonists
Neurologic disorders— e.g., cord compression, cauda equina syndrome

Diabetes mellitus or insipidus
Restricted mobility
Infection— urinary tract infection (UTI)
Psychiatric disorders— e.g., depression
Stool impaction

B. **Chronic urinary incontinence**
   1. **Urge incontinence. Detrusor hyperreflexia** (i.e., involuntary detrusor contraction due to an underlying neurologic disorder) or **instability** (i.e., involuntary detrusor contraction without an underlying neurologic disorder) is characterized by the sudden urge to void.
   2. **Stress incontinence.** Weakening of the pelvic floor muscles can result from **aging, multiparity,** or **surgical** or **neurologic impairment of the bladder neck.** These patients experience incontinence when their intra-abdominal pressure increases (e.g., when they laugh or cough).
   3. **Overflow incontinence.** Bladder outlet obstruction (e.g., as a result of **prostate enlargement)** or decreased detrusor contraction (e.g., as a result of **diabetic neuropathy)** causes the bladder to fill to distention and then overflow.

HOT

KEY

The elderly often have mixed incontinence (i.e., multiple mechanisms contribute).

III **APPROACH TO THE PATIENT**

A. Patient history

    1. Acute urinary incontinence. The goal of history-taking is to rule out precipitating causes.

    2. Chronic urinary incontinence. Attempt to classify the patient's incontinence as urge incontinence, stress incontinence, or overflow incontinence.

B. Physical examination. Special attention should be given to the following areas:

    1. Abdominal examination. Palpate for bladder distention.

    2. Rectal examination. Look for stool impaction and assess rectal tone.

    3. Pelvic examination. Look for genital atrophy (evidenced by dryness and loss of pubic hair); bladder, rectal, or uterine prolapse; and pelvic masses.

    4. Neurologic examination

        a. A motor and sensory examination and gait testing should be performed to assess for underlying neurologic disorders (e.g., stroke, multiple sclerosis).

        b. A mental status evaluation may reveal cognitive problems that could impair the patient's ability to recognize the need to void.

HOT

KEY

Spinal cord compression (e.g., from metastatic cancer) should always be considered in patients with acute urinary incontinence.

    5. Provocative stress test. With a full bladder, the patient is asked to cough while in the standing or lithotomy position. Instant urinary incontinence is diagnostic of stress urinary incontinence, while delayed or persis-

TABLE 49-1. Pharmacological Therapy of Urinary Incontinence

Type of Incontinence	Agent	Dosing Regimen
Urge incontinence	Oxybutynin	2.5–5.0 mg at bedtime, may increase to three times daily
	Propantheline	7.5–30 mg, 3–5 times daily
	Imipramine	Start with 10–25 mg at bedtime; increase as needed to 25–150 mg at bedtime
	Estrogens (oral, transdermal or topical)	See regimens given for stress incontinence
Stress incontinence	Phenylpropanolamine	25–50 mg, up to 4 times daily
	Estrogens (oral, transdermal, or topical)	Conjugated estrogen, 2 g intravaginally daily for 14 days, then twice weekly
		OR
		Conjugated estrogen, 0.3–1.25 mg orally daily (with a progesterone in women who have not had a hysterectomy)*
	Imipramine	Start with 10–25 mg at bedtime; increase as needed to 25–150 mg at bedtime
Overflow incontinence	Bethanechol	20–100 mg, 4 times daily
	Terazosin	1–10 mg daily†
	Prazosin	3–12 mg, divided, 2 or 3 times daily‡

*Many other regimens are available.
†Increase dose as tolerated.
‡Patient should take first dose (1 mg) while still supine.

tent urinary incontinence suggests detrusor instability (i.e., urge urinary incontinence).

C. **Laboratory studies**
   1. **Urinalysis.** Urine should be evaluated for white blood cells (WBCs), bacteria, glucose, occult blood, and protein.
   2. **Blood work.** Evaluate the blood urea nitrogen (BUN), creatinine and glucose levels.

D. **Post-void residual (PVR) study.** A PVR study is usually performed in patients with suspected overflow incontinence [e.g., an elderly man with benign prostatic hyperplasia (BPH)]. A PVR of less than 50 ml is normal, while a PVR greater than 200 ml is considered abnormal. Intermediate values (i.e., a PVR of 50–200 ml) may be abnormal and must be interpreted on an individual basis.

IV TREATMENT

A. **Nonpharmacologic therapy**
   1. **Scheduling regimens** (i.e., behavioral therapy) are primarily used for patients with **urge urinary incontinence.** Patients are advised to void at regular intervals to avoid excessive filling of the bladder.
   2. **Pelvic floor muscle exercises (Kegel exercises)** are primarily used for patients with **stress urinary incontinence.** Patients are taught to contract the periurethral, perianal, and perivaginal muscles simultaneously. A typical regimen is 20 contractions four times daily.
   3. **Urinary collection devices.** Patients who remain symptomatic despite other therapies may benefit form urinary collection devices (e.g., condom catheters, special undergarments).

B. **Pharmacologic** therapy is summarized in Table 49-1.

V FOLLOW-UP AND REFERRAL. Patients should be referred to a urologist in the following situations:

A. Failure of medical therapy
B. Hematuria, when a cause cannot be identified
C. Cause of incontinence unclear
D. Comorbidities related to urinary incontinence (e.g., recurrent UTI, persistent irritative voiding symptoms)

References
Urinary Incontinence Guideline Panel: Urinary incontinence in adults: clinical practice guideline (AHCPR Pub. No. 92–0038). Rockville, MD, Agency for Health Care Policy and Research, Public Health Service, United States Department of Health and Human Services, March, 1992.

50. Contraception

I INTRODUCTION

A. Many different methods of contraception are available. In order to help patients who seek contraception make the most appropriate choice, primary care physicians must be familiar with the risks and benefits associated with each method. Whenever there is uncertainty about the most appropriate choice, consultation with a gynecologist is recommended.

B. Physicians should assume an active role in counseling and should not rely on patients to introduce the topic of contraception. The value of preventing unwanted pregnancy and sexually transmitted diseases (STDs) cannot be overemphasized.

II CONTRACEPTIVE METHODS.
Table 50-1 lists the common methods of reversible contraception along with the failure rates, advantages, and disadvantages associated with each. The methods of birth control can be remembered using the mnemonic "COITUS."

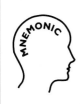

Birth Control Methods ("COITUS")

Condoms and other barrier methods
Oral contraceptives and other hormonal methods
Intrauterine device (IUD)
Timing methods
Unprotected (coitus interruptus)
Surgical methods

A. Barrier methods

1. **Condoms.** Latex condoms offer significant protection against STDs (including HIV), and should be recommended to all sexually active patients who are not in a monogamous relationship where both partners are known to be free of STDs.

   a. Condoms made from animal intestines do not offer the same protection against STDs.

   b. The female condom has a higher failure rate than

TABLE 50-1. Contraceptive Methods

Method	Mechanism of Action	Failure rate* Typical Use	Perfect Use	Disadvantages	Advantages
No method	. . .	85%	. . .	. . .	. . .
Periodic abstinence	Avoidance of coitus during presumed fertile days	20%	. . .	. . .	. . .
Spermicide alone	Inactivation of sperm	21%	6%	Vaginal irritation	May protect against some STDs
Cervical cap with spermicide	Mechanical barrier, inactivation of sperm	18%	12%	Cervical irritation, may be difficult to fit, Pap smear abnormalities	Protection against STDs
Diaphragm with spermicide	Mechanical barrier, inactivation of sperm	18%	6%	Cervical irritation, increased risk of urinary tract infection	Protection against STDs

Method	Mechanism			Disadvantages	Advantages
Condom	Mechanical barrier				
Male		12%	3%	Allergic reactions	Protection against STDs
Female		21%	5%	Difficult to insert, poor acceptability	Protection against STDs, protection of the external genitalia
Oral contraceptives					
Combined	Suppression of ovulation, changes in cervical mucus and endometrium	3%	0.1%	Thromboembolism and stroke (rare), myocardial infarction in older smokers, nausea, headache, depression	Protection against ovarian and endometrial cancer, PID, fibrocystic breast disease, ovarian cysts, iron-deficiency anemia, and dysmenorrhea
Progestin-only	Changes in cervical mucus and endometrium, possibly suppression of ovulation	3%	0.5%	Irregular, unpredictable bleeding in some	Protection against PID, iron-deficiency anemia, and dysmenorrhea

continued

TABLE 50-1. Contraceptive Methods

Method	Mechanism of Action	Failure rate* Typical Use	Perfect Use	Disadvantages	Advantages
Intrauterine devices Progesterone T (Progestastert)	Inhibition of sperm migration, fertilization, and ovum transport	2%	1.5%	Increased incidence of ectopic pregnancy	Decrease in menstrual blood loss and dysmenorrhea
Copper T 380A (ParaGard)	Same mechanism of action as progesterone T device	0.8%	0.6%	Uterine perforation (rare), increase in menstrual blood loss	Can be left in place for 10 years
Medroxyprogesterone acetate (Depo-Provera)	Suppression of ovulation, changes in cervical mucus and endometrium	0.3%	0.3%	Menstrual irregularities, headache, weight gain, acne	Effective for 3 months
Levonorgestrel subdermal implants (Norplant)	Similar to progestin-only oral contraceptives	0.09%	0.09%	Menstrual irregularities, headache, weight gain, acne, removal problems	Ease of use, reversibility, effective for 5 years

Modified with permission from The Medical Letter: Choice of contraceptives. *Med Lett Drugs Ther* 37 (941):9, 1995.
PID = pelvic inflammatory disease; STDs = sexually transmitted diseases.
*Percent accidental pregnancy during first year of use. Modified from RA Hatcher, et al: *Contraceptive Technology,* 16th ed. New York, Irvington, 1994, p 113.

the male condom, but does protect the external female genitalia from STDs.

2. **Diaphragms** and **cervical caps** must be fitted by a trained physician. Proper use is associated with a decreased risk of STDs, although failure rates are considerably higher than with many other methods.

   a. Spermicide must be applied to the cervical side of the barrier.

   b. The device should be left in place for 6–8 hours after intercourse.

B. **Hormonal methods**

1. **Oral contraceptive pills.** Physicians should be familiar with the many different types of oral contraceptive pills (Table 50-2). Patients respond to these medications differently, and it may be necessary to change to a different type of oral contraceptive pill to minimize unwanted side effects.

   a. **Mechanism of action.** Oral contraceptive pills are available in **two main formulations:** combination (estrogen plus progesterone) or progesterone-only.

      (1) **Combination pills** prevent ovulation by suppressing the mid-cycle luteinizing hormone (LH) surge. The progesterone component increases the viscosity of the cervical mucus and changes the characteristics of the endometrium to decrease implantation.

         (a) Combination pills are available in triphasic formulations, which vary the dose of estrogen, progesterone, or both throughout the cycle with the goal of decreasing the total hormone dose without decreasing efficacy.

         (b) Newer, more potent progestins (e.g., norgestimate, desogestrel) are being used in combination pills in lower doses and may be associated with fewer side effects.

      (2) **Progesterone-only pills** are as efficacious as combination pills, but they do not prevent ovulation and therefore may be associated with higher rates of ectopic pregnancy.

   b. **Side effects**

      (1) **Nausea, breast tenderness,** and **fluid retention** are often associated with the estrogen component. **Increased appetite, depression, fatigue, acne,** and **hirsutism** may be associated with the progestin component.

TABLE 50-2. Selected Oral Contraceptive Pills

Type	Brand Names	Estrogen Dose	Progestin Dose	Comments
Combination Pills				
Monophasic formulations	Ortho-Novum 1/35, Norinyl 1 + 35	35 μg	1 mg norethindrone	Now less commonly used due to the development of newer pills containing lower doses of progesterone
	Nordette, Levlen	30 μg	0.15 mg levonorgestrel	
	Lo/Ovral	30 μg	0.3 mg norgestrel	
Triphasic formulations	Triphasil, Tri-Levlen	30 μg	0.5 mg levonorgestrel (days 1–6)	Fewer progesterone-associated side effects† (as compared with monophasic formulations); multiple pill types may make dosing more confusing
		40 μg	0.075 mg levonorgestrel (days 7–11)	
		30 μg	0.125 mg levonorgestrel (days 12–21)	
	Ortho-Novum 7/7/7	35 μg	0.5 mg norethindrone (days 1–7)	

		35 μg	0.75 mg norethindrone (days 8–14) 1 mg norethindrone (days 15–21)	
Formulations containing the new progestins	Ortho-Cept, Desogen Ortho-Cyclen	30 μg 35 μg	0.15 mg desogestrel 0.25 mg norgestimate	Least androgenic of the combination pills (may cause less acne and hirsutism)
Progesterone-only pills	Micronor, Nor-QD Ovrette	. . . . . .	0.35 mg norethindrone 0.075 mg norgestrel	Associated with more breakthrough bleeding, but fewer of the estrogen-dependent side effects‡

*Estrogen component is ethinyl estradiol.
†Progesterone-associated side effects include increased appetite, depression, fatigue, acne, and hirsutism.
‡Estrogen-associated side effects include nausea, breast tenderness, and fluid retention.

       (2) Breakthrough bleeding commonly occurs with both combination and progesterone-only pills during the first 3 months of use. The breakthrough bleeding usually becomes much less frequent with combination pills, but may persist with progesterone-only pills. If irregular bleeding persists beyond 3 months, patients should be evaluated for other causes of abnormal bleeding (see Chapter 46).

       (3) Increased blood pressure. The patient's blood pressure should be monitored for the first few months after the patient begins to take oral contraceptive pills, and annually thereafter.

       (4) Headache. Oral contraceptive pill use may be associated with an increased frequency of headaches in some women. Patients presenting with headache require a thorough evaluation. Patients with persistent headaches may do better with another form of birth control or a switch to progesterone-only pills.

  c. **Advantages.** Oral contraceptive pills are associated with a number of important health benefits, in addition to having a low failure rate.

       (1) Both combination and progesterone-only pills decrease dysmenorrhea and the amount of uterine bleeding, leading to decreased iron-deficiency anemia among users. In addition, oral contraceptive use lowers the risk of ectopic pregnancy and pelvic inflammatory disease (PID).

       (2) Combination oral contraceptive pills are associated with a decreased risk of ovarian cancer, endometrial cancer, and fibrocystic breast disease.

  d. **Risks**

       (1) Studies that have examined the risk of **breast cancer** in users of oral contraceptive pills have yielded contradictory results. Women at high risk for breast cancer may wish to use another method of contraception.

       (2) Oral contraceptive pills should not be prescribed to women older than 35 years who smoke, because these women are at risk for **myocardial infarction.** Oral contraceptive pills in the currently used formulations are generally not thought to increase the risk of cardiovascular disease among patients who do not smoke.

e. **Contraindications.** Major contraindications to oral contraceptive pill use include:

   (1) A history of thromboembolic disorder, stroke, myocardial infarction, breast cancer, estrogen-dependent tumors, liver disease, or gallbladder disease

   (2) Pregnancy and breast-feeding

2. **Medroxyprogesterone acetate (Depo-Provera) injections** are a very effective means of contraception.

   a. **Mechanism of action.** Medroxyprogesterone acetate suppresses ovulation, thickens the cervical mucus, and alters the endometrial lining to prevent pregnancy.

   b. **Administration.** Medroxyprogesterone acetate (150 mg subcutaneously) is administered once every 12 weeks.

      (1) Although the injections are effective for 14 weeks, they are generally given every 12 weeks so that the woman has a 2-week "grace period" if she misses her appointment.

      (2) The injection should take place within 5 days of the onset of menses. Women who are more than 2 weeks late for their injections should have pregnancy excluded before re-injection.

   c. **Side effects**

      (1) **Irregular bleeding** and **spotting** occurs in almost all women using medroxyprogesterone acetate. After several months of use, the incidence of spotting decreases, and **amenorrhea** is common.

HOT

KEY

The amenorrhea associated with medroxyprogesterone acetate use can cause anxiety for patients, who may believe they are pregnant.

---

      (2) **Weight gain** of 2–7 pounds (1–3 kilograms) is common, and **headache, bloating, fatigue, depression,** and **decreased libido** have also been reported.

HOT

KEY

Fertility may be delayed for as long as 1 year after stopping medroxyprogesterone acetate injections.

       d. **Risks.** Medroxyprogesterone acetate injections are not known to increase the risk of breast, ovarian, or endometrial cancer.

   3. **Levonorgestrel subdermal implants (Norplant)**

       a. **Mechanism of action.** Norplant is a device consisting of six Silastic implants that slowly release levonorgestrel over 5 years, providing excellent contraceptive efficacy.

       b. **Side effects.** The major side effect is **irregular bleeding** and **spotting,** which occurs initially in most patients, but becomes less common after the first year.

       c. **Risks.** The risk of gynecologic malignancy in Norplant users is not known.

 C. **Intrauterine devices (IUDs)** are one of the most effective contraceptive methods available.

   1. The **copper T 380A device** causes a sterile inflammatory response in the endometrium that is thought to be spermicidal. It is approved for 10 years of use.

   2. The **progesterone T device** alters the endometrial lining and thickens the cervical mucus and is approved for 1 year of use.

HOT

KEY

IUDs should not be used in patients who are at risk for bacterial endocarditis because they may cause transient bacteremia.

 D. **Surgical methods** include **vasectomy** and **tubal ligation.** Vasectomy is a less invasive procedure and is associated with fewer complications. Both are very effective methods of **permanent sterilization.** Patients should be advised about the availability of reversible contraception, and should clearly understand the permanency of these procedures.

III   FOLLOW-UP AND REFERRAL

A. **After initiating any new method of contraception, all patients** (including those who have chosen barrier methods) **should have scheduled follow-up,** generally within 2–12 weeks. **Improper use of contraceptives is one of the most common reasons for failure.**

B. Patients who are having **persistent side effects** caused by a hormonal method of contraception may benefit from consultation with a gynecologist.

C. Patients who opt for **Norplant** or an **IUD** must see a physician who is trained in the insertion of these devices.

References

Kaunitz AM, Illions EH, Jones JL, et al: Contraception: a clinical review for the internist. *Med Clin North Am* 79(6):1377–1405, 1995.

The Medical Letter: Choice of contraceptives. *Med Lett Drugs Ther* 37 (941):9–12, 1995.

PART VIII

Orthopedics and Rheumatology

51. Approach to Joint Aspiration and Joint Injections

I INTRODUCTION

A. **Joint aspiration (arthrocentesis).** Aspiration of fluid from an inflamed joint can be both diagnostic and therapeutic. Arthrocentesis is the best way to differentiate among infectious, traumatic, inflammatory, degenerative, and metabolic causes of joint disease.

B. **Joint injection.** Intra-articular injection of steroids — once infection has been excluded — can provide substantial pain relief. Most rheumatologists limit patients to four joint injections per joint per year, although there is little evidence that more frequent injections are harmful.

II TECHNIQUE

A. **Preliminary steps**
   1. **Sterile preparation of the area.** Clean the overlying skin with antiseptic, then palpate the area through a sterile gauze pad. Sterile gloves are not necessary.
   2. **Anesthesia** is optional. If desired, **ethyl chloride vapo-coolant** can be applied topically, or **1% lidocaine** can be administered subcutaneously.

B. **Joint aspiration**
   1. **Assemble your materials.**
      a. **Needles.** A 20-gauge, 1.5-inch needle is sufficient for most aspirations, although aspiration of pus may require a larger (i.e., 18-gauge) needle.
      b. **Syringes** with a capacity of 2–20 milliliters are preferable. Larger syringes are more cumbersome and are not as effective at removing fluid.
   2. **Quickly introduce the needle, aspirating gently until synovial fluid begins to flow.**
      a. If the needle hits cartilage or bone, withdraw the needle partially and reposition it.
      b. Aspirate as much fluid as possible; if necessary, milk fluid toward the needle from another site.
   3. **Send the aspirated joint fluid for cell count, Gram staining, culture,** and **crystal analysis.** If no obvious

fluid is obtained, save the material from the needle lumen for culture and crystal analysis.

HOT

KEY

Joint infection as a result of arthrocentesis is extremely rare; nevertheless, worsening pain and swelling after arthrocentesis should raise the concern of an infection.

C. **Therapeutic steroid injection**
   1. **Steroid preparations** include **triamcinolone** (the longest acting preparation), **prednisolone,** and **methyl-prednisolone.**
      a. The dose depends on the size of the joint. For example, 20–40 mg are used for a large joint such as a knee; less is used for smaller joints.
      b. A local anesthetic, such as 1–2 ml of 1% lidocaine or 1–2 ml of 0.5% bupivacaine, can be added to the steroid to provide immediate relief of pain until the anti-inflammatory properties of the steroid takes effect.
   2. **Technique.** Care must be taken to avoid injecting the steroid into tendons or ligaments. Injection should require very little pressure. If resistance is met, withdraw the needle and reposition it until the steroid flows freely into the joint.

HOT

KEY

Many patients complain of a pain flare that lasts for several hours following steroid injection. Such flares are self-limited and may be mitigated by massaging the joint with ice.

III **ANATOMIC APPROACHES** (Figure 51-1)

HOT

KEY

Synovial sacs are most superficial on extensor surfaces, where there are no major nerves or vessels.

1. **Interphalangeal joints.** Aspirate from the superolateral or superomedial aspect, staying dorsal to the digital vessels and lateral to the extensor tendon (see Figure 51-1A). Use a small needle (22- to 25-gauge) to minimize trauma.

2. **Wrist.** Passively flex the joint 20°–30° to open the joint space on the dorsal aspect of the wrist. Direct the needle into the space distal to the radius, ulnar to the extensor pollicis longus tendon, and radial to the extensor tendon for the index finger (see Figure 51-1B).

3. **Elbow**
   a. Position the arm in 45° flexion. Approach the joint laterally, and enter the joint lateral to the olecranon process and 1 centimeter inferior to the lateral epicondyle (see Figure 51-1C).
   b. An alternative approach is to insert the needle just proximal to the head of the radius (see Figure 51-1D).

4. **Shoulder**
   a. To aspirate the **glenohumeral joint,** have the patient sit with her arm relaxed in her lap. Approach the joint anteriorly, holding the needle horizontally. Insert the needle medial to the head of the humerus and below the tip of the coracoid process (see Figure 51-1E).
   b. To aspirate the **subacromial bursa,** insert the needle laterally under the acromion, directly into the bursa (see Figure 51-1F).

5. **Hip.** Aspiration of the hip is difficult and should only be performed by those experienced with the procedure. An anterior approach is used.
   a. Insert a 2.5-inch needle 2 centimeters lateral to the femoral pulse, and 3–4 centimeters inferior to the anterior superior iliac spine.
   b. Direct the needle at a 60° angle posteromedially through the tough capsular ligaments to the bone, then withdraw it slightly and aspirate (see Figure 51-1G).

6. **Knee.** Have the patient lie supine with his knee extended but relaxed. Either a medial or a lateral approach may be used. Direct the needle posterior to the patella and anterior to the femoral condyle (see Figure 51-1H).

7. **Ankle.** Position the patient's foot in slight plantar flexion. Approach the tibiotalar joint slightly medial to the extensor hallucis longus tendon, approximately 1 centimeter above and 1 centimeter lateral to the medial malleolus (see Figure 51-1I).

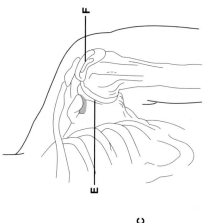

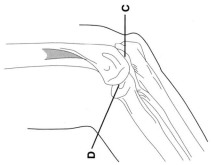

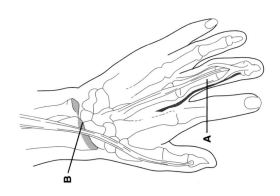

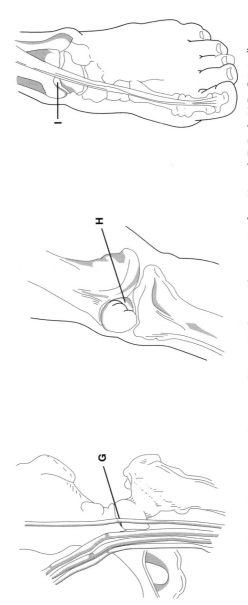

FIGURE 51-1. Approaches to commonly aspirated joints. (Redrawn with permission from Kenneth E. Sack, M.D. Originally appeared in Sack KE and Miller CJ: Needle aspiration of joints. *Houston Medical Journal* 1:25 and 27, 1985.)

52. Acute Ankle Pain

INTRODUCTION. Acute ankle pain is one of the most common musculoskeletal complaints. Although most patients presenting with acute ankle pain have a minor injury, as many as one-third of patients experience residual symptoms.

A. Anatomy (Figure 52-1). The ankle is a **hinge joint:** articulations between the distal tibia and fibula form an arch (mortise) that overlies the talus. Stability of the joint is provided by **multiple ligaments.**

B. Mechanisms of injury

1. **Inversion injuries.** Inversion of the foot may result in injury of the **lateral ligaments** (i.e., the **anterior talofibular, posterior talofibular,** and **calcaneofibular ligaments).**

HOT

Inversion injuries involving the lateral ligaments are the most common ankle injuries.

KEY

---

2. **Eversion injuries** are much less common than inversion injuries. Because the deltoid ligament (i.e., the ligament that attaches the medial malleolus to the talus) is strong, it is not as prone to rupture as the lateral ligaments. The most common eversion injury is actually a fracture of the lateral malleolus. Therefore, both inversion and eversion injuries usually involve the lateral ankle.

DIFFERENTIAL DIAGNOSIS

A. Ankle sprains. Most ankle injuries are **ligamentous sprains,** usually sustained while playing a sport: basketball, volleyball, and football players are at highest risk. Although sprains are usually related to vigorous activity, any sudden stress on a ligament (such as may occur when stepping off a curb) can result in injury.

1. The patient may hear a "pop" followed by the sudden onset of acute pain.

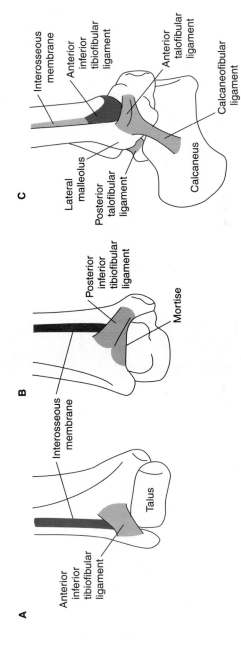

FIGURE 52-1. Distal tibiofibular joint and tibiotalar joint. (A) Anterior view. (B) Posterior view. (C) Lateral view. (Redrawn with permission from Steinberg GC, Baran DT, Akins CM: *Ramamurti's Orthopaedics in Primary Care*, 2e. Baltimore, Williams & Wilkins, 1992.)

2. Symptoms correlate with the severity of the injury. Usually, the patient is unable to bear weight initially, followed by a feeling of the ankle "giving way" and the development of marked ecchymosis around the ankle.

3. Sprains are usually assigned one of three grades (Table 52-1).

B. **Ankle fracture.** The most common fractures (in order of decreasing frequency) are fracture of the lateral malleolus of the fibula, fracture of the medial malleolus of the tibia, bimalleolar fractures, and fractures of the talus.

C. **Bone contusion.** Trauma may lead to contusion of the lateral or medial malleolus.

D. **Syndesmosis injuries** may accompany severe inversion or eversion injuries and involve the inferior and transverse tibiofibular ligaments. In some cases, the proximal interosseous membrane is involved as well.

E. **Peroneal tendon injuries** include **subluxation, tendinitis,** and **rupture.**

F. **Achilles tendon** injuries include **rupture** and **tendinitis.** Abrupt dorsiflexion of the foot (such as might occur following a jump) is the usual cause of tendon rupture.

TABLE 52-1. Classification of Ankle Sprains

Grade	Criteria
First degree	Stretching of the ligament No instability or impairment of functional ability Mild tenderness and pain on stress
Second degree	Partial tear of the ligament Mild to moderate instability and impaired functional ability Moderate swelling and tenderness on initial examination
Third degree	Complete rupture of the ligament Marked instability of the joint resulting in minimal functional ability Marked swelling, tenderness, and ecchymosis on initial examination

▐▐▐ APPROACH TO THE PATIENT

A. Patient history

1. What were the circumstances surrounding the injury?
2. How long ago did the injury occur?
3. Was the patient able to bear weight immediately after the injury occurred?

B. Physical examination

1. Document any ecchymosis or swelling.
2. Assess peripheral sensation.
3. Palpate the pedal and posterior tibial pulses.
4. Palpate the bones, tendons, and ligaments of the ankle and foot. Pay particular attention to the:
    a. Medial and lateral malleoli (especially the posterior edges)
    b. Lateral ligaments
    c. Achilles and peroneal tendons
    d. Navicular and cuboid bones
    e. Base of the fifth metatarsal bone
5. Determine whether the patient is able to bear weight and take four steps.
6. Perform specific tests as necessary (Figure 52-2).
    a. **Anterior drawer test** (see Figure 52-2A). Position the patient so that she is sitting or lying down with her knee slightly flexed. Make sure the ankle is positioned at a 90° angle to the leg. With one hand on the tibia and the other hand on the back

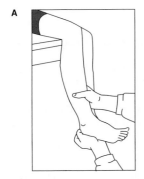 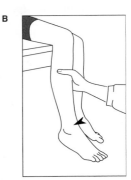

FIGURE 52-2. (A) Anterior drawer test. Instability when the foot is pulled forward suggests rupture of the anterior talofibular ligament. (B) Squeeze test. Pain in the distal ankle (*arrow*) suggests injury of the syndesmotic ligaments.

of the heel, try to draw the foot forward. Rupture of the anterior talofibular ligament (i.e., the first lateral ligament injured by an inversion injury) is indicated by instability.

   b. Squeeze test (see Figure 52-2B). Squeeze the tibia and fibula together at midcalf, then assess for pain in the distal ankle. A positive test suggests injury of the **syndesmotic ligaments.**

HOT

A syndesmosis injury should be suspected in patients with chronic pain after an ankle sprain.

KEY

---

   c. Thompson test. Position the patient so that she is prone, with her foot extending off the edge of the table, and squeeze the gastrocnemius-soleus complex. Normally, this maneuver results in plantar flexion, but in patients with **Achilles tendon rupture,** the foot will not flex.

   d. Peroneal tendon examination should be performed when there is pain or a "snapping" sensation over the lateral malleolus. Tendon injury is suggested by subluxation when the patient everts her foot against resistance.

C. Imaging studies

   1. Radiography

      a. Indications. Radiographs are obtained for patients who meet the criteria described in the **Ottawa rules.**

         (1) Ankle films should be ordered to rule out an ankle fracture if pain is present near either malleolus and the patient:

            (a) Cannot bear weight immediately after the injury and for four steps during the evaluation, **or**

            (b) Has bone tenderness at the posterior or inferior edge of either malleolus

         (2) Foot films should be ordered to rule out a foot fracture if pain is present at the midfoot and the patient:

            (a) Cannot bear weight immediately after

the injury and for four steps during the
evaluation, **or**

(b) Has bone tenderness at the navicular bone,
the cuboid bone, or the base of the fifth
metatarsal bone

HOT

KEY

Studies that have been done to validate the Ottawa rules
have demonstrated that their sensitivity is high (95%–100%)
but their specificity is low (15%–40%). Thus, if all three of
the criteria are **not** met one can be comfortable ruling out
an ankle fracture, but many patients who do meet one of
the criteria do not have an ankle fracture.

---

b. **Views**
   (1) **Ankle films**
      (a) **Anteroposterior, lateral,** and **oblique
          views** are the standard views. The main
          objective is to rule out fracture, and if one
          is found to determine whether or not
          there has been displacement of bone.
      (b) **Stress anteroposterior ankle films** may be
          obtained if no fracture is seen but signifi-
          cant swelling and tenderness are present
          on examination. Widening of the ankle
          mortise suggests a tear in either the me-
          dial deltoid ligament or the lateral collat-
          eral ligament (or both).

HOT

KEY

Suspect a talar dome fracture in a patient with persistent
pain after a sprain. These fractures are characterized radiographically by a small necrotic fragment of bone on the
articular surface of the talus.

---

   (2) **Foot films.** Standard views include **antero-
       posterior, internally rotated oblique,** and **lat-
       eral views.**
   (3) **Fibula films** should be obtained to evaluate
       the possibility of a high fibular fracture in pa-
       tients suspected of having a syndesmosis in-
       jury.

2. **Magnetic resonance imaging (MRI)** is often performed to confirm a suspected peroneal tendon injury.

IV TREATMENT
A. Ankle sprains

Treatment of an Acute Ankle Sprain ("PRICE")

Protection of the area
Rest
Ice
Compression
Elevation

1. Ice should be applied for 15–20 minutes every 1–2 hours, and the ankle should be immobilized by wrapping it with an elastic bandage. This treatment should be continued for 24–48 hours.
2. Patients with second- or third-degree sprains should be seen by an orthopedist within 24–48 hours.

B. Ankle fractures
1. Fractures of either malleolus that are small and undisplaced can be treated with a short leg walking cast. The ankle should be immobilized for 8 weeks.
2. Undisplaced fractures of both malleoli, the calcaneus, or the base of the fifth metatarsal bone and single malleolar fractures that show displacement should be immobilized in a short leg sugar-tong splint and the patient should be referred to an orthopedist for treatment.
3. Fractures that involve dislocation of the talus require emergent reduction. The patient should be referred to an orthopedist as soon as possible.

HOT

KEY

Ankle fracture-dislocation is an orthopedic emergency because blood flow may be compromised and avascular necrosis of the navicular bone can occur. Immediate reduction is recommended.

C. Syndesmosis injuries
1. When complete ruptures are present, **surgery** may be necessary.
2. For less severe injuries, **nonsurgical treatment** is often used. Because these injuries can take as long as 12 weeks to heal, aggressive therapy with a **pneumatic brace** and the use of **crutches** for 1–2 weeks is often recommended.

D. Peroneal tendon subluxation. Patients require orthopedic surgery for reduction and immobilization.

E. Achilles tendon injuries
1. **Achilles tendinitis** can be treated conservatively with rest, heat, stretching exercises, and nonsteroidal anti-inflammatory drugs (NSAIDs).
2. **Achilles tendon rupture** warrants referral to an orthopedist for immediate surgical repair.

VI FOLLOW-UP AND REFERRAL

A. Most patients with first-degree sprains can be managed in a primary care setting, and usually can resume normal activities after about 4 weeks.

B. Patients with second- or third-degree sprains, fractures, or tendon rupture must be evaluated by an orthopedic surgeon within 48 hours. Any patient with signs of neurovascular compromise should see an orthopedist immediately.

References

Auleley GR, Ravaud P, Giraudeau B, et al: Implementation of the Ottawa ankle rules in France: a multicenter randomized controlled trial. *JAMA* 277(24):1935–1939, 1997.

Lucchesi GM, Jackson RE, Peacock WF, et al: Sensitivity of the Ottawa rules. *Ann Emerg Med* 26(1):1–5, 1995.

53. Acute Knee Pain

I **INTRODUCTION.** The anatomy of the knee is shown in Figure 53-1.

II **DIFFERENTIAL DIAGNOSIS** (Table 53-1)

A. Fractures. The **patella, tibial plateau,** and **fibular head** can all sustain fractures following trauma.

B. Joint space disorders include **infection, inflammatory arthritis,** and **degenerative joint disease (DJD).**

C. Ligament injuries (sprains)
   1. The **medial (tibial) collateral ligament, lateral (fibular) collateral ligament, anterior cruciate ligament,** and **posterior cruciate ligament** are all susceptible to sprains.
      a. **Collateral ligament injuries** are usually caused by stress in the medial or lateral direction (e.g., a blow to the lateral aspect of the knee could result in medial collateral ligament rupture).
      b. **Cruciate ligament injuries** are usually caused by hyperextension stress.
   2. **Classification.** Sprains are usually graded as **first-degree** (no laxity), **second-degree** (some laxity), or **third-degree** (complete disruption).

D. Meniscal tears may be traumatic or atraumatic. A history of injury while the knee was flexed and twisting is typical.

E. Patellar tendinitis ("jumper's knee"), often seen in patients who play basketball or participate in track and field, occurs when overuse results in microscopic tears of the patellar tendon.

F. Bursitis usually results from **direct trauma** or **overuse** and can affect the **prepatellar, pes anserinus, superficial intrapatellar,** or **deep intrapatellar bursae.**

H. Patellofemoral syndrome is often seen in runners. The syndrome usually results from malalignment of the femur, patella, and tibia. Patellofemoral syndrome can lead to patellar chondromalacia.

APPROACH TO THE PATIENT

A. **Patient history.** A careful history gives important clues to the anatomic source of pain. Be sure to answer the following questions:

   1. What was the mechanism of injury?
   2. Where is the pain located?
   3. Is there effusion, and if so, how soon did it appear?
   4. Do any activities exacerbate the pain (e.g., twisting, squatting, ascending or descending stairs)?

HOT

KEY

Complaints of the knee "buckling" or "giving out" are common, and are actually not specific as to the location of the injury. These symptoms may simply be indicative of quadriceps muscle weakness.

B. **Physical examination**

   1. **Inspection.** Loss of the infrapatellar indentations signals an effusion. Compare the appearance of the affected knee with the unaffected knee.
   2. **Palpation**
      a. Check for joint line and bony tenderness.
      b. Evaluate for effusions by pushing down on the kneecap.
      c. Tenderness outside of the knee joint may suggest bursitis or tendinitis.
   3. **Range of motion assessment.** Evaluate the knee's range of motion while feeling for crepitus. True "locking" of the knee (i.e., a sudden inability to completely extend the knee) usually indicates a meniscus tear, a cruciate ligament rupture, an osteochondral fracture, or a loose body.

HOT

KEY

A true locked knee is an emergency! Arthroscopy is necessary for definitive diagnosis.

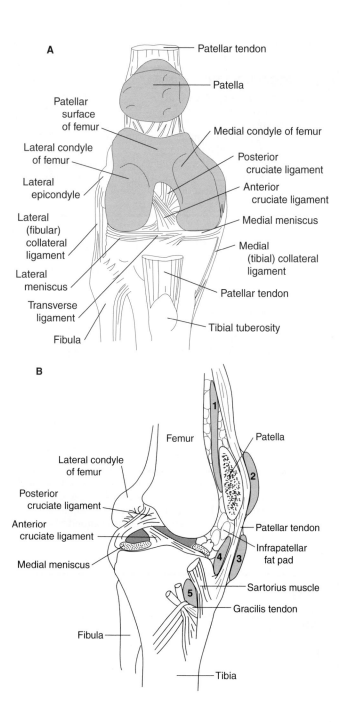

A

Patellar tendon

Patella

Patellar surface of femur

Medial condyle of femur

Lateral condyle of femur

Posterior cruciate ligament

Lateral epicondyle

Anterior cruciate ligament

Lateral (fibular) collateral ligament

Medial meniscus

Medial (tibial) collateral ligament

Lateral meniscus

Patellar tendon

Transverse ligament

Tibial tuberosity

Fibula

B

Femur

Patella

Lateral condyle of femur

Posterior cruciate ligament

Anterior cruciate ligament

Patellar tendon

Infrapatellar fat pad

Medial meniscus

Sartorius muscle

Gracilis tendon

Fibula

Tibia

TABLE 53-1. Clinical Manifestations of Disorders That Can Cause Acute Knee Pain

Disorder	Clinical Manifestations
Fracture	Tenderness, inability to bear weight on limb, effusion (tibial plateau fractures)
DJD	Chronic pain, bland effusion
Infection	Joint erythema, warmth, and effusion
Inflammatory arthritis	Joint erythema, warmth and effusion
Ligament injury	Laxity on stress testing
Meniscal tear	Pain with twisting motion, locking, joint line tenderness, positive McMurray's test, positive Apley test (with compression)
Patellar tendinitis	Tenderness at the superior or inferior pole of the patella
Bursitis	Tenderness, often accompanied by erythema, warmth, and swelling
Patellofemoral syndrome	Anterior knee pain at rest, crepitus, pain while ascending stairs, pain with compression of the patella, positive apprehension test (i.e., patient resists lateral movement of the patella)

DJD = degenerative joint disease.

FIGURE 53-1. Anatomy of the knee. (*A*) Anterior view, emphasizing the collateral ligaments. (*B*) Sagittal view with the medial condyle removed. The bursae are numbered: *1* = suprapatellar; *2* = prepatellar; *3* = superficial infrapatellar; *4* = deep infrapatellar; *5* = pes anserinus. (Part *A* redrawn with permission from Moore KL, Agur AMR: *Essential Clinical Anatomy.* Baltimore, Williams & Wilkins, 1995, p 270. Part *B* redrawn with permission from Byank RP, Beatie WE: Exercise-related musculoskeletal problems. In *Principles of Ambulatory Medicine,* 4th ed. Edited by Barker LR, Burton JR, Zieve PD. Baltimore, Williams & Wilkins, 1995, p 899.)

4. **Special maneuvers**
   a. **Evaluation for patellar tendinitis.** With the knee
      fully extended, evaluate for tenderness at the su-
      perior or inferior pole of the patella.
   b. **Valgus** and **varus stress testing** can be used to
      evaluate the **collateral ligaments.** With the knee
      slightly flexed (to about 10°) place one hand
      above and the other below the knee and then
      "bend" the knee laterally and medially. Laxity
      suggests a collateral ligament injury.

HOT

KEY

Laxity with straight-leg valgus and varus testing suggests
multiple ligament tears.

   c. **Drawer** and **Lachman's tests.** These tests are
      used to evaluate the **cruciate ligaments.** Have the
      patient lie supine with his knee flexed at either a
      20° angle (Lachman's test) or a 90° angle (drawer
      test). Place both of your hands just below the
      knee and pull, as if you were opening a drawer.
      Anterior movement of the tibia indicates an an-
      terior cruciate ligament disruption.

HOT

KEY

Lachman's test is more sensitive than the drawer test for a
ligament tear.

   d. **McMurray's test.** This test can be used to evalu-
      ate a **meniscal tear.** With the patient supine, flex
      and extend her knee, first with the foot internally
      rotated and then with it externally rotated, while
      palpating with the opposite hand for popping or
      locking of the knee.
   e. **Apley compression-distraction test.** This test can
      be used to evaluate the knee for **meniscus** and
      collateral ligament injuries.

    (1) Meniscus injury. With the patient prone and the knee flexed at a 90° angle, apply a gradual downward force on the leg and then internally and externally rotate the foot. Pain with compression suggests meniscus injury.

    (2) Collateral ligament injury. Repeat the maneuver while applying upward traction on the leg rather than downward pressure. Pain with this maneuver suggests a collateral ligament injury.

  C. Laboratory studies. Diagnostic joint aspiration (see Chapter 51) should be performed in patients with an effusion.

HOT

Aspiration of gross blood suggests a serious injury (usually a fracture or ligament tear).

KEY

  D. Imaging studies. A plain film of the knee in the setting of acute injury should be ordered if the patient meets any one of the following criteria, known as the **Ottawa rules:**

    1. Patient is 55 years or older

    2. Patient has tenderness at the head of the fibula

    3. Patient has isolated tenderness of the patella

    4. Patient unable to flex the knee to 90°

    5. Patient unable to bear weight on the limb immediately after the injury and at the time of evaluation

IV TREATMENT

  A. General measures. Rest, ice, and **elevation** often help to relieve swelling, which can delay recovery.

HOT

In patients with large or bloody effusions, aspirating the effusion may alleviate some of the patient's symptoms.

KEY

B. Specific therapies
   1. Fractures. Patients should be referred to an orthopedist after the fracture has been immobilized.
   2. DJD (osteoarthritis)
      a. Acetaminophen is as effective as nonsteroidal anti-inflammatory drugs (NSAIDs) for relieving the pain of osteoarthritis and is preferred due to its better side effect profile.

HOT **KEY**

Because NSAIDs may exacerbate certain medical conditions (e.g., peptic ulcer disease, renal insufficiency, bleeding diatheses), consider a patient's history before prescribing an NSAID.

---

      b. Weight loss in overweight patients can help prevent disease progression. Patients should also be advised to **avoid kneeling, squatting,** and **high-impact exercises.**
   3. Ligament injuries. Treatment depends on the patient's level of activity. Most patients with these types of injuries should see an orthopedic surgeon or sports medicine specialist.
      a. Anterior cruciate ligament injuries may be treated conservatively in an inactive person but early surgical repair is recommended in an athletic individual.
      b. Posterior cruciate ligament injuries are usually associated with other ligament injuries, and surgery is usually required.
      c. Medial and **lateral collateral ligament tears** commonly require only immobilization followed by rehabilitation.
   4. Meniscal tears may heal spontaneously if they are peripheral, but **many require surgical repair.** Most patients should be referred to an orthopedist after the knee is immobilized.
   5. Bursitis
      a. Rest, heat, and **NSAIDs** are usually used to treat bursitis.
      b. Antibiotics should be used if infection is suspected (e.g., prepatellar bursitis often results from infection).

HOT

KEY

The application of direct pressure to the bursae should be avoided; patients with pes anserinus bursitis should be advised to sleep with a pillow between their legs.

  6. **Patellar tendinitis** is difficult to treat. Patients should be advised to reduce their activity level and perform exercises designed to stretch and strengthen the quadriceps and hamstring muscles.

 FOLLOW-UP AND REFERRAL. Patients with persistent undiagnosed knee pain should be referred to an orthopedist or sports medicine specialist for diagnosis and treatment.

References

Stiell IG, Greenberg GH, Wells GA, et al: Derivation of a decision rule for the use of radiography in acute knee injuries. *Ann Emerg Med* 26(4):405–413, 1995.

54. Shoulder Pain

I INTRODUCTION

A. Incidence. Approximately 1 in 5 adults experiences shoulder pain during his or her lifetime.

B. Anatomy (Figure 54-1). The clinically relevant components of the shoulder joint can be remembered as "4-3-2-1."

Anatomy of the Shoulder Joint ("4-3-2-1")

4 muscles—supraspinatus, infraspinatus, teres minor, subscapularis (rotator cuff)
3 joints—acromioclavicular, sternoclavicular, glenohumeral
2 tendons—supraspinatus, biceps
1 bursa—subacromial

Muscles of the Shoulder Joint ("SITS")

Supraspinatus
Infraspinatus
Teres minor
Subscapularis

II DIFFERENTIAL DIAGNOSIS

A. Subacromial bursitis and **supraspinatus tendinitis** result in essentially the same clinical illness. Repetitive overhead motion (e.g., serving in tennis or throwing a baseball) is the usual cause.

B. Adhesive capsulitis ("frozen shoulder") usually results from prolonged immobility due to pain from another disorder (e.g., subacromial bursitis).

C. Rotator cuff tears can occur in young adults who subject the joint to extreme overuse (e.g., in baseball pitchers). In older adults, even minor trauma to the shoulder can cause a rotator cuff tear.

D. Degenerative joint disease (DJD) usually affects the

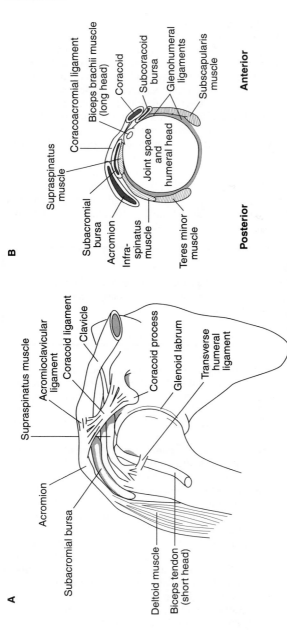

FIGURE 54-1. Anatomy of the shoulder joint. (A) Anterior view. (B) Sagittal view. (Part A redrawn with permission from Kern DE: Shoulder Pain. In *Principles of Ambulatory Medicine*, 4th ed. Edited by Barker LR, Burton JR, Zieve PD. Baltimore, Williams & Wilkins, 1995, p 849. Part B modified with permission from Pansky B: *Review of Gross Anatomy.* New York, Macmillan, 1979.)

acromioclavicular joint; much more rarely, the glenohumeral joint is affected.

E. Bicipital tendinitis results from overuse (e.g., repeated
flexion-extension or pronation-supination of the elbow).

F. Glenohumeral instability is subluxation or dislocation of
the glenohumeral joint secondary to prior trauma.

G. Referred pain. Cervical disk disease, an apical lung tumor, pleural disease, myocardial ischemia or infarction,
and subdiaphragmatic processes (e.g., gallbladder disease, abscess, free air) should all be considered as possible causes of shoulder pain.

 APPROACH TO THE PATIENT. Approximately 85% of cases
of shoulder pain can be diagnosed by history and physical examination alone. Clinical findings for each of the common
causes are given in Table 54-1.

HOT

  Most cases of shoulder pain are caused by subacromial
bursitis, supraspinatus tendinitis, rotator cuff tear, or adhesive capsulitis.

KEY

A. Patient history. Key points include the following.

1. What is the **patient's age?** Rotator cuff tears are more
   common in patients older than 50 years.

2. Was the **onset sudden?**
   a. A **sudden "pop"** while lifting overhead suggests
      a **rotator cuff tear.**
   b. The **onset of pain** is usually **gradual** in **subacro-
      mial bursitis** and **supraspinatus tendinitis.**

3. Are there any **aggravating factors?**
   a. **Difficulty brushing one's hair** or **nocturnal pain**
      caused by rolling over onto the shoulder may sig-
      nify the **impingement syndrome** (i.e., repetitive
      friction between the acromion and the greater
      tuberosity of the humerus leads to inflammation
      of the rotator cuff and bursa). **Subacromial bur-
      sitis, supraspinatus tendinitis,** or **small rotator
      cuff tears** can all cause the impingement syn-
      drome and therefore have similar clinical presen-
      tations.
   b. **Pain as a result of curling the arm** (e.g., lifting a

pot away from the stove) suggests **bicipital ten-dinitis.**

    c. **Pain that occurs when the patient reaches behind herself** (e.g., to put on a coat or fasten a bra) may signify **adhesive capsulitis.**

B. Physical examination

    1. Palpation. Palpate the acromioclavicular joint, the subacromial bursa, the glenohumeral joint, and the bicipital groove for tenderness, which may be a sign of DJD, bursitis, adhesive capsulitis, or bicipital tendinitis, respectively.

    2. Range of motion assessment

        a. Active range of motion

            (1) Have the patient reach behind his head and touch the opposite shoulder to test abduction and external rotation.

            (2) Ask the patient to reach behind his back with his hand in the "hitchhiker" position and touch the ipsilateral shoulder blade to test adduction and internal rotation. Note the highest spinous process reached for future comparisons.

        b. Passive range of motion. If the active range of motion is decreased, test the passive range of motion.

            (1) In **impingement disorders,** the active range of motion is decreased due to pain, but the passive range of motion is preserved.

            (2) In **adhesive capsulitis,** both the active and the passive range of motion are decreased.

    3. Special maneuvers

        a. Impingement sign. Have the patient elevate her arm with the elbow flexed (like a military salute) against resistance. Pain with this motion indicates the **impingement syndrome.**

        b. Drop arm test. Have the patient hold the affected arm in 90° of abduction. Place downward force on the patient's outstretched arm at the wrist and note any pain or weakness. In patients with severe pain, it may be necessary to inject the subacromial bursa with lidocaine prior to performing this test.

            (1) Weakness is indicated by arm drop and suggests a **significant rotator cuff tear.**

            (2) Pain without weakness usually indicates **supraspinatus tendinitis** or **subacromial bursitis.**

TABLE 54-1. Clinical Manifestations of the Common Causes of Shoulder Pain

Disorder	History	Physical Examination	Imaging
Subacromial bursitis and Supraspinatus tendinitis	Pain with overhead activity (e.g., shampooing hair) Nocturnal pain that interferes with sleep	Point tenderness over the subacromial area Painful arc (60°–120°) with active range of motion Positive impingement sign No weakness	None necessary
Adhesive capsulitis	Diffuse, dull ache Decreasing function (e.g., difficulty putting on coat)	Diffuse tenderness Decreased active and passive range of motion	None usually necessary; arthroscopy can detect decreased capsular volume
Rotator cuff tear	Patient may describe hearing or feeling a sudden "pop" Pain with overhead activity; patient may be unable to lift arm without assistance Nocturnal pain	Point tenderness over subacromial area Painful arc (60°–120°) with active range of motion Positive impingement sign Weakness	MRI

Bicipital tendinitis	Anterior shoulder pain, exacerbated by lifting or curling (e.g., lifting a pan off the stove top)	Tenderness over bicipital groove Pain with resisted forearm supination	None necessary
DJD of the acromioclavicular joint	Pain over the acromio-clavicular joint	Tenderness over the acromioclavicular joint Pain with crossed-chest adduction test	Plain films may show narrowed joint space and osteophyte formation
Glenohumeral instability	Severe pain after acute event Patient often holds arm close to body with unaffected hand	Neurovascular compromise in some patients	Plain films are diagnostic
Referred pain	Diffuse, progressive pain that overlaps anatomic boundaries Pain can radiate below elbow	Preserved range of motion Other findings depend on the cause	Plain film of shoulder and chest Additional studies guided by clinical suspicion

DJD = degenerative joint disease.

        c. **Resisted supination test.** Have the patient attempt supination while you apply resistance at the wrist. Pain with this test suggests **biceps tendinitis.**

        d. **Head compression test.** With the patient seated, apply firm downward pressure on the top of her head. Neck pain or radicular symptoms suggest **cervical disk disease.**

    4. **Neuromuscular examination** is important for patients with glenohumeral instability. Evaluate the brachial and medial pulses and the sensory and motor function of the forearm, wrist, and hand.

C. Imaging studies

    1. **Plain film radiography.** Radiographs are essential in patients with a **history of trauma** to rule out a humeral head fracture, acromioclavicular joint separation, or shoulder dislocation.

        a. Usually, an anteroposterior view in internal and external rotation, a lateral view, and a scapular view are obtained.

        b. Calcium densities are often seen, but their clinical significance is unclear.

    2. **Arthrography**

        a. Long considered the **gold standard** for detecting **rotator cuff tears** (especially when the supraspinatus muscle is involved), arthrography is gradually being replaced by magnetic resonance imaging (MRI) as the test of choice for diagnosing this condition.

        b. Arthrography can also be used to diagnose **adhesive capsulitis;** reduced contrast capacity of the joint space is suggestive.

    3. **MRI** is noninvasive, readily available, and is as accurate as arthrography for diagnosing partial and complete **rotator cuff tears.**

    4. **Ultrasonography** is rarely used in the assessment of shoulder pain, but can be useful for diagnosing a **large rotator cuff tear.**

IV TREATMENT

A. Impingement syndromes and **bicipital tendinitis.** Therapy is only moderately effective for these patients. Fewer than 50% of patients undergoing multimodal therapy will be asymptomatic after 1 year.

1. **Pharmacologic therapy**
   a. **Nonsteroidal anti-inflammatory drugs (NSAIDs)** should be tried initially. Common regimens include ibuprofen, 400–800 mg orally, three times daily for 2 weeks, or naproxen, 250–500 mg orally twice daily for 2 weeks.
   b. **Corticosteroid injections** (see Chapter 51 II C) may be used if NSAID therapy fails or is contraindicated. Injections may be slightly more effective than NSAIDs, but in the absence of definitive data on safety and efficacy, they should be administered no more than four times a year.
2. **Exercise**
   a. **Passive range of motion exercises** should be **initiated immediately.** The patient should be shown how to perform pendulum and other passive range of motion exercises at home. Patient-oriented literature is available to demonstrate and reinforce the importance of practicing these exercises.
   b. **Active range of motion exercises.** Physical therapy involving a combination of **isometric exercises** (performed with elastic tubing), **shoulder shrugs,** and **wall push-ups** can be **started 2 weeks after initiating NSAID therapy** or administering a corticosteroid injection. These exercises strengthen the rotator cuff muscles.
3. **Monitoring.** The patient should return 2–4 weeks after beginning active range of motion exercises so that the physician can assess the patient's progress and the effectiveness of pharmacologic therapy.

B. **Rotator cuff tears**
   1. **Small rotator cuff tears** are managed conservatively, as described in IV A. Small, uncontrolled trials that have examined the safety and efficacy of steroid injections in the treatment of small rotator cuff tears have suggested that steroid therapy is moderately beneficial and not deleterious in these patients.
   2. **Moderate** to **large rotator cuff tears** are best managed with **surgery** (arthroscopic or open techniques may be used). Aggressive and supervised **physical therapy** is necessary after surgery; rehabilitation can take 6–9 months.

C. **Adhesive capsulitis.** The recovery from adhesive capsulitis is slow and requires persistent physical therapy.
   1. As in the treatment of impingement syndromes,

NSAIDs and **exercise** are the mainstays of therapy. The patient should begin immediately with passive range of motion exercises (e.g., pendulum exercises) and advance to active range of motion exercises (e.g., wall push-ups).

    2. The role of **corticosteroid injections** in the treatment of adhesive capsulitis is controversial. Studies in a small number of patients showed that intra-articular steroids may improve range of motion without causing demonstrable harm.

    3. Shoulder manipulation under anesthesia can be considered for patients with recalcitrant disease.

D. Glenohumeral instability. The primary care provider should temporarily immobilize the shoulder with a **splint** and refer the patient to an **orthopedic specialist.**

E. DJD

    1. Conservative management with **physical therapy** and **acetaminophen** or **NSAIDs** should be tried.

    2. Mixed injections of **lidocaine** and **short-acting steroids** can also provide relief.

HOT

Conservative therapy is appropriate for all patients with shoulder pain, except for those with moderate to large rotator cuff tears or glenohumeral instability.

KEY

V FOLLOW-UP AND REFERRAL

A. Referral to an **orthopedist** is appropriate for patients with moderate to large rotator cuff tears or glenohumeral instability. Patients who fail to obtain significant relief of symptoms after 4 weeks of conservative therapy should also be referred to an orthopedist, regardless of the cause of the shoulder pain.

B. A **physical therapist** can integrate the home exercises described in the patient literature with a more formal exercise program. Consultation with a physical therapist also helps to ensure patient compliance.

References

Smith DL, Campbell SM: Painful shoulder syndromes: diagnosis and management. *J Gen Intern Med* 7(3):328–339, 1992.

55. Elbow Pain

I **INTRODUCTION.** The elbow allows positioning of the hand in space via flexion-extension and pronation-supination. Pain or dysfunction can originate in any structure of the elbow (i.e., bone, ligaments, tendons, nerves, bursae, joint space).

II **DIFFERENTIAL DIAGNOSIS.** Elbow disorders can be caused by trauma, overuse, nerve compression, infection, or systemic disease.

A. **Fractures** of the distal humerus, radial head, or olecranon (proximal ulna) are usually caused by direct trauma. Older patients with osteoporosis are much more susceptible to elbow fractures.

B. **Dislocations.** Elbow dislocations are relatively common. Posterior displacement of the radius and ulna accounts for most elbow dislocations and usually results from falling on an extended, abducted arm.

C. **Ligament injuries** are typically seen in athletes, especially those who are required to throw a ball.
   1. The **medial (ulnar) collateral ligament** is affected most often.
   2. The **pain** is **usually medial** and located just **below the epicondyle.** The pain worsens when valgus stress is applied while the elbow is held in the flexed position.

D. **Lateral epicondylitis (tennis elbow, tendinitis)** most commonly results from **overuse** of the extremity. The **pain** is **usually lateral** and located just **below the epicondyle.**

HOT KEY

Overuse injuries usually involve the patient's dominant extremity.

E. **Nerve entrapment.** The **ulnar nerve** is affected more often than the radial or medial nerves.

365

1. Pressure over the cubital tunnel (during intoxication or coma or from trauma) or cumulative injury from repeated elbow flexion and extension can result in ulnar neuropathy.
2. Clinical manifestations include medial elbow or forearm pain and hand clumsiness that worsens with activity.

F. Olecranon bursitis can result from **trauma** or **infection.** Clinical manifestations include pain and "goose egg" swelling as a result of fluid collection.

G. Arthritis. Infectious arthritis, inflammatory arthritis (e.g., rheumatoid arthritis, gout, pseudogout), and degenerative joint disease (DJD) can all affect the elbow joint. Patients complain of effusion and acute elbow pain that increases with movement.

III APPROACH TO THE PATIENT

A. Patient history. Answers to the following questions can help to narrow the differential diagnosis.
   1. Was the **onset of symptoms** abrupt or gradual? The abrupt onset of pain and a "popping" sound are worrisome for a ligament tear.
   2. Where is the **pain located?**
   3. Are there **associated symptoms** (e.g., numbness, swelling, loss of function)?
   4. What is the patient's **exercise** and **work history?** Overuse injuries are common.
   5. Is there a **history of trauma?**
   6. Is there a **history of arthritis at other joints?**

B. Physical examination
   1. **Inspection**
      a. **Olecranon bursitis** is suggested by a **tender, localized fluid collection** over the olecranon (i.e., the "funny bone").
      b. **Rheumatoid arthritis**
         (1) **Rheumatoid nodules** may be seen on the extensor surface of the elbow.
         (2) Always examine the hands and feet for **signs of systemic arthritis.**
      c. **Elbow dislocation.** Patients with elbow dislocations usually hold the **limb close to the body at a 45° angle.**
   2. **Palpation**
         (1) Tenderness **just below the lateral epicondyle** may suggest **lateral epicondylitis.**
         (2) Tenderness **1–2 centimeters below the lateral epicondyle** may suggest **elbow joint arthritis.**

3. **Range of motion assessment.** The elbow's range of motion, including **flexion-extension** and **pronation-supination,** should be evaluated.
   a. Septic arthritis usually results in severe pain that limits the patient's range of motion.
   b. In patients with lateral epicondylitis, passive flexion-extension of the elbow is painless, but forced pronation-supination is painful.
4. **Neurologic examination** is necessary to rule out entrapment syndromes.
   a. **Weakness, atrophy,** or **sensory deficits** imply nerve involvement.
   b. **Tinel's sign.** Tapping over the ulnar nerve in the cubital tunnel between the medial epicondyle and the olecranon may elicit shock-like pain in a patient with nerve compression.
5. **Distal neurovascular examination** is mandatory for a patient with a dislocated elbow to rule out nerve entrapment (common) and circulatory compromise (rare). The brachial and radial pulses and the sensory and motor function of the fingers and wrist should be evaluated.

C. **Laboratory studies.** When clinical suspicion warrants it, aspiration and analysis of joint or bursal fluid should be carried out as described in Chapter 51. The joint fluid should be sent for a cell count, Gram staining, culture, and crystal analysis to rule out infection or crystal-induced arthritis.

D. **Imaging studies**
   1. **Radiography.** In the setting of trauma, plain radiographs of the elbow should be obtained to rule out fracture or dislocation. Anteroposterior views of the elbow in the neutral position and in supination, as well as a lateral view with the elbow held at a 90° angle, are most useful.
   2. **Magnetic resonance imaging (MRI)** of the elbow may be useful if a ligament tear is suspected.

E. **Nerve conduction studies** are used to confirm a diagnosis of nerve entrapment, especially when a more proximal lesion (e.g., radiculopathy, plexopathy) cannot be excluded on the basis of the physical examination.

IV TREATMENT

A. **Fractures and dislocations**
   1. **Simple, nondisplaced fractures** of the radius or olecranon can be splinted. The patient should see an orthopedic surgeon within 1 week.

2. **Displaced fractures, dislocations,** or **fractures associated with nerve palsy** require expedient orthopedic referral.

B. **Ligament tears** are best treated with **rest.** Operative repair is possible but challenging, and is usually attempted only in competitive athletes or in the setting of a complete tear.

C. **Lateral epicondylitis** is treated with **rest** and **nonsteroidal anti-inflammatory drugs (NSAIDs).**

   1. A **counterforce brace** placed circumferentially on the proximal forearm may improve pain by alleviating strain on the affected tendon.

   2. **Injection of corticosteroids** adjacent to, but not in, the tendon sheath may be used if necessary.

   3. **Operative treatment** is rarely required.

D. **Nerve entrapment** is treated initially with **rest** and **elbow padding** during activity. **Operative decompression** and **transposition of the ulnar nerve** is considered when the pain lasts longer than 6 weeks or evidence of motor denervation exists.

E. **Olecranon bursitis**

   1. **Infectious bursitis** is treated with repeated **aspiration** of the bursal fluid and oral **antibiotics** (e.g., cephalexin or dicloxacillin, 250–500 mg orally three times daily for 7–10 days).

   2. **Traumatic bursitis** is treated with **aspiration, immobilization,** and **NSAIDs. Local corticosteroid injections** (see Chapter 51) can also be used once infection has been excluded.

      a. Ibuprofen, 400–800 mg orally three times daily for 5–7 days, is often used.

      b. Maintaining the elbow in flexion opposes the two walls of the bursa and aids healing.

F. **Arthritis** is treated according to its cause.

   1. **Septic arthritis.** Patients require **intravenous antibiotic therapy** and **repeat aspirations** of infected joint fluid. Orthopedic referral and arthroscopic decompression may be required if cell counts, pain, and swelling do not resolve in 2–3 days.

   2. **Inflammatory arthritis.** Symptomatic relief most commonly includes **NSAIDs, acetaminophen,** or intra-articular injections of **corticosteroids.**

   3. **DJD. Elbow arthroscopy** with removal of osteochondral fragments is an option for patients with severely damaged joints.

References

Caldwell GL, Safran MR: Elbow problems in the athlete. *Orthop Clin North Am* 26(3):465–485, 1995.

56. Wrist and Hand Pain

....

I **APPROACH TO THE PATIENT.** All patients with wrist injuries must be carefully evaluated because in many cases, the diagnosis of a serious disorder must be made on the basis of clinical, rather than radiographic, evidence.

A. **Patient history.** Important features of the history include when the trauma occurred, the position of the wrist at the time of injury, and a complete recreational and occupational history.

B. **Physical examination**
1. Assess vascular perfusion, neurologic function, and muscle tone, bulk, and strength of the affected hand.
2. In examining the wrist, pay particular attention to focal pain, tenderness, or swelling, and any maneuvers that exacerbate the pain. Muscle atrophy is a sign of chronic disease.

C. **Radiographic evaluation.** Anteroposterior and lateral views should be obtained for all patients with wrist injuries. Special views (e.g., oblique or carpal tunnel views) may be obtained as clinical suspicion warrants.

HOT **KEY** The space between each carpal bone should be approximately equal to the other carpal-carpal spaces; enlargement of a space may indicate a ligament injury, while closure of a space may indicate a displaced carpal bone.

II **WRIST FRACTURES.** The bones of the wrist are shown in Figure 56-1.

A. **Types of fractures.** Table 56-1 summarizes the clinical features and treatment of each type of wrist fracture.
1. **Scaphoid fractures** account for 80% of all carpal injuries.
2. **Triquetrum fractures** are second in incidence to scaphoid fractures.

HOT

KEY

Fractures of the hamulus ("hook") of the hamate are often misdiagnosed as sprains.

  B. **Treatment**
      1. **Conservative therapy** entails **rest, immobilization, ice, elevation,** and **nonsteroidal anti-inflammatory drugs (NSAIDs).**
      2. **Physical therapy** is an important adjunct to successful rehabilitation.
  C. **Follow-up and referral.** When in doubt, it is always a safe policy to either obtain immediate orthopedic evaluation, or, when this is unavailable, to immobilize the wrist with a splint or short arm cast and have the patient follow up with an orthopedist the following day.

III   **LIGAMENT INJURIES.** Figure 56-2 shows the ligaments of the wrist and their relation to the scaphoid, lunate, capitate, radius, and ulna. The clinical findings and treatment of ligament injuries of the wrist are summarized in Table 56-2.

  A. **Scaphoid dislocations** usually result from falling on an outstretched and hyperextended wrist.
  B. **Lunate dislocations** occur when the lunate is displaced in a volar direction. **Carpal tunnel syndrome** can be a complication of lunate dislocations.
  C. **Perilunate (capitate) dislocations** are characterized by dorsal displacement of the capitate, while the lunate remains in correct alignment with the radius. Perilunate dislocations are often accompanied by **scaphoid fractures.**
  D. **Ulnar or radial dislocations** result from disruption, degeneration, or tearing of the **triangular fibrocartilage** as a result of chronic mechanical stress or inflammation. The triangular fibrocartilage, a thick band of connective tissue that connects the ulnar-radial articulation to the first carpal row, provides stability during wrist weight-bearing and grasping.

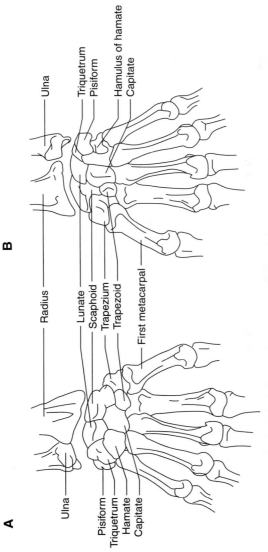

FIGURE 56-1. Bones of the wrist.

TABLE 56-1. Wrist Fractures

Bone	Mechanism of Injury	Signs and Symptoms	Radiographic Findings	Complications	Treatment
Scaphoid	Falling on an outstretched and dorsiflexed hand	Tenderness in the anatomical snuff-box	Loss of the scaphoid fat pad stripe	Nonunion and avascular necrosis	Thumb spica cast for 14 days; follow-up with ortho-pedist in 1–2 weeks
Lunate	Compression; chronic stress	Chronic wrist pain; often patient has no recollection of incipient event	Fragmentation of the lunate with distal collapse	Avascular necrosis of fragment	Conservative ther-apy; arthroplasty may be necessary for severe fractures
Triquetrum	Falling on an outstretched, dorsiflexed, ulnar-deviated hand	Swelling and tender-ness of the dorsal–ulnar wrist	Dorsally displaced fractures on oblique films	Ulnar nerve injury	Short arm cast for 4 weeks; follow-up with an ortho-pedist in 2 weeks
Pisiform	Direct, high-velocity trauma to the hypo-thenar eminence	Pain, tenderness, and swelling at the hypothenar eminence	Transverse, commin-uted, or avulsion fracture line	Often accom-panied by fractures of other carpal bones	Short arm cast or splint for 4–6 weeks

Trapezium	Direct trauma to the thenar eminence with the hand outstretched and the thumb in adduction	Pain and swelling at the base of the thumb; immobility of the thumb in some cases	Fracture lines seen on routine views	Displacement	Short arm cast for 4 weeks; displaced fractures must be reduced by an orthopedist
Capitate	Falling on an outstretched hand with slight radial deviations or direct trauma to the volar wrist	Pain, tenderness, and swelling in the mid-volar aspect of the wrist	Instability of the "stacked" arrangement of the capitate, lunate, and radius on lateral views (with dislocation)	Avascular necrosis	Short arm cast and immediate follow-up with an orthopedist (fracture usually requires open reduction)
Hamate	Falling on an outstretched hand or direct trauma to the volar wrist	Pain and swelling over the hypothenar eminence; pain increases with gripping or swinging a gripped object	Anteroposterior films may demonstrate loss of the cortical ring	Ulnar neuropathy and flexion tendon rupture	Cast for 4 weeks (only when patient cannot tolerate symptoms) and follow-up with an orthopedist in 2 weeks; surgical excision for fractures of the hamulus ("hook")

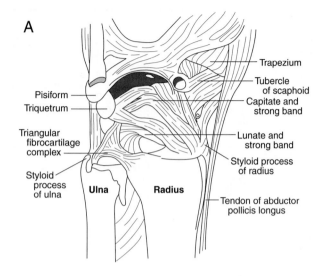

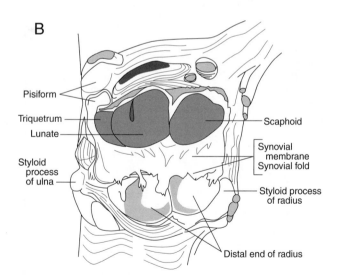

FIGURE 56-2. (A) Ligaments of the distal radioulnar, radiocarpal, and intercarpal joints, anterior view. (B) Dissection of the right radiocarpal joint, opened anteriorly. (Redrawn with permission from Moore KL: *Clinically Oriented Anatomy,* 3rd ed. Baltimore, Williams & Wilkins, 1992, p 627.)

TABLE 56-2. Ligamentous Injuries of the Wrist

Dislocation	Signs and Symptoms	Diagnosis	Treatment
Scaphoid	Pain with dorsiflexion and point tenderness at the scaphoid–lunate joint	Anteroposterior films demonstrate a gap between the scaphoid–lunate joint of more than 3 mm	Volar wrist splinting and surgical consultation within 24–72 hours
Lunate or perilunate (capitate)	Minimal swelling and tenderness, chronic wrist pain, patient usually has no recollection of incipient event	Lateral films show disruption of the normal "stacked" alignment of the capitate, lunate, and radius	Volar wrist splinting and surgical consultation within 24–72 hours
Triangular fibro-cartilage complex	Pain at the volar–ulnar side of the wrist	Excessive mobility of the wrist on performing the "shuck" test*; wrist arthrography or MRI are definitive	Conservative therapy (i.e., splinting) and follow-up with an orthopedist in 1–2 weeks; physical therapy

MRI = magnetic resonance imaging.
*"Shuck" test: The examiner stabilizes the radial side of the wrist, while moving the ulnar wrist in an anteroposterior direction. Excessive mobility of the wrist implies triangular fibrocartilage disruption, degeneration, or tear.

HOT

KEY

While some patients with fractures need immediate ortho-pedic evaluation, all patients with ligament injuries need early referral for surgical therapy. Early recognition and re-ferral is often the difference between successful correction and long-term wrist instability and disability.

IV TENDON INJURIES of the wrist and hand are summarized in Table 56-3.

   A. DeQuervain's tenosynovitis is thickening and narrowing of the tendon sheath of the extensor brevis and abductor longus pollicis muscles as a result of repetitive gripping.

   B. Acute calcific tendonitis, which is caused by hydroxyap-atite deposition in the tendons, may mimic DeQuervain's tenosynovitis and is treated similarly.

   C. Intersection syndrome ("squeaker's wrist") is inflam-mation surrounding the tendon sheaths as they pass un-der the first and second compartments of the wrist (peri-tendinitis).

   D. Tendon rupture rarely occurs in the wrist, except in as-sociation with hamulus of the hamate fractures. Frac-tures of the hamulus can fray the flexor digiti minimi tendon.

   E. Myxoid cyst (synovial cyst, synovial ganglion). A myxoid cyst is a synovial cyst on the dorsal surface of the wrist or hand. These cysts originate from either a tendon or a joint and usually result from trauma or overuse.

HOT

KEY

Carpometacarpal osteoarthritis, characterized by dorsal wrist pain that increases with wrist flexion and extension, can present as a tendinitis-like syndrome.

V NEUROVASCULAR INJURIES

   A. Vascular injury is rare. The usual cause is repetitive trauma at the ulnar aspect of the wrist, leading to the for-mation of an ulnar artery aneurysm and subsequent thrombosis or spasm of the artery. Baseball catchers,

TABLE 56-3. Tendon Disorders of the Wrist

Disorder	Signs and Symptoms	Diagnosis	Treatment
DeQuervain's tenosynovitis	Pain in the extensor and abductor tendons of the thumb	Pain on Finkelstein's test*	Conservative therapy with splinting, NSAIDs, and avoidance of repetitive gripping motions; refractory cases may require injection of lidocaine and steroids at the radial styloid
Intersection syndrome	Pain and crepitus with gripping and flexion of the wrist	(Pain is more proximal than that seen with DeQuervain's tenosynovitis); considerable dorsal swelling	Conservative therapy
Tendon rupture	Pain and weakness of the involved tendon	History of trauma and weakness on exam	Splinting and orthopedic referral within 24–72 hours
Myxoid cyst	Firm cyst that is usually not tender on the dorsal surface of the wrist; patient may report mild pain over the dorsal ganglion	Jelly-like material on aspiration	Aspiration with a large-bore needle followed by steroid injection; surgical excision usually required to prevent recurrence

NSAIDs = nonsteroidal anti-inflammatory drugs.
*Finkelstein's test: Examiner folds the patient's thumb onto his palm and deviates the wrist in an ulnar direction.

handball players, and waitstaff who repeatedly receive
blows to the wrist from swinging kitchen doors are typical
patients.
  1. **Clinical findings.** Symptoms are related to arterial in-
     sufficiency (e.g., cold digits, mottling, pain, paresthe-
     sias). A mass (i.e., the aneurysm) may be palpable.
  2. **Diagnosis.** Arteriography is the diagnostic test of
     choice.
  3. **Treatment.** Immediate referral to a vascular surgeon
     is indicated.
B. **Carpal tunnel syndrome (median neuropathy)** is discussed in Chapter 67.
C. **Ulnar nerve entrapment** is rare and is usually seen in association with sports or occupational activities that require
   power gripping with weight-loading on the hypothenar
   eminence (e.g., power lifting, gripping a baseball bat).
  1. **Clinical findings.** Paresthesias of the fourth and fifth
     digits are usually seen. Interosseous wasting may be
     seen in long-standing injury.
  2. **Diagnosis.** The diagnosis is usually made clinically.
     Radiographs are needed for patients who have a his-
     tory of trauma to exclude hamate fracture or disloca-
     tion.
  3. **Treatment** entails wrist padding. Surgical decom-
     pression may be required for patients with refractory
     disease.

References
Cohen MS: Fractures of the carpal bones. *Hand Clin* 13(4):587–599, 1997.
Mastey RD, Weiss AP, Akelman E: Primary care of hand and wrist athletic injuries. *Clin Sports Med* 16(4):705–724, 1997.
Morgan RL, Linder MM: Common wrist injuries. *Am Fam Physician* 55(3): 857–868, 1997.
Watson HK, Weinzweig J: Physical examination of the wrist. *Hand Clin* 13(1):17–34, 1997.

57. Degenerative Joint Disease (Osteoarthritis)

I **INTRODUCTION.** Degenerative joint disease (DJD, osteo-arthritis) is characterized by the progressive degeneration of articular cartilage and is a common disorder with aging.

    A. DJD may be either **monoarticular** or **polyarticular.** The most frequently affected joints include the:
        1. Distal interphalangeal (DIP) joints
        2. Proximal interphalangeal (PIP) joints
        3. Thumb [i.e., the metacarpophalangeal (MCP) and carpometacarpal (CMC) joints]
        4. Knee
        5. Hip
        6. Spine

    B. DJD may be either **primary** or **secondary** (i.e., occurring in damaged or abnormal joints). **Predisposing factors** include the following:
        1. Increasing age
        2. Female gender
        3. Obesity
        4. Major joint trauma
        5. Repetitive joint stress
        6. Chronic inflammatory arthritis
        7. Congenital and developmental joint defects
        8. Metabolic and endocrine disorders (e.g., hemochromatosis, Wilson's disease, acromegaly, diabetes mellitus, hyperparathyroidism, hypothyroidism)
        9. Type II collagen mutations

II **DIFFERENTIAL DIAGNOSIS.** Other causes of monoarticular and polyarticular arthritis must be ruled out, (see Chapters 59 and 60) including:

    A. Crystal-induced arthritides [e.g., gout, calcium pyrophosphate deposition disease (CPPD)]
    B. Joint infection (bacterial, spirochetal, or viral)
    C. Inflammatory arthritides (i.e., seropositive polyarthritis and seronegative spondyloarthropathies)
    D. Joint trauma
    E. Neoplasia

HOT

KEY

DJD is usually only associated with minimal joint warmth and swelling and generally affects weight-bearing joints. If the clinical picture does not fit this pattern, consider other causes of monoarticular or polyarticular arthritis.

APPROACH TO THE PATIENT. The patient history and physical examination findings establish the diagnosis.

A. **Patient history.** DJD is characterized by the gradual onset of joint pain and stiffness.

B. **Physical examination**
   1. Local findings include **decreased range of motion, crepitus, small effusions, minimal local warmth and tenderness,** and **bony enlargement.**
   2. **Heberden's nodes** and **Bouchard's nodes** are hard, nontender nodules that represent bony outgrowths of the DIP joints and PIP joints, respectively.

C. **Radiographic studies.** Plain films may demonstrate joint space narrowing, subchondral bone sclerosis, and osteophytes.

D. **Laboratory studies** are usually unremarkable but may help identify the underlying cause in patients with secondary DJD. Synovial fluid analysis typically reveals a white blood cell (WBC) count of less than 2000/mm^3 with a mononuclear predominance. (see Table 59-1)

TREATMENT. No treatment has been shown to slow the progression of DJD. Management strategies focus on controlling pain and minimizing disability.

A. **Pharmacologic therapies**
   1. **Acetaminophen** is as effective as NSAIDs and is easier for patients to tolerate.
   2. **NSAIDs** should be used with caution; these agents may exacerbate peptic ulcer disease, renal insufficiency, and bleeding diatheses.
   3. **Corticosteroid injections** provide temporary relief but may result in articular cartilage breakdown. Injections should generally not be given more than four times per year (per joint).

B. Nonpharmacologic therapies
  1. **Weight loss** or the use of a **cane, crutches,** or a **walker** can help to reduce the load on the joint.
  2. **Orthoses** or **braces** can be used to correct body malalignment.
  3. **Physical therapy.** Moderate activity is indicated to maintain muscle strength and range of motion. Aggravation of involved joints should be avoided.

C. Surgical therapies
  1. **Knee arthroscopy** can be used to remove loose cartilage fragments.
  2. **Joint arthroplasty** is indicated for patients with debilitating disease that is refractory to medical therapy.
  3. **Spinal laminectomy, fusion,** or **both** is indicated for patients with intractable pain resulting from DJD and spinal stenosis.

IV FOLLOW-UP AND REFERRAL

A. All patients should be referred to an occupational and physical therapist for assistance in developing an exercise regimen.

B. Patients with debilitating disease should be referred to an orthopedic surgeon or neurosurgeon.

References

Bradley JD, Brandt KD, Katz BP, et al: Comparison of an antiinflammatory dose of ibuprofen, an analgesic dose of ibuprofen, and acetaminophen in the treatment of patients with osteoarthritis of the knee. *N Engl J Med* 325(2):87–91, 1991.

Kraus VB: Pathogenesis and treatment of osteoarthritis. *Med Clin North Am* 81(1):85–112, 1997.

58. Gout

I **INTRODUCTION.** Gout is a disease of disordered purine metabolism that results in elevation of the serum uric acid level and attacks of arthritis. The clinical presentation ranges from occasional attacks of monoarticular arthritis to a debilitating chronic polyarticular arthritis accompanied by erosive bony changes.

   A. Pathogenesis. Gout stems from the episodic or constant elevation of the serum uric acid to a level that exceeds 7.0 mg/dl. At this concentration, the serum is saturated with monosodium urate, and the excess is deposited in both articular and extra-articular tissue. Deposition of urate in the tissues leads to inflammation.

HOT **KEY** Pseudogout [calcium pyrophosphate deposition disease (CPPD)] is often difficult to distinguish from gout clinically. Pseudogout tends to be accompanied by chondrocalcinosis that is visible radiographically and patients usually have normal uric acid levels.

   B. Epidemiology. Gout characteristically affects men older than 30 years and women after menopause. The mean age of onset in men is 48 years.

II **CLINICAL MANIFESTATIONS OF GOUT**
   A. Articular manifestations
      1. **Arthritis.** Typically, the involved joint is **swollen, warm, erythematous,** and **extremely tender.** The onset of symptoms is **acute,** usually evolving over 24–48 hours. If untreated, acute attacks resolve within 7–10 days.
         a. The arthritis is typically **monoarticular,** or **oligoarticular** and **asymmetric.**
            (1) The **first metatarsophalangeal (MTP) joint of the foot** is the most common site for first attacks. Other sites commonly involved include the **instep of the foot,** the **ankle,** and the **knee.**

(2) If untreated, the disease may result in an asymmetric arthritis with shortened pain-free periods and involvement of more joints, including those of the upper extremities.

b. Precipitants include trauma, surgery, exposure to cold, infection, diuretic use, and alcohol consumption.

HOT

75% of patients experience a recurrent attack within 2 years of the initial attack.

KEY

---

2. **Tophaceous gout** is characterized by the development of yellowish-white nodular collections of urate crystals in the subcutaneous tissue, bone, cartilage, and joints.
   a. The tophi are usually painless, but lead to erosive destruction of cartilage and bone.
   b. Tophaceous gout usually develops approximately 10 years after the initial attack; however, some patients may present initially with tophi.
B. **Renal manifestations**
   1. **Urolithiasis.** Radiolucent uric acid kidney stones may precede gouty arthritis. Uric acid stones may serve as a nidus for other types of kidney stones.
   2. **Uric acid nephropathy** is reversible acute renal failure that is caused by the precipitation of crystals in the renal tubules and collecting ducts. Uric acid nephropathy often occurs when a dramatic increase in uric acid production (e.g., as a result of tumor lysis in patients receiving chemotherapy for leukemia) elevates the urinary uric acid levels.
   3. **Urate nephropathy** is chronic renal insufficiency secondary to interstitial deposits of uric acid. Urate nephropathy occurs in the setting of severe gout.

III **CAUSES OF GOUT.** Gout results from **hyperuricemia,** which can be caused by decreased urate excretion or increased urate production.

A. **Decreased urate excretion** is the cause of hyperuricemia in **90% of patients.** Causes include renal disease, alcohol, and drugs (e.g., low-dose salicylates, diuretics). However, in most patients, the cause of decreased urate excretion is unclear.

B. Urate overproduction. Causes include inborn errors of metabolism (e.g., Lesch-Nyhan syndrome), myelo- and lymphoproliferative diseases, hemolysis, alcohol, psoriasis, obesity, and therapy with chemotherapeutic agents.

Ⅳ APPROACH TO THE PATIENT

A. Patient history and **physical examination findings** are described in II A 1.

HOT

A presumptive diagnosis of acute gout can be made on the basis of suggestive clinical findings, hyperuricemia, and a rapid response to a therapeutic trial of colchicine.

KEY

B. Laboratory studies

1. **Serum uric acid level.** Although approximately 95% of patients have a serum uric acid level of more than 7.5 mg/dl when serial measurements are taken during an attack, as many as 25% of patients have normal uric acid levels on a single measurement. Note that hyperuricemia alone is not sufficient for the diagnosis.

2. **Joint fluid analysis.** In a patient with acute arthritis, joint fluid analysis is the most reliable way of diagnosing gout and excluding other diagnoses. During acute attacks, joint aspiration has a sensitivity of approximately 85%.

   a. The fluid sample should be sent for crystal analysis, Gram stain and culture, and a total leukocyte count with differential. (See Table 59-1.)

   b. In patients with gout, the fluid is **predominantly neutrophilic** with at least some **intracellular monosodium urate crystals.** The crystals are **needle-shaped** with **negative birefringence** under polarized microscopy (i.e., they appear yellow when aligned parallel to the plane of polarized light and blue when perpendicular to it).

HOT KEY

Crystals in **p**seudogout appear rhomboid and have **p**ositive birefringence (i.e., the crystals parallel to the light appear blue and those perpendicular to it appear yellow.)

3. **Tophi aspiration.** A wet mount may reveal clusters of urate crystals.
4. **Urinalysis.** A 24-hour urine collection can be used to classify patients as urate overproducers or underexcreters. Overproducers will demonstrate uric acid excretion of more than 800 mg/day on a regular diet, whereas underexcreters will show uric acid excretion of less than 800 mg/day on a regular diet.

C. **Radiographic studies.** Radiographs are usually normal early in the disease. Later, the bone has "punched out" erosions with sclerotic borders and an overhanging margin. The articular surface tends to be relatively well preserved.

V TREATMENT

A. **Asymptomatic hyperuricemia** does not warrant therapy because most of these patients never develop gout.
B. **Acute gouty arthritis**
1. **Bed rest** and **warm soaks** provide symptomatic treatment.
2. **Pharmacologic therapy**
   a. **Nonsteroidal anti-inflammatory drugs (NSAIDs)** are the drugs of choice for the treatment of acute gouty arthritis. The NSAID should be prescribed at the highest approved dose until inflammation has resolved (e.g., indomethacin, 25–50 mg orally every 8 hours).
   b. **Colchicine** can be used for patients who cannot tolerate NSAIDs.
      (1) To be effective, colchicine must be taken early during an attack.
      (2) The dose is 0.6 mg orally every hour until symptoms resolve, gastrointestinal side effects occur, or a total dose of 6 mg has been administered. (Gastrointestinal side effects are dose-limiting in as many as 80% of patients.)

   c. Glucocorticoids

   (1) Intra-articular corticosteroid injection (e.g., **triamcinolone,** 10–40 mg, depending on the size of the joint) is a good alternative to NSAID therapy for patients with monoarticular arthritis.

   (2) Systemic corticosteroid therapy (e.g., **prednisone** starting at 40 mg orally daily and tapered over 7–10 days) is an alternative for patients with multiple joint involvement who are not good candidates for NSAID therapy.

C. Intercritical gout (i.e., between acute attacks)

   1. Uric acid-lowering therapy is indicated for those with hyperuricemia and recurrent attacks of arthritis, chronic tophaceous gout, or nephropathy. **The goal is to lower the serum uric acid level to less than 6.0 mg/dl.**

   a. Lifestyle modifications include **weight loss, decreased alcohol consumption,** and **avoidance of diuretics** and **purine-rich foods** (e.g., meat, seafood, legumes).

   b. Pharmacologic therapy should be started only after all signs of an acute attack have resolved. The choice of drugs may be made empirically or based on the results of a 24-hour urine collection.

   (1) Allopurinol is a xanthine oxidase inhibitor that decreases the production of uric acid.

   (a) Indications. Allopurinol is the drug of choice for patients who meet any of the following conditions:

   (i) Urate overproduction

   (ii) Chronic tophaceous gout

   (iii) Renal disease with a serum creatinine level that exceeds 2.0 mg/dl or a creatinine clearance of less than 80 ml/min

   (iv) History of urinary stones

   (b) Dose. The initial dose is 100 mg daily for 7 days; this dose is then titrated up to 300 mg every day.

   (i) The dose should be limited to 100 mg per day for those with creatinine clearance less than 40 ml/min and 200 mg per day for those with a creatinine clearance of 60–80 ml/min.

   (ii) Concomitant use of 6-mercaptopurine or azathioprine warrants a re-

duction of the dose of those drugs to 25% of the usual dose.

    (c) Side effects. If a patient who requires allopurinol develops a mild rash, desensitization is a possibility. However, desensitization is not warranted for those with severe reactions, such as exfoliative dermatitis, hepatitis, or interstitial nephritis.

  (2) Uricosuric agents can be used for patients with evidence of decreased uric acid excretion, lack of urinary stones, and relatively normal renal function (i.e., a serum creatinine level of less than 2 mg/dl).

    (a) Probenecid can be given at an initial dose of 250 mg orally twice daily; the dose can be increased as needed up to a maximum dose of 2.0 g per day.

    (b) Sulfinpyrazone can be given at an initial dose of 50 mg orally twice daily; the dose can be increased to a maximum of 300–400 mg per day in 3–4 divided doses.

  2. **Prophylaxis against recurrent attacks** is indicated for at least 6 months on initiating uric acid-lowering therapy.

    a. **Colchicine** is the drug of choice. The usual dose is 0.6 mg orally twice daily. In the setting of renal insufficiency, 0.6 mg orally once daily should be used.

    b. **NSAIDS** may also be used for prophylaxis.

References

Emmerson BT: The management of gout. *N Engl J Med* 334(7): 445–451, 1996.

Fam AG, Lewtas J, Stein J, et al: Desensitization to allopurinol in patients with gout and cutaneous reactions. *Am J Med* 93(3):299–302, 1992.

59. Monoarticular Arthritis

I **INTRODUCTION.** When a patient presents with joint complaints, the list of possible causes seems enormous. However, the number of possibilities can be lowered considerably by answering the following questions:

A. Is the arthritis monoarticular or polyarticular?
B. Which joints are involved? For example:
  1. **Distal interphalangeal (DIP) joint involvement** is often attributable to degenerative joint disease (DJD) or psoriatic arthritis.

HOT

▶ **D**IP involvement = **D**JD and **P**soriatic arthritis

KEY

---

  2. **Wrist involvement** is often attributable to rheumatoid arthritis.
  3. **First metatarsophalangeal (MTP) joint inflammation** is usually caused by gout or DJD.

II **CAUSES OF MONOARTICULAR ARTHRITIS.** It is important to diagnose a monoarticular arthritis quickly in order to prevent permanent joint damage and, in some cases, sepsis. The mnemonic "If I Make The Diagnosis, No More Harm" will help you recall the most important causes of monoarticular arthritis.

Causes of Monoarticular Arthritis ("If I Make The Diagnosis, No More Harm")

Infection of the joint
Inflammatory disease
Metabolic disorders
Trauma
DJD
Neoplasia
Miscellaneous causes (foreign body synovitis, avascular necrosis)
Hemarthrosis

A. **Infection of the joint** must be considered first because it is potentially life-threatening. Commonly implicated organisms include *Streptococcus, Staphylococcus* and *Neisseria gonorrhoeae.*

B. **Inflammatory disorders** (e.g., **psoriatic arthritis, rheumatoid arthritis, Reiter's syndrome,** and other **collagen vascular diseases).** Although these diseases usually are polyarticular (see Chapter 60), they may begin as a monoarticular swelling and thus have to be considered after other causes have been ruled out.

C. **Metabolic disorders** include **gout** and **pseudogout** (calcium pyrophosphate deposition disease; CPPD). These disorders are discussed in Chapter 58.

D. **Trauma** to a joint (e.g., torn ligament, bone fracture) can lead to hemarthrosis or internal joint derangement. The patient should always be asked about a history of trauma to the affected joint.

E. **DJD** can cause monoarticular or polyarticular arthritis.

F. **Neoplasia** is a rare cause of monoarticular swelling but should be considered. Examples include **osteoid osteoma** and **pigmented villonodular synovitis.**

F. **Miscellaneous causes** include **foreign body synovitis** and **avascular necrosis.**

G. **Hemarthrosis.** Bleeding into a joint, when not related to trauma, is usually associated with **clotting disorders** (e.g., hemophilia) or **anticoagulant therapy.**

III **APPROACH TO THE PATIENT**

A. **Patient history**

   1. A history of joint complaints would imply a crystal-induced or other noninfectious etiology.

   2. Identifying sexual risk factors is important, especially in young patients.
B. Physical examination. The physical examination is useful for:
   1. Determining which joints are involved
   2. Excluding periarticular processes that may mimic arthritis (e.g., cellulitis, bursitis, tendinitis)
   3. Discerning signs that suggest specific causes (e.g., skin evidence of psoriasis)
C. Other diagnostic modalities
   1. Plain radiographs of the affected joint are sometimes helpful (e.g., when DJD, pseudogout, or fracture is the cause of the joint pain), but generally, radiographs are not useful.
   2. Arthrocentesis and **joint fluid analysis** is the **mainstay of diagnosis** and should be performed in most patients, especially if infection is a consideration (Table 59-1).

HOT Because the synovial fluid white blood cell count (WBC) may be low early in the disease course, always consider infection, regardless of the joint fluid analysis results. Re-aspiration of the joint after 24 hours is indicated if infection is suspected and the initial joint fluid analysis is inconclusive.
KEY

---

   3. Synovial biopsy and **arthroscopy** should be considered if the diagnosis is still unclear.

IV **TREATMENT** depends on the underlying disease.

A. Joint infection
   1. Arthrocentesis. Serial aspirations should be obtained for 5–7 days to decrease pain, minimize the risk of joint damage, and minimize the risk of failed antibiotic treatment.
   2. Empiric antibiotic therapy should be directed against the most common pathogens. Gram stain and culture are used to guide further treatment.
      a. If the Gram stain is negative, **ceftriaxone** (1 g intravenously daily) or **cefotaxime** (1 g intravenously every 8 hours) can be administered.
      b. If the Gram stain reveals Gram-positive cocci, **nafcillin** (2 g intravenously every 4 hours) should be used.

TABLE 59-1. Joint Fluid Analysis*

	Normal	Noninflammatory	Inflammatory	Septic
WBCs/mm³	< 200	200–10,000	10,000–100,000	> 100,000
%PMN	< 25%	< 25%	50%–90%	50%–100%
Possible causes	· · ·	DJD, trauma, aseptic necrosis	Collagen–vascular diseases, crystal-induced disease, TB, mycotic infections	Pyogenic bacterial infections

DJD = degenerative joint disease; PMNs = polymorphonuclear neutrophils; TB = tuberculosis; WBCs = white blood cells.
*Results in different diseases may be variable.

      3. Surgical intervention is required for nonresolving infections to ensure adequate drainage of the infected joint.

B. Gout. The treatment of gout is discussed in Chapter 58 V.

C. Inflammatory disorders

      1. Rheumatoid arthritis. The treatment of rheumatoid arthritis is discussed in Chapter 60 IV A.

      2. Ankylosing spondylitis. The treatment of ankylosing spondylitis is discussed in Chapter 60 IV C.

D. DJD. The treatment of DJD is discussed in Chapter 57 III.

V FOLLOW-UP AND REFERRAL

A. Referral to a **rheumatologist** is indicated when the diagnosis remains in question despite initial testing.

B. Referral to a **surgeon** is indicated for patients with infection that is not responsive to needle aspiration and therapy with appropriate antibiotics.

References

American College of Rheumatology Ad Hoc Committee on Clinical Guidelines: Guidelines for the initial evaluation of the adult patient with acute musculoskeletal complaints. *Arthritis Rheum* 39(1):1–8, 1996.

Baker DG, Schumacher HR: Acute monarthritis. *N Engl J Med* 330(11):769–774, 1994.

60. Polyarticular Arthritis

I **INTRODUCTION.** In order to organize the many causes of polyarticular arthritis, classify them as belonging to one of three main categories: classic seropositive, classic seronegative, or miscellaneous (Table 60-1).

A. **Autoimmune — classic seropositive.** These disorders are characterized by **symmetric swelling** and the presence of **autoantibodies.**

B. **Autoimmune — classic seronegative.** All of the seronegative disorders are characterized by an **asymmetric polyarthritis** affecting either the spine or large peripheral joints, a strong association with **HLA-B27,** the **early onset of disease** (usually before the age of 40 years), and an **absence of autoantibodies** (hence the term "seronegative").

C. **Miscellaneous causes.** Many other illnesses present with polyarthritis. These can easily be remembered in the following manner: one gonorrheal, two spirochetal, three viral, four infiltrative, and five "other."

II **CAUSES OF POLYARTICULAR ARTHRITIS**

A. **Autoimmune — classic seropositive**

1. **Rheumatoid arthritis** is a chronic systemic inflammatory disease primarily involving the synovial membranes of multiple joints.

   a. **Epidemiology.** The disease affects women twice as often as men, and the usual age at the time of onset is 20–40 years.

   b. **Clinical manifestations.** In order to diagnose rheumatoid arthritis, four of seven diagnostic criteria must be present (i.e., You must **AMASS** 4 of 7 to **RX** a patient with rheumatoid arthritis):

      (1) **Major symptoms** include malaise, fever, morning stiffness, and progressive symmetric swelling of the small joints. The onset of symptoms is insidious.

TABLE 60-1. Common Causes of Polyarticular Arthritis

Autoimmune—classic seropositive
Rheumatoid arthritis
Systemic lupus erythematosus (SLE)
Systemic sclerosis
Polymyositis
Overlap syndrome
Autoimmune—classic seronegative
Ankylosing spondylitis
Psoriatic arthritis
Reiter's syndrome
Arthritis related to enteric disorders (e.g., inflammatory bowel
   disease, Whipple's disease, enteric infection)
Miscellaneous
   1 Gonorrheal—disseminated gonococcal infection
   2 Spirochetal—Lyme disease, secondary syphilis
   3 Viral—HIV, hepatitis B, parvovirus
   4 Infiltrative—sarcoidosis, amyloidosis, hemochromatosis,
      tophaceous gout
   5 Other—degenerative joint disease (DJD), Still's disease,
      inflammatory bowel disease, rheumatic fever, vasculitis

Criteria for the Diagnosis of Rheumatoid Arthritis
("AMASS RX")

Arthritis in 3 or more joint areas
Morning stiffness lasting 1 hour or more
Arthritis of the hand joints
Symmetric arthritis
Serum rheumatoid factor (RF) present

Rheumatoid nodules
X-ray changes consistent with rheumatoid arthritis
(e.g., erosions)

   (2) Extra-articular findings may include subcuta-
        neous nodules, polyserositis, lymphadenopa-
        thy, and splenomegaly.
   (3) Radiographic findings classically include pe-
        riarticular osteoporosis, joint erosions, and,

occasionally, subluxation of the upper cervical spine.

(4) Laboratory findings. Eighty-five percent of patients are **RF-positive.**

2. **Systemic lupus erythematosus (SLE)** is a multisystemic autoimmune disorder.

   a. **Epidemiology.** Eighty-five percent of all patients are women 20–40 years of age.

   b. **Clinical manifestations.** The criteria for diagnosis are helpful to remember because they include the major clinical manifestations of the disease. The presence of 4 of the 11 criteria makes the diagnosis. In our medical school, in order to pass, we needed to know the 11 criteria for SLE; therefore, we were all in "P-MOAD"—7 Ps and M O A D. The first two Ps are positive lab tests; the next five Ps are arranged from head to toe. Let's go through it:

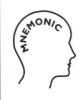

Criteria for the Diagnosis of SLE ("P-MOAD")

Positive antineutrophil antibody (ANA) test: seen in 95% of patients

Positive other immunologic test [antibody (Ab) to double-stranded DNA, Ab to Smith, lupus erythematosus (LE) cell preparation, or false-positive syphilis serology]

Psychosis, seizures, or other neurologic abnormalities

Photosensitivity rash

Polyserositis (pleuritis, pericarditis, or peritonitis)

Proteinuria or renal involvement

Pancytopenia or single-cell line "penia" (anemia, thrombocytopenia, leukopenia)

Malar rash

Oral ulcers

Arthritis

Discoid rash

---

3. **Systemic sclerosis (scleroderma)** is characterized by fibrosis of the skin and internal organs leading to dysphagia, pulmonary fibrosis, and cardiac and renal disease.

a. **Clinical manifestations**
  (1) **Symptoms.** Raynaud's disease (seen in 90% of patients) and arthralgias are usually early symptoms.
  (2) **Laboratory findings.** Antibodies that are specific for scleroderma include anti-topoisomerase (Scl-70), anti-nucleolar antibody, and anti-centromere antibody.
b. There are **two forms** of systemic sclerosis.
  (1) **Diffuse systemic sclerosis** affects 20% of patients.
  (2) **Limited systemic sclerosis (CREST syndrome).** **CREST** syndrome is the syndrome of **c**alcinosis, **R**aynaud's phenomenon, **e**sophageal motility dysfunction, **s**clerodactyly, and **t**elangiectasia. Those with CREST syndrome have a decreased risk of renal involvement, a higher risk of pulmonary hypertension, increased incidence of anti-centromere antibodies, and a better prognosis.

B. Autoimmune—classic seronegative
  1. **Ankylosing spondylitis** is characterized by the gradual onset of back pain in those younger than 40 years, progressive limitation of anterior flexion of the lumbar spine, and radiographic evidence of sclerosis of the sacroiliac joint. HLA-B27 is present in more than 90% of patients.
  2. **Psoriatic arthritis,** occurring in as many as 20% of patients with psoriasis, is characterized by a destructive arthritis of the distal interphalangeal (DIP) joints, nail pitting, and onycholysis.
  3. **Reiter's syndrome** is classically characterized by the clinical triad of **conjunctivitis, urethritis,** and **arthritis**—the patient cannot "see, pee, or bend at the knees."

C. Miscellaneous causes
  1. **Gonorrheal infection.** Disseminated gonococcal infection (caused by *Neisseria gonorrhoeae*) may result in migratory polyarthralgias of the large joints, tenosynovitis, fever, and/or a pustular rash.
  2. **Spirochetal infection**
    a. **Lyme disease** (caused by *Borrelia burgdorferi*) is characterized by flu-like symptoms, erythema migrans, neurologic problems (e.g., facial nerve palsy, meningitis), cardiac disease, and/or a chronic or recurrent large joint arthritis.
    b. **Secondary syphilis** can involve almost any part of the body, including the joints.

3. **Viral infection.** The three common viral causes of polyarticular arthritis include **HIV, hepatitis B virus,** and **parvovirus.**
4. **Infiltrative disorders** include **sarcoidosis, amyloidosis, hemochromatosis,** and **tophaceous gout;** biopsy of the joint or other affected organs is usually necessary to make the diagnosis.
5. **Other disorders**
   a. **Degenerative joint disease (DJD)** may be the most common cause of polyarticular arthritis and is discussed in detail in Chapter 57.
   b. **Still's disease** is a form of juvenile rheumatoid arthritis that also affects adults. It is characterized by spiking fevers, arthritis, and an evanescent, salmon-colored rash.
   c. **Inflammatory bowel disease** is associated with polyarthritis. Ten to twenty percent of patients with Crohn's disease or ulcerative colitis develop arthritis. Articular symptoms tend to flare concomitantly with the activity of the bowel disease.
   d. **Rheumatic fever** is a delayed sequela of pharyngitis caused by a group A streptococcus. Classic clinical manifestations include a migratory polyarthritis, fever, carditis, chorea, and subcutaneous nodules.
   e. **Vasculitis** is discussed in Chapter 87.

III **APPROACH TO THE PATIENT.** Because polyarticular arthritis has many causes, clinical, laboratory, and radiographic features are used to establish a diagnosis.

A. Patient history
1. A history of symmetric large- and small-joint arthritis with morning stiffness suggests classic seropositive or seronegative arthritis.
2. Asymmetric, additive, or migratory arthralgias are suggestive of an infectious or crystal-induced arthritis.

HOT

  Infectious or crystal-induced arthritis is usually monoarticular.

KEY

   3. A history of exposure to ticks or sexually transmitted
   disease, or the presence of a rash or fever increases
   the likelihood of infectious arthritis.
B. Physical examination. The physical examination is useful
for:
   1. Determining which joints are involved
   2. Evaluating extra-articular manifestations of disease
   (e.g., oral ulcers, alopecia, and rash may suggest SLE;
   calcinosis, sclerodactyly, and telangiectasias may suggest CREST syndrome)
C. Laboratory studies
   1. Serologic studies
      a. RF, ANA, Ab to double-stranded DNA, and ex-
      tractable nuclear antibodies [i.e., Smith, Ro, La,
      anti-centromere, anti-histone, or anti-ribonuclear
      protein (anti-RNB)] are appropriate when a sym-
      metric polyarthritis is present and clinical findings
      suggest rheumatoid arthritis or SLE.
      b. Anti-topoisomerase (Scl-70), anti-nucleolar, and
      anti-centromere antibody tests are indicated if
      scleroderma or CREST is the suspected diagnosis.
      c. Antibodies to *Borrelia burgdorferi* and the Vene-
      real Disease Research Laboratory (VDRL) test
      can be used to evaluate for Lyme disease and
      syphilis, respectively.

HOT

  Patients with SLE may have false-positive VDRL test results.

KEY

---

   2. Genetic testing for HLA-B27. Eighty to ninety
   percent of patients with ankylosing spondylitis are
   HLA-B27 positive. However, genetic testing is not
   generally helpful because 7% of people of western
   European descent without ankylosing spondylitis test
   positive.

 TREATMENT depends on the underlying disease.

A. Autoimmune — classic seropositive
   1. Rheumatoid arthritis
      a. Nonsteroidal anti-inflammatory drugs (NSAIDs)

are the mainstay of treatment. Aspirin (1 g three times daily) or ibuprofen (400–800 mg every 6 hours) may be used.

   b. **"Disease-modifying agents"** (e.g., prednisone, gold salts, hydroxychloroquine, methotrexate, azathioprine, cyclosporine, and penicillamine) alter autoimmunity, thereby slowing disease progression. These agents should be given only after consultation with a rheumatologist.

2. **SLE.** Like rheumatoid arthritis, SLE is treated with NSAIDs and immunosuppressive agents (e.g., hydroxychloroquine, cyclophosphamide, or azathioprine). Immunosuppressive agents should only be prescribed after consultation with a rheumatologist.

3. **Systemic sclerosis.** Because the disease is refractory to most immunosuppressive therapies, treatment is aimed at relieving symptoms.

   a. D-Penicillamine, glucocorticoids, or colchicine have been used to treat severe cases.

   b. Treatment should be tailored to the patient. Consultation with a rheumatologist is recommended.

B. **Autoimmune—classic seronegative**
1. **Ankylosing spondylitis**

   a. **Physical therapy** is indicated to preserve the patient's range of motion.

   b. **NSAIDs** (e.g., indomethacin) and **sulfasalazine** are used for pain relief and disease control. Initially, 500 mg of sulfasalazine may be given daily. The dose can be increased in 500-mg increments each week until the patient's symptoms improve or a maximum dose of 3 g (divided into two or three doses daily) is reached.

HOT **KEY**

Because sulfasalazine can lead to neutropenia and thrombocytopenia, the blood counts of patients taking this medication should be monitored frequently.

---

2. **Psoriatic arthritis** is treated with NSAIDS, colchicine, intra-articular steroid injections, gold salts, methotrexate, azathioprine, or sulfasalazine.

C. **Miscellaneous causes.** The treatment strategy usually entails addressing the underlying cause (e.g., antibiotics for infectious arthritis, phlebotomy for hemochromatosis, glucocorticoids for sarcoidosis, allopurinol for tophaceous gout). The treatment of DJD is discussed in Chapter 57, and the treatment of vasculitis is discussed in Chapter 87.

V **FOLLOW-UP AND REFERRAL.** Referral to a rheumatologist is indicated when:

A. The diagnosis remains in question despite initial testing

B. Immunosuppression is required to control joint symptoms refractory to NSAIDs

C. There is any evidence of ongoing joint damage

References

American College of Rheumatology Ad Hoc Committee on Clinical Guidelines: Guidelines for the initial evaluation of the adult patient with acute musculoskeletal complaints. *Arthritis Rheum* 39(1):1–8, 1996.

Pinals RS: Polyarthritis and fever. *N Engl J Med* 330(11):769–774, 1994.

61. Low Back Pain

I INTRODUCTION. As many as 90% of adults experience low back pain at some time.

A. Low back pain is second only to upper respiratory tract infection as the most common reason to visit an internist.

B. The cost of back pain in terms of work hours lost exceeds that of ischemic heart disease.

II CLINICAL MANIFESTATIONS

A. Fewer than 5% of patients with low back pain have **sciatica** (i.e., pain that radiates into the buttock and down one leg to below the knee). This symptom complex is seen with nerve root compression, a form of radiculopathy (i.e., nerve root disease). The distribution is dermatomal.

B. Fewer than 1% of patients have **cauda equina syndrome,** an acute radiculopathy characterized by bowel and bladder disturbances (usually urinary retention), saddle anesthesia, and bilateral neurologic deficits.

HOT

KEY

Cauda equina syndrome is a surgical emergency! Patients with signs or symptoms of cauda equina compression require emergent magnetic resonance imaging (MRI) or computed tomography (CT) scanning and surgical evaluation.

III DIFFERENTIAL DIAGNOSIS

A. Back pain as a result of disorders of the vertebrae and disks. Disorders of the vertebrae and disks account for most cases of low back pain. The pain is usually related to one of the following processes.

1. Spondylosis is degenerative changes of the disks and facet joints.

2. Spondylolisthesis is forward displacement of a lumbar vertebra onto the one below it.

3. **Disk herniation** usually occurs posterolaterally and can result in nerve root compression. Ninety-five percent of disk herniations occur at disk L4-L5 (affecting the L5 root) or disk L5-S1 (affecting the S1 root). Massive midline herniation can cause cauda equina compression.

4. **Spinal stenosis.** Degenerative changes of the facet joints and the ligamentum flavum cause narrowing of the spinal canal, resulting in compression of the spinal cord. The classic symptom of spinal stenosis is **neurogenic claudication (pseudoclaudication),** which is characterized by poorly localized buttock and leg pain that is exacerbated by walking. Walking downhill is worse than walking uphill because flexion typically alleviates the compression caused by the spinal stenosis.

HOT

In patients with spinal stenosis, walking **down** causes pain levels to go **up.**

KEY

B. **Back pain as a result of systemic disease**
1. **Malignancy. Metastatic disease** from breast, lung, or prostate cancer is the most common form of malignancy-related back pain. **Primary tumors, multiple myeloma,** and **lymphoma** should also be considered. Patients with a malignancy often experience unrelenting nocturnal pain.
2. **Infection.** Local infections, such as **osteomyelitis, diskitis,** and **epidural abscess,** can cause low back pain.
3. **Inflammatory spondyloarthropathies,** such as **ankylosing spondylitis,** can cause low back pain. Typically, patients are younger than 40 years and have symptoms on awakening that decrease with activity.
4. **Vertebral compression fractures** as result of **osteoporosis** can cause low back pain in elderly patients and those who take steroids for long periods.
C. **Referred visceral pain.** Low back pain can be a symptom of:
1. **Aortic aneurysm**
2. **Urologic disorders** (e.g., calculi, pyelonephritis, prostatitis)

3. **Gastrointestinal disorders** (e.g., colorectal or peptic ulcer disease, pancreatitis)
4. **Gynecologic disorders** [e.g., endometriosis, pelvic inflammatory disease (PID)]

IV **APPROACH TO THE PATIENT** (Figure 61-1)

A. **Patient history.** Care should be taken to evaluate the patient's risk factors for a **systemic cause** (e.g., malignancy, infection) of the low back pain. Risk factors include:
1. Age greater than 50 years
2. History of cancer or intravenous drug abuse
3. Signs or symptoms of systemic disease (e.g., fever, weight loss, lymphadenopathy)

B. **Physical examination**
1. **Spinal examination.** Inspect the spine for deformity, palpate for point tenderness, and assess the patient's range of motion.
2. **Neurologic examination.** A directed neurologic examination can be used to screen for radiculopathy.
   a. **Straight-leg raising test.** With the patient supine, lift the patient's leg with the knee extended. If radicular pain occurs when the leg is elevated 30°–60° off the table, the test is positive.
      (1) This test is sensitive for identifying **nerve root irritation,** but not very specific.
      (2) A positive crossed straight-leg raising test (i.e., sciatica is reproduced in the affected leg by lifting the opposite leg) is much more specific for **herniated disk,** but is not very sensitive.
   b. **Screening motor examination.** More than 95% of disk herniations occur at the L4-L5 disk (affecting the L5 root) or the L5-S1 disk (affecting the S1 root) and the remaining 2%–5% occur at the L2-L3 disk or the L3-L4 disk (affecting the L3 and L4 roots, respectively). A screening motor examination should be performed in all patients.
      (1) Have the patient rise from the chair and do a heel walk and a toe walk. Check extensor hallucis longus function (by testing the big toe strength) and evaluate the ankle jerk and knee jerk.
      (2) Table 61-1 reviews the neurologic findings associated with impingement of these roots.

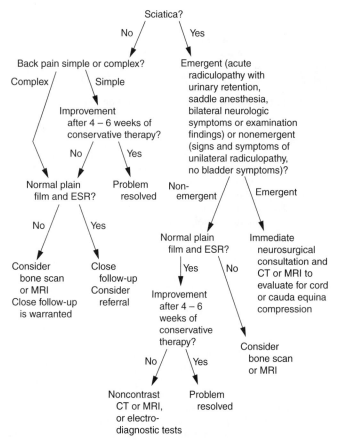

FIGURE 61-1. Approach to the patient with low back pain. *CT* = computed tomography; *ESR* = erythrocyte sedimentation rate; *MRI* = magnetic resonance imaging. (Modified with permission from Wipf JE, Deyo RA: Low back pain. In Branch WT (ed): *Office of Practice of Medicine*, 3rd ed. Philadelphia, WB Saunders, 1994, p 654.)

HOT KEY If the patient has bilateral symptoms or bowel or bladder retention or incontinence, the physical examination should also include a careful perineal sensory examination and evaluation of rectal tone and the sacral reflexes to evaluate for possible cauda equina syndrome.

TABLE 61-1. Neurologic Findings In Disk Herniation

Affected Nerve Root	Motor Findings	Sensory Findings*	Reflexes
L3, L4	Difficulty rising from chair (loss of knee extensor function) or performing heel walk	Anterior knee and medial calf	Decreased or absent knee jerk reflex
L5	Difficulty performing heel walk; decreased strength in foot and big toe dorsiflexion	Medial forefoot (first web space)	Reflexes intact
S1	Difficulty performing toe walk; foot eversion and plantar flexion	Lateral foot	Decreased or absent ankle jerk reflex

*Decreased sensation or paresthesias.

   3. **General examination.** If the history has raised the possibility of back pain as a result of a **systemic disorder** or **referred visceral pain,** a more general examination should be performed. For example:
      a. **Abdominal examination** (to rule out aneurysm in an elderly patient with known vascular disease)
      b. **Joint examination** (if the history suggests an inflammatory spondyloarthropathy)
      c. **Lymph node examination** and a more thorough **evaluation for masses** (if malignancy is suspected)
C. **Laboratory studies.** Most patients do not require routine laboratory tests. An **erythrocyte sedimentation rate (ESR)** may be helpful if there is high suspicion for infection, inflammatory disease, or malignancy.
D. **Imaging studies**
   1. **Plain films.** Degenerative changes are ubiquitous in patients older than 40 years and lumbar films yield 20 times the radiation of a chest radiograph; therefore, radiographs are indicated only for the following patients:
      a. Those with risk factors for a systemic cause of low back pain (see IV A)
      b. Those who have sustained significant trauma
      c. Those in whom the history suggests ankylosing spondylitis
      d. Those who take steroids or have advanced osteoporosis
      e. Those with significant neuromotor deficits
      f. Selected patients who have failed to respond to conservative therapy
   2. **Bone scan.** If plain films increase the suspicion for cancer or infection, a bone scan is indicated.

HOT

Bone scans are normal in patients with multiple myeloma.

KEY

---

   3. **MRI** and **CT with myelogram** must be selectively ordered because these studies are associated with a high incidence of **false-positive results.**
      a. An MRI or CT with myelogram should be performed immediately in patients with suspected

malignancy or infection, or any evidence of cauda equina syndrome.

b. These tests are appropriate for the pre-operative assessment of patients who require surgery for persistent or progressive radiculopathy.

E. **Classification.** Most cases of low back pain cannot be assigned a precise pathoanatomic diagnosis. Nevertheless, it is important to classify the patient's low back pain as either simple or complex on the basis of the clinical findings because this distinction affects the recommended work-up (see Figure 61-1).

1. **Simple low back pain.** Two-thirds of patients have simple low back pain (i.e., no risk factors for or signs of underlying pathology and a normal neurologic examination).

2. **Complex low back pain.** Patients either have an abnormal neurologic examination, or they have risk factors for a systemic cause of low back pain.

V TREATMENT

A. **Conservative therapies.** For most patients, even those with radiculopathy, symptoms improve with conservative therapy within 4–6 weeks.

1. **Bed rest.** Bed rest is generally not beneficial for patients with suspected disk herniations. A gradual return to normal activity should take place within 1–2 weeks.

2. **Pharmacologic therapy**
   a. **Analgesics**
      (1) **Nonsteroidal anti-inflammatory drugs (NSAIDs)** are effective (e.g., ibuprofen, 800 mg orally as needed, up to 3 times daily). **Acetaminophen** or **aspirin** may also be tried.
      (2) **Opioids** should be used sparingly. They have no clear benefit over NSAIDs in most patients, are associated with central nervous system (CNS) side effects, and may lead to dependency.
   b. **Muscle relaxants.** In selected patients, a muscle relaxant (e.g., cyclobenzaprine, 10 mg twice daily) may be useful, but use should be limited to 1–2 weeks.
   c. **Steroid injections** are controversial.

3. **Education.** Patients should be educated about the cause of back pain and reassured about the expected course and recovery.

    4. Other approaches
        a. Physical therapy. Patients with prolonged symptoms may benefit from an exercise program.
        b. Chiropractic manipulation may be helpful for patients with simple mechanical low back pain, but should be avoided in patients with radiculopathy.
        c. Traction is probably not useful.

B. Surgery is better for relieving radicular symptoms than for relieving back pain. Relief of symptoms is more rapid with surgery, but long-term outcomes of both surgery and conservative therapy often are similar. Indications for surgery in patients with herniated disks include:

1. **Cauda equina syndrome**
2. **Severe** or **progressive neurologic deficit**
3. **Persistent neuromotor deficit** after 4–6 weeks of conservative therapy
4. **Persistent sciatica, sensory deficit,** or **reflex loss** in a patient with a **positive straight-leg raising test, consistent clinical findings,** and **favorable psychosocial circumstances** (e.g., realistic expectations and no evidence of depression, substance abuse, or excessive somatization)

References
Acute low back problems in adults. Guideline overview. Agency for Health Care Policy and Research. Rockville, Maryland. *J Natl Med Assoc* 87(5):331–333, 1995.
Wipf JE, Deyo RA: Low back pain. *Med Clin North Am* 79(2):231, 1995.

PART IX

Neurology

62. Headache

I **INTRODUCTION.** Headaches affect more than 90% of the population and are one of the most common reasons for office and emergency room visits. Although most headaches are symptoms of self-limited conditions, it is crucial to identify the small percentage of headaches that signal life-threatening disease.

II **DIFFERENTIAL DIAGNOSIS.** The mnemonic for recalling the differential diagnosis of headache, "Take Care to Diagnose My Symptoms; I don't want to be MAIMED," conveniently divides the differential into "common" and "less common" causes.

Differential Diagnosis for Headache ("Take Care to Diagnose My Symptoms; I don't want to be MAIMED")

Tension headache
Cluster headache
Drugs or **D**ental pain
Migraine headache
Sinusitis or **S**ystemic illness

Mass lesion
Arteritis or **A**cute angle glaucoma
Ischemia
Meningitis
Encephalitis or **E**levated intracranial pressure (ICP)
Dural venous sinus thrombosis

A. Common causes
 1. Tension headache. Patients often describe a "band-like" sensation of tightening around the head. The pain is likely muscular in origin, and it may be precipitated by stress. Tension headaches are generally differentiated from migraines by the absence of associated symptoms (e.g., nausea, vomiting, aura).

2. **Cluster headaches** occur almost exclusively in middle-aged men. These headaches are usually unilateral, centered around the orbit, and described as sharp, stabbing, and severe. The headache often occurs at the same time each day and generally lasts 30–60 minutes. The headaches last for several months, resolve spontaneously, and then recur (hence the name "cluster").

3. **Drugs.** Nitroglycerin, histamine-2 (H_2) blockers, nonsteroidal anti-inflammatory drugs (NSAIDs), nifedipine, atenolol, digoxin, and theophylline can all cause headache.

4. **Dental pain.** Patients with abscesses, caries, or infections of the gingiva may complain of a headache.

5. **Migraine headaches** show a strong familial pattern. The pain is usually described as unilateral, pulsating, and exacerbated by physical activity. Patients commonly have photophobia, phonophobia, nausea, and vomiting. An aura (i.e., premonitory symptoms such as visual abnormalities, vertigo, or taste sensations) may be present (migraines are classified as occurring with or without aura).

6. **Sinusitis** characteristically causes a frontal or retro-orbital headache that is exacerbated by leaning forward (see Chapter 11).

7. **Systemic conditions.** Many systemic illnesses can cause headaches (e.g., **common cold, malignant hypertension, fever, carbon monoxide poisoning).**

B. **Less common causes**

1. **Mass lesions.** The presentation varies, but new symptoms, progressive symptoms, or neurologic abnormalities are suggestive features.

   a. **Tumors** often produce a subacute, progressive, unilateral pain. The classic symptoms of morning headache, vomiting, and increased pain with the Valsalva maneuver are seen only in a minority of patients.

   b. **Abscesses** are usually associated with fever and an abnormal neurologic examination.

   c. **Subdural hematoma.** Although a history of trauma in the previous weeks is suggestive, the patient may not recall the incident (this is especially true with elderly patients).

   d. **Intraparenchymal** or **subarachnoid hemorrhage** usually results from the rupture of a berry aneurysm or an arteriovenous malformation (AVM). Patients classically report the "worst headache of my life."

2. **Arteritis and other connective tissue diseases**

   a. **Temporal arteritis** should be considered in patients older than 50 years who present with temporal headache, unilateral visual abnormalities (e.g.. flashing lights, amaurosis fugax), or jaw claudication.

   b. **Other connective tissue diseases** [e.g., systemic lupus erythematosus (SLE), polyarteritis nodosa, Wegener's granulomatosis] can be associated with arteritis (e.g., cerebral vasculitis) and headache.

3. **Acute angle glaucoma** should be considered in an older patient who presents with a new, frontal headache.

4. **Ischemia.** Stroke and transient ischemic attacks (TIAs) should be considered in patients with risk factors for these conditions.

5. **Meningitis.** Patients may initially present with a headache. Fever, mental status changes, and meningeal signs (e.g., neck pain with neck flexion or hip flexion) may also be present.

6. **Encephalitis** almost always is associated with mental status changes.

7. **Elevated ICP** (as a result of **pseudotumor cerebri** or a **mass lesion)** may cause headache. Papilledema or abnormal neurologic signs are suggestive.

8. **Dural venous sinus thrombosis** is usually associated with a predisposing condition (e.g., pregnancy, malignancy, other hypercoagulable disorders).

III **APPROACH TO THE PATIENT.** A thorough history and physical examination can establish the diagnosis in most patients. The goal is to avoid missing any potentially life-threatening cause of headache.

A. **Patient history.** A detailed history of all symptoms associated with the current and past headaches is required. The presence of any of the following symptoms raises "NEW FEARS" and suggests a need for more intensive evaluation.

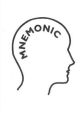

Worsome Symptoms Associated with Headache
("NEW FEARS")
NEW or different headache (especially in patients older than 40 years)

Fever
Exertional headache (e.g., headache with exercise, cough, sexual activity)
Abnormal mental status or personality changes
Recent history of trauma
Severe symptoms

B. Physical examination. A full physical examination is required.
   1. **Papilledema** suggests increased ICP.
   2. **Increased intraocular pressure** is associated with glaucoma.
   3. **Meningismus** (i.e., pain with passive forward neck flexion) suggests meningeal irritation, which can be caused by meningitis or subarachnoid hemorrhage.
   4. A **petechial rash** that is noted first on the lower extremities may be seen with meningococcal meningitis.

HOT

KEY
A dangerous cause for the headache is likely if the headache is accompanied by a neurologic abnormality.

C. Laboratory studies. Patients who have no worrisome historical or physical examination findings generally do not require laboratory testing.
   1. A **complete blood count (CBC), serum chemistries,** and an **erythrocyte sedimentation rate (ESR)** should be obtained for patients with an unclear diagnosis or with worrisome features. The ESR is almost always elevated in patients with temporal arteritis, although many other inflammatory disorders can also increase the ESR.
   2. **Cerebrospinal fluid (CSF) analysis** is indicated for patients with suspected meningitis or subarachnoid hemorrhage.

HOT

A lumbar puncture should not be performed in patients with focal neurologic signs until a head computed tomography (CT) scan has been performed to rule out increased ICP.

KEY

D. **Imaging studies.** Head CT or magnetic resonance imaging (MRI) are indicated when clinical and laboratory evaluation do not yield a diagnosis.

HOT

In patients with suspected subarachnoid hemorrhage, a negative CT scan does not rule out the disorder, and lumbar puncture should be performed.

KEY

IV TREATMENT

A. **Tension headaches** can usually be managed with mild analgesics (e.g., acetaminophen, 650 mg every 4–6 hours or ibuprofen, 400–800 mg every 6 hours). Exercise, avoidance of stress, and relaxation techniques may be useful.

B. **Cluster headaches**
   1. **Acute therapy.** An acute attack can often be arrested by administering **inhaled oxygen** (6 L/min for 10 minutes). **NSAIDs, ergotamine,** and **sumatriptan,** as used for the treatment of migraine headaches (see IV C 1), are also effective.
   2. **Chronic therapy.** A course of **steroids** (e.g., prednisone, 60 mg daily tapered over 2 weeks) may terminate cluster headaches in some patients.

C. **Migraine headaches**
   1. **Abortive therapy** (Table 62-1) is required during the episode.
   2. **Prophylactic therapy** (Table 62-2) may be considered for patients with frequent attacks (i.e., attacks occurring more than twice a month) or attacks that interfere with the patient's lifestyle. **β Blockers** (e.g., atenolol), **tricyclic antidepressants** (e.g., amitriptyline), and **calcium channel blockers** (e.g., verapamil) can be used in the prophylactic treatment of migraine.

TABLE 62-1. Selected Abortive Treatments for Migraine Headache

Severity of Migraine	Medications	Dose	Cautions
Mild to moderate	Naproxen	500–750 mg orally every 12 hours	May cause gastrointestinal ulceration or bleeding
	Aspirin	650 mg orally every 4–6 hours	Avoid in pregnant women, patients younger than 18 years, and patients with gastrointestinal bleeding or bleeding disorders
	Acetaminophen	500–1000 mg orally every 6 hours	Maximum dose is 1.5 g/day in patients with liver disease, best to avoid use of this drug in these patients
Moderate to severe	Ergotamine	2 mg orally or sublingually, then 1 mg every 30 minutes up to a maximum dose of 6 mg/24 hours OR 2 mg per rectum	Contraindicated in patients with coronary artery disease (CAD), peripheral vascular disease, or pregnancy Should not be used in combination with sumatriptan

Drug	Dose	Comments
Sumatriptan	6 mg subcutaneously; may repeat after 1 hour; maximum dose is 12 mg/day	Contraindicated in patients with CAD Prinzmetal's angina, hypertension, or pregnancy Should not be given concomitantly with ergotamine May cause flushing, neck pain, or chest tightness; first dose should be medically supervised
Severe and unresponsive		
Dihydroergotamine	1 mg intramuscularly; can be repeated twice at 1-hour intervals	Side effects and contraindications are similar to those of ergotamine Should not be given if ergotamine has been used in the past 4 days
Metoclopramide	10 mg intravenously every 4 hours as needed	May cause dystonia, hypotension, nausea, and vomiting
Prochlorperazine	10 mg intravenously over 2 minutes	May cause tardive dyskinesia, hypotension, nausea, and vomiting
Meperidine	25-mg increments intravenously every hour as needed; maximum dose is 1–1.8 mg/kg	May be habituating; use infrequently for severe attacks

TABLE 62-2. Selected Prophylactic Therapy for Migraine Headache

Medication	Dose	Side Effects
Atenolol*	50–100 mg orally daily	Depression, fatigue, hypotension
Amitriptyline	10–150 mg orally at bedtime	Xerostomia, urinary retention, drowsiness, cardiac arrythmias
Verapamil	80–360 mg orally daily	Constipation, hypotension, bradycardia

*Use with caution in patients with reactive airway disease

- **D. Sinusitis.** Treatment of the sinusitis should resolve the headache (see Chapter 11 VI).
- **E. Mass lesions.** Patients must be referred to a neurosurgeon immediately.
- **F. Temporal arteritis.** If the diagnosis is suspected on clinical grounds, patients should be started on prednisone (1 mg/kg/day) and scheduled for urgent temporal artery biopsy in order to make a definitive diagnosis. Untreated temporal arteritis may lead to permanent blindness.
- **G. Ischemia.** The treatment of cerebrovascular disease is discussed in Chapter 64 V.
- **H. Meningitis**
    - **1. Antibiotics.** Any patient with suspected meningitis should receive intravenous antibiotics without delay, even before a lumbar puncture or CT scan is performed. A reasonable initial choice is **ceftriaxone** (2 g every 12 hours) **plus ampicillin** (50 mg/kg every 6 hours).
    - **2. Steroids.** Although the practice is controversial, many authorities also recommend administering steroids to patients with suspected meningitis prior to confirming the diagnosis with a lumbar puncture. **Dexamethasone** (0.4 mg/kg every 12 hours) is often used.
- **I. Encephalitis.** Patients with suspected encephalitis should be started on empiric therapy for herpes simplex virus (HSV) [e.g., **acyclovir,** 10 mg/kg intravenously over 1 hour every 8 hours]. A neurologist and an infectious disease specialist should be consulted.

J. Pseudotumor cerebri or **hydrocephalus.** These patients require consultation with a neurologist.

V FOLLOW-UP AND REFERRAL

A. Patients with life-threatening causes of headache must be referred to a neurologist, a neurosurgeon, or both. Neurology referral may also be useful for patients with severe migraine headaches or headaches that do not respond to conservative therapy.

B. Patients with non-life-threatening causes of headache should be seen for a repeat examination within 1 month and then as needed, unless symptoms recur.

References

Maizels M: The clinician's approach to the management of headache. *West J Med* 168(3):203–212, 1998.

Pryse-Phillips WE, Dodick DW, Edmeads JG, et al: Guidelines for the diagnosis and management of migraine in clinical practice. Canadian Headache Society. *CMAJ* 156(9):1273–1287, 1997.

63. Vertigo

....

I INTRODUCTION

A. **Dizziness** is a term used to describe an unusual head sensation or gait unsteadiness. Faintness and vertigo are two types of dizziness.

B. **Faintness** is usually described as a sense of **light-headedness** and is usually caused by an insufficient supply of oxygen, blood, or glucose to the brain. Faintness often occurs with hyperventilation or hypoglycemia, or just before a syncopal event.

C. **Vertigo,** the topic of this chapter, is the illusion of **movement (usually spinning).** The patient may perceive that he is moving while the environment is still, or vice versa.

1. **Pathophysiology.** Vertigo is caused by a defect in one of three systems:

   a. **Vestibular system** (most common)

   b. **Visual system**

   c. **Somatosensory system**

2. **Classification.** Prognostically, the important distinction to make is between **central** and **peripheral** vertigo. Central vertigo usually has a poorer prognosis than peripheral vertigo.

II CLINICAL MANIFESTATIONS OF VERTIGO. Both central
and peripheral vertigo can be associated with nausea, vomiting, gait unsteadiness, and ataxia, and both are exacerbated by head movement. However, several features distinguish central vertigo from peripheral vertigo.

A. **Central vertigo**

1. **Brain stem, cerebellar,** or **cerebral hemispheric signs,** such as headache, limb ataxia, true weakness, paresthesias, dysarthria, and diplopia, often accompany central vertigo.

2. **Nystagmus** may be present and can take any form (i.e., horizontal, vertical, or multidirectional).

3. **Tinnitus** or **hearing loss** are **usually not associated with central vertigo.**

B. **Peripheral vertigo** tends to cause more patient distress, although the episodes are briefer. [The central nervous system (CNS) tends to adapt, shortening episodes in patients with peripheral vertigo.]

1. There are **no brain stem, cerebellar,** or **cerebral hemispheric signs.**
2. **Nystagmus,** which is **invariably present,** occurs unidirectionally, is horizontal, and has its fast component toward the side of the normal ear. The nystagmus is inhibited by visual fixation (this is not the case in central vertigo).
3. **Tinnitus** or **hearing loss** are often associated with peripheral vertigo.

III DIFFERENTIAL DIAGNOSIS

A. **Central vertigo.** The most common causes of central vertigo can be remembered with the mnemonic, "SPIN."

Causes of Central Vertigo ("SPIN")

Sclerosis (i.e., multiple sclerosis)
Pretty bad migraine (especially basilar)
Ischemia or CNS lesions [especially basilar transient ischemic attack (TIA)]
Neuroma (i.e., acoustic neuroma)

---

1. **Multiple sclerosis** should be considered in patients with suggestive neurologic symptoms or signs. Episodic vertigo, chronic imbalance, and unilateral hearing loss are occasionally seen in patients with multiple sclerosis.
2. **Migraine,** especially when severe, may be associated with focal neurologic deficits, visual disturbances, aphasia, and vertigo.
3. **Ischemia.** Transient ischemia of the vertebrobasilar artery can cause ataxia, diplopia, dysarthria, blurred vision, vertigo, and bilateral leg weakness.
4. **Acoustic neuroma.** This common tumor of the cerebellopontine angle usually arises from the vestibular division of the eighth cranial nerve.

B. **Peripheral vertigo** is usually a result of processes that involve the **labyrinth** (inner ear) or **eighth cranial nerve.** The most common causes of peripheral vertigo can be remembered with the mnemonic, "AMPLI-TUDE."

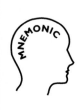

Common Causes of Peripheral Vertigo ("AMPLITUDE")

Acoustic neuroma
Meniere's disease (endolymphatic hydrops)
Positional vertigo
Labyrinthitis
Infection of the middle or inner ear
Trauma (head)
Usychogenic
Drugs
Endocrine disorders

1. **Acoustic neuroma** can cause central vertigo as well as peripheral vertigo.
2. **Meniere's disease** is caused by distention of the endolymphatic compartment within the inner ear. Characteristics include sensorineural hearing loss, "blowing" tinnitus, aural pressure, and episodic vertigo. The disease is usually idiopathic but may result from head trauma or syphilis.
3. **Benign paroxysmal positional vertigo (BPPV)** causes very brief episodes of vertigo, which usually last less than 1 minute and are brought on by head movement. BPPV often follows ear trauma or infection.
4. **Labyrinthitis** can occur following an upper respiratory tract infection and is characterized by acute, severe vertigo; nausea and vomiting; and hearing loss and tinnitus. Symptoms may last for days to weeks.
5. **Infection** of the middle or inner ear is a rare cause of vertigo but should be considered in those with evidence of infection (e.g., fever, chills).
6. **Trauma.** Recent head trauma can cause a labyrinthine concussion, producing vertigo that may last as long as 1 month.
7. **Psychogenic causes** should be considered in patients with a normal neurologic examination who do not have nystagmus.
8. **Drugs.** Aminoglycosides are the most common culprits.
9. **Endocrine disorders,** such as hypothyroidism and diabetes mellitus, can be associated with vertigo.

IV APPROACH TO THE PATIENT

A. **Patient history.** The cause of the vertigo can be discerned from the history alone in more than 70% of patients.

B. Physical examination should focus on the ears, eyes, and nervous system.

   1. Note the presence or absence of ear infection, nystagmus, or neurologic deficits.

   2. The **Nylen-Bárány maneuver** is important in the assessment of BPPV. Have the seated patient turn her head to one side while quickly lying down, so that her head hangs over the edge of the table. If vertigo is reproduced (along with nystagmus), BPPV is the likely diagnosis.

C. Laboratory studies are usually not necessary.

   1. A **thyroid-stimulating hormone (TSH) level** should be ordered if thyroid disease is suspected.

   2. A **serum glucose level** should be ordered if diabetes mellitus is suspected.

D. Other studies

   1. **Audiometric testing** is useful to evaluate for Meniere's disease or acoustic neuroma in patients with hearing loss or tinnitus.

   2. **Brain magnetic resonance imaging (MRI)** is usually indicated if peripheral causes seem unlikely or if the patient has neurologic abnormalities.

   3. **Caloric stimulation, electronystagmography,** and **brain stem auditory evoked potential studies** may be used to distinguish peripheral from central vertigo, or to reach a diagnosis in patients with persistent vertigo.

V **TREATMENT** is generally cause-specific.

A. Central vertigo

   1. **Multiple sclerosis.** Therapy with high-dose steroids, immunosuppressants, β-interferon, or copolymer 1 may be useful.

   2. **Acoustic neuroma.** These tumors can often be removed surgically if they are small enough.

   3. **Basilar TIA**

      a. **Pharmacologic therapy**

         (1) **Aspirin** (325 mg daily) is first-line therapy.

         (2) **Ticlopidine** (250 mg twice daily) can be used for those who cannot tolerate aspirin; however, close monitoring of the white blood cell (WBC) count is necessary because of the risk of agranulocytosis.

         (3) **Warfarin.** Some clinicians use warfarin for patients who are symptomatic despite therapy with aspirin or ticlopidine. The target international normalized ratio (INR) is 2–3.

    b. Surgery. Selected patients with evidence of concomitant carotid distribution disease may benefit from **carotid endarterectomy.**

  4. Migraine. For patients with both migraine headaches and vertigo, **β blockers** (e.g., propranolol, 80–240 mg once or twice daily to a maximum dose of 240 mg/day) and **ergots** (e.g., ergotamine, 1 mg four times daily) may be helpful.

B. Peripheral vertigo

  1. General symptomatic therapy

    a. Pharmacologic therapy. Medications may prevent CNS adaptation to peripheral vertigo and should not be used for long periods.

      (1) Diazepam (2.5–5 mg intravenously once) may terminate the attack and may be appropriate for patients with severe vertigo.

      (2) Meclizine (25 mg orally four times daily), **dimenhydrinate** (25–50 mg orally four times daily), or **chlordiazepoxide** (5–25 mg orally three times daily) may benefit those with less severe vertigo.

      (3) Scopolamine patches (0.5 mg/day transdermally) are useful for those with recurrent vertigo.

    b. Exercise. A mild exercise program can help the adaptation process and improve symptoms.

  2. Meniere's disease. Treatment is aimed at lowering the endolymphatic pressure.

    a. Conservative methods include a **low-salt diet** and **diuretics** (e.g., hydrochlorothiazide, 25–100 mg daily).

    b. Surgical therapy to decompress the endolymphatic sac may be considered for those who remain severely symptomatic despite medications.

VI FOLLOW-UP AND REFERRAL

A. Follow-up. Patients with severe symptoms should be seen frequently (e.g., once or twice a week) until their symptoms subside.

B. Referral

  1. When the initial work-up suggests central vertigo, the patient should be referred to a neurologist.

2. If brain imaging suggests an acoustic neuroma, consultation with a neurosurgeon is appropriate.

References
Bernard ME, Bachenberg TC, Brey RH: Benign paroxysmal positional vertigo: the canalith repositioning procedure. *Am Fam Physician* 53(8): 2613–2616, 2621, 1996.
Luxon LM: The medical management of vertigo. *J Laryngol Otol* 111(12):1114–1121, 1997.

64. Transient Ischemic Attacks

I. INTRODUCTION

A. Transient ischemic attacks (TIAs) are **focal losses of neurologic function** that **reverse completely within 24 hours** and are **caused by vascular disease.**

B. Approximately 50,000 people experience TIAs each year in the United States, and **approximately one third of these patients develop strokes.**

C. Role of the primary care physician. The primary care physician must:

1. Identify patients at risk for TIAs and initiate appropriate preventive measures
2. Identify patients with new or recurrent symptoms suggestive of TIAs and arrange for appropriate diagnostic studies and referrals
3. Counsel patients regarding the risks and benefits of the various treatment options
4. Assist in preoperative risk assessment of patients being considered for surgical intervention

II. CAUSES OF TRANSIENT ISCHEMIC ATTACKS (TIAS)

A. Extracranial atherosclerotic causes of TIA are responsible for more than 50% of all TIAs and include **carotid artery disease** and **vertebrobasilar disease.** Carotid artery disease is the more common of the two.

B. Intracranial causes of TIA include:

1. **Atherosclerosis** of the **cerebral blood vessels**
2. **Inflammation** of the **cerebral blood vessels** [e.g., as a result of systemic lupus erythematosus (SLE), syphilis, or giant cell arteritis]
3. **Hypercoagulable** and **hyperviscosity syndromes** (e.g., antiphospholipid antibody syndrome, polycythemia vera)

C. Cardiogenic emboli as a result of arrhythmias, valvular disease, myocardial infarction, or endocarditis can lead to TIAs.

D. Paradoxical emboli [i.e., embolization through a patent foramen ovale or atrial septal defect (ASD)] can result from venous thrombosis, leading to TIAs.

CLINICAL MANIFESTATIONS OF TRANSIENT ISCHEMIC ATTACKS. The onset of symptoms is **sudden** and without warning, and the **median duration** of the attack is approximately **10 minutes.** Symptoms should resolve within 1 hour; the longer the symptoms last, the more likely the person is to develop a stroke.

A. **Extracranial atherosclerotic causes**
   1. **Carotid artery disease.** Symptoms include:
      a. Unilateral visual changes, such as blurring, graying, or vision loss (amaurosis fugax)
      b. Weakness or clumsiness
      c. Numbness of the limbs or face
      d. Confusion or other cognitive changes
   2. **Vertebrobasilar disease.** Symptoms include:
      a. Ataxia
      b. Dysarthria
      c. Dizziness or vertigo
      d. Diplopia, visual field cut, or bilateral vision loss
B. **Intracranial causes** and **emboli.** Patients with TIA as a result of an intracranial disorder or embolus will have symptoms similar to those seen in patients with carotid artery or vertebrobasilar disease, depending on the intracranial distribution of disease or the location of the embolus. For example, if the area of disease is in a carotid artery distribution, then the patient's symptoms will mimic those of carotid artery disease.

HOT

TIAs are rarely associated with syncope.

KEY

 DIFFERENTIAL DIAGNOSIS. The following entities must be differentiated from TIAs.

A. **Focal seizures** are often accompanied by abnormal movements (e.g., clonic movements of a limb). These movements are not associated with weakness, and they typically start distally in a limb and spread or "march" proximally, occasionally progressing to generalized tonic-clonic seizures. Electroencephalographic changes may be seen.

B. Central nervous system (CNS) mass lesions (e.g., tumors, hemorrhage) mimic the symptoms of a TIA in a very small percentage of patients.

C. Classic migraines (i.e., migraines with aura) can usually be distinguished from TIAs by the premonition (often visual) of the episode and by associated symptoms (e.g., headache, autonomic arousal with nausea).

HOT

KEY
Headache accompanied by a neurologic abnormality signals a serious CNS disorder until proven otherwise.

D. Hypo- or hyperglycemic episodes occasionally masquerade as a TIA in patients with diabetes, with hypoglycemia a more common culprit than hyperglycemia.

HOT

KEY
The adage, "A stroke is not a stroke until a patient has received 50 grams of 50% dextrose" underscores the importance of considering and even empirically treating for hypoglycemia in any patient with TIA or stroke symptoms that have not yet resolved.

IV APPROACH TO THE PATIENT. Evaluation is aimed at excluding other diagnoses and, when TIA is suspected, at identifying the source of the ischemia.

A. Patient history
　　1. Delineating the **nature** and the **onset of the symptoms** is important, both for ruling out other conditions and for assessing the urgency of the work-up. Like patients with coronary ischemia and unstable angina, patients with cerebral ischemia and "unstable TIAs" (i.e., those at highest risk for developing a stroke) should be strongly considered for admission. "Unstable TIAs" are suggested by:

      a. Symptoms that are recent in onset (i.e., within 24 hours)

      b. Symptoms of prolonged duration

      c. Symptoms that implicate a large vascular territory

      d. Multiple episodes

   2. Be sure to query the patient about potentially modifiable risk factors for TIA (e.g., cigarette smoking, cocaine use).

B. Physical examination. Key features include the following:

HOT KEY

Marked hypertension with bradycardia (Cushing response) may indicate a cerebrovascular accident (CVA) accompanied by increased intracranial pressure (ICP).

---

   1. Blood pressure assessment. Hypertension is a risk factor for TIAs.

   2. Cardiovascular examination

      a. Listen for an **irregular heart rate** and **murmurs** (which may indicate valvular disease or ASD), and evaluate for the **peripheral stigmata of endocarditis** (e.g., Janeway lesions, Osler's nodes, Roth's spots).

      b. Note that generally, the presence or absence of a **carotid bruit** is a poor predictor of the extent of carotid artery disease.

   3. Neurologic examination. By the time a patient with a suspected TIA receives medical attention, the neurologic examination is usually normal, so abnormal findings should prompt an expedient and thorough work-up. Abnormal findings may include:

      a. Signs of upper motor neuron lesions, such as hyperreflexia, increased tone, or an extensor plantar response

      b. Sensory changes, such as decreased sensation to light touch, pin prick, or two-point discrimination

      c. Brain stem findings, such as cranial nerve deficits or gait disturbances

      d. Visual field defects

C. Laboratory studies

   1. General studies

      a. A **complete blood count (CBC) with platelets**

should be obtained to rule out hyperviscosity (from polycythemia) or hypercoagulability (from thrombocytosis).

    b. A **blood glucose level** is particularly important to obtain in patients with known diabetes who are taking insulin or oral hypoglycemic agents.

    c. The **prothrombin time (PT)** and **partial thromboplastin time (PTT)** should be obtained to screen for rare hypercoagulable states (e.g., lupus anticoagulant). It is also important to have baseline measurements of these parameters for patients who are being considered for anticoagulation therapy.

    d. A **lipid profile** should be obtained to assess for hypercholesterolemia, a modifiable risk factor.

  2. **Other studies** may be appropriate to screen for certain conditions if the history or physical examination findings are suggestive.

    a. A **rapid plasmin reagin (RPR)** or **Venereal Disease Research Laboratory (VDRL) test** can be used to screen for syphilis.

    b. An **erythrocyte sedimentation rate (ESR)** can be used to screen for collagen vascular diseases.

    c. A **toxicology screen** should be obtained if cocaine use is a possibility.

D. Imaging studies

  1. **General studies**

    a. An **electrocardiogram (EKG)** is important for detecting atrial fibrillation, and for looking for evidence of prior myocardial infarction.

    b. **Head computed tomography (CT)** or **magnetic resonance imaging (MRI)** should be performed in all patients suspected of having TIAs because a nonvascular cause for the TIA-like symptoms (i.e., a tumor or hemorrhage) is discovered in approximately 1% of patients.

    c. **Carotid duplex ultrasonography** can accurately identify patients with high-grade stenoses who might benefit from surgical carotid endarterectomy.

  2. **Other studies** may be appropriate, depending on the clinical situation.

    a. **Magnetic resonance angiography (MRA)** of the head and neck is a noninvasive technique that is being used more frequently to image the vertebrobasilar circulation and intracranial large vessels.

    b. **Transcranial Doppler ultrasound** can also be used to image the intracranial large vessels.

    c. **Transthoracic echocardiography (TTE)** or **transesophageal echocardiography (TEE)** may be used to detect valvular vegetations, atrial or ventricular thrombi, ASD, and patent foramen ovale.

    d. **Cerebral arteriography** is mainly used as an adjunct to carotid duplex ultrasonography to delineate more precisely the extent of carotid disease prior to surgical intervention. This technique is associated with serious complications (usually stroke) and the outcome is very operator-dependent. The complication rate is approximately 0.5%–1.0%.

V **TREATMENT** focuses on **stroke prevention.**

A. Risk factor modification

    1. **Control of hypertension.** Both systolic and diastolic hypertension are independent risk factors for the development of stroke.

        a. Antihypertensive therapy is discussed in Chapter 16 IV.

        b. The long-term goal of therapy is to control the patient's blood pressure; however, in the setting of an acute unresolved TIA, antihypertensive therapy should be delayed until a major stroke has been ruled out. Lowering the blood pressure during an acute stroke could result in cerebral hypoperfusion.

    2. **Cigarette smoking cessation** reduces the risk of stroke.

    3. **Control of hyperlipidemia.** Hyperlipidemia is likely to be a risk factor for the development of stroke. The current recommendation is to use the patient's risk factors for coronary artery disease (CAD) as the basis for deciding whether or not to begin therapy aimed at lowering the cholesterol level (See Chapter 17).

    4. **Discontinuation of oral contraceptives** is recommended for women who smoke. In addition, even women who have had a TIA and do not smoke should probably avoid this method of contraception.

B. Medical therapy

    1. **Aspirin** has been shown to decrease the risk of stroke in patients with TIAs.

        a. **Indications.** Aspirin therapy should be initiated in every patient with a TIA who does not require anticoagulation therapy (see V B 3), barring any contraindications to aspirin.

    b. The recommended **starting dose** is usually 325 mg daily; a maximum dose of 650 mg twice daily may be given in patients with recurrent TIAs.

2. Ticlopidine is an anti-platelet agent that has proven beneficial effects in preventing strokes in patients with TIAs.

    a. Although ticlopidine is not associated with gastrointestinal bleeding, it is associated with **neutropenia** (2%–3% of patients, usually within 3 months of initiating therapy) and **severe diarrhea** (10%–15% of patients). In addition, it is **significantly more expensive than aspirin.**

    b. The **starting dose** is 250 mg orally, twice daily.

HOT

Patients who begin ticlopidine therapy should have frequent CBCs to monitor for neutropenia.

KEY

---

3. Heparin or **warfarin** is used for **anticoagulation therapy.**

    a. Indications

        (1) Anticoagulation therapy is indicated for patients who have a **presumed cardiac source of emboli** (except for those with endocarditis) and who have no contraindications to anticoagulation therapy.

        (2) Anticoagulation therapy may prevent stroke in patients with **vertebrobasilar disease** and in those who experience **recurrent TIAs despite aspirin therapy.**

    b. Regimen (for patients who have experienced a stroke as a result of cardiogenic emboli)

        (1) Heparin should be started as an intravenous drip, targeting a goal PTT of 2–3 times the upper limit of normal. The typical dose is 18 units/kg. The PTT should be checked 6 hours after heparin therapy is initiated, or whenever there is a change in dose.

        (2) Warfarin can be started once the PTT is in the therapeutic range for 24 hours. Typical starting doses are 5–10 mg orally daily. The international normalized ratio (INR) should be followed daily; the goal is an INR of 2–3. Once the INR is in this range, heparin therapy can be stopped.

    c. Contraindications to anticoagulation therapy may include:

      (1) Bleeding disorders or a recent history of gastrointestinal bleeding

      (2) Uncontrolled hypertension (e.g., a blood pressure greater than 200/110 mm Hg)

      (3) A high risk for falling

C. Surgical management. The decision to perform surgery in a patient with TIAs is based on the distribution of the patient's symptoms (i.e., carotid or vertebrobasilar), the severity of the vascular stenosis, and the patient's surgical risk.

    1. Carotid endarterectomy. The risk of death or disabling stroke for patients who undergo carotid endarterectomy is approximately 5% in experienced centers. Therefore, certain subsets of patients with TIAs have worse outcomes with surgery than with medical management.

      a. Patients with **stenoses of 70%–99%** generally fare better when treated by carotid endarterectomy.

      b. Patients with **stenoses of 30%–69%** may benefit from endarterectomy if their symptoms are worsening despite maximal medical therapy; however, endarterectomy should not be the initial treatment strategy.

      c. Patients with **stenoses of less than 30%** have increased mortality when treated surgically.

    2. Vertebrobasilar surgery. Limited information and a lack of easy surgical accessibility has forced surgical treatment of vertebrobasilar disease to be reserved for select patients. Patients must be excellent candidates for surgery, have very refractory symptoms despite maximal medical therapy, and be willing to undergo a risky and unproven procedure.

VI FOLLOW-UP AND REFERRAL

A. Neurologic consult

    1. In a patient with a **new TIA,** a neurologist can assist in tailoring the diagnostic work-up and assessing the urgency with which the work-up should be completed, as well as in recommending appropriate therapy.

      2. Specific issues that should prompt **immediate consultation** with a neurologist include:

        a. Multiple or **recurrent TIAs**

        b. TIAs of long duration (i.e., more than 5–10 minutes)

        c. TIAs in a young patient

B. Surgical consult. Consultation with a surgeon is appropriate for patients who meet the following requirements:

    1. Good surgical candidate

    2. Willing to undergo surgery

    3. Carotid stenoses greater than 70% or refractory symptoms on maximal medical therapy

References

Feinberg WM, Albers GW, Barnett HJ, et al: Guidelines for the management of transient ischemic attacks. From the Ad Hoc Committee on Guidelines for the Management of Transient Ischemic Attacks of the Stroke Council of the American Heart Association. *Circulation* 89(6):2950–2965, 1994.

65. Dementia

I **INTRODUCTION.** Dementia is a syndrome of multiple acquired cognitive deficits that are not attributable to a transient confusional state.

A. Patients exhibit a **decline in cognitive abilities,** resulting in **functional impairment.**

B. Intellectual deterioration occurs in **memory,** as well as in at least one of the following areas: **language, executive function, judgement, praxis, calculation, visuospatial ability,** or **abstraction.**

II **CLINICAL MANIFESTATIONS OF DEMENTIA.** Patients with dementing disorders most commonly present with **changes in cognition, function, personality,** or **behavior.** A family member may voice concern, or clinical suspicion may be raised if the patient:

A. Complains of memory loss

B. Reports getting lost, causing an automobile accident, or burning a pot on the stove

C. Fails to keep an appointment

D. Answers questions with increasing vagueness or inaccuracy

E. Has difficulty managing finances, procuring adequate meals, or taking medication as directed

F. Has new depressive or psychotic symptoms

G. Has a disorder commonly associated with dementia (e.g., cerebrovascular disease, parkinsonism, alcoholism)

III **DIFFERENTIAL DIAGNOSIS**

A. **Delirium** is a change in mental status characterized by a disturbance of consciousness, impairment of cognition, and fluctuating signs and symptoms that develop over hours to days and can be attributed to an underlying medical condition or drug intoxication. One way to remember the causes of delirium is to consider the **"reversible dementias"** (i.e., conditions that improve or resolve when treated). Causes of delirium ("reversible dementia") include:

1. **Drugs,** such as opiates, benzodiazepines, antihistamines, and cocaine

   2. **Emotional disorders,** such as mania
   3. **Metabolic or endocrine disorders,** such as hypo- or hyperglycemia, hypercalcemia, uremia, hepatic encephalopathy, hypoxia, and hypercarbia
   4. **Ear or eye dysfunction**
   5. **Nutritional deficiencies,** such as vitamin B_{12}, folate, or thiamine
   6. **Neurologic disorders,** such as normal pressure hydrocephalus
   7. **Trauma** (e.g., leading to a subdural hematoma)
   8. **Tumor**
   9. **Ischemia** as a result of cerebrovascular disease
   10. **Infections,** such as syphilis, meningitis, and systemic infections
   11. **Alcohol**

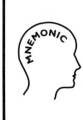

Reversible Dementias ("DEMENTIA")

Drug effects
Emotional disorders
Metabolic or endocrine disorders
Ear or **E**ye dysfunction
Nutritional deficiencies or **N**eurologic disorders
Trauma or **T**umor
Ischemia or **I**nfection
Alcohol

B. Dementia
   1. **Alzheimer's disease.** Patients are **usually older than 60 years,** and the **dementia** is of **insidious onset** and **gradual progression.**
      a. Although the definitive diagnosis is based on neuropathologic findings, the diagnosis can be presumed on the basis of clinical findings in 90% of patients.
      b. Other neurologic, psychiatric, or systemic diseases that could explain the patient's signs and symptoms must be ruled out.
   2. **Multi-infarct (vascular) dementia** may be associated with a significant cerebrovascular accident (CVA), or it may result from multiple small strokes. Most patients have neurologic signs on physical examination and findings of extensive small vessel disease on neuroimaging.
   3. **Dementia of the Lewy body type** is a syndrome in

which the patient exhibits at least one of the following:

a. Parkinsonism developing concurrently with cognitive loss

b. Visual hallucinations early in the dementia

c. A changing level of attention and alertness

HOT

KEY

Patients with dementia of the Lewy body type exhibit hypersensitivity to neuroleptic agents.

IV APPROACH TO THE PATIENT

A. Rule out delirium.

1. A thorough **history** and **physical examination** should be performed, searching for causes of "reversible dementia."

2. **Laboratory studies**

  a. General studies. The following studies should be obtained:

   (1) Complete blood count (CBC)

   (2) Electrolyte panel (including glucose and calcium levels)

   (3) Blood urea nitrogen (BUN) and creatinine levels

   (4) Liver function tests

   (5) Thyroid-stimulating hormone (TSH) level

   (6) Vitamin B_{12} and folate levels

   (7) Syphilis serologies

   (8) HIV serology

   (9) Prothrombin time (PT) and partial thromboplastin time (PTT)

   (10) Arterial blood gases (ABGs), possibly including carboxyhemoglobin level

   (11) Toxicology screen

   (12) Urinalysis

  b. Other studies may be appropriate, such as:

   (1) Electrocardiography

   (2) Chest radiography

   (3) Lumbar puncture (with an opening pressure)

   (4) Head computed tomography (CT) or magnetic resonance imaging (MRI)

3. **Empiric interventions.** Several agents can be given empirically in an attempt to reverse an acute episode of delirium:

   a. **Thiamine administration.** Malnutrition and alcoholism predispose to thiamine deficiency, which can lead to behavioral changes. Patients suspected of having **Wernicke-Korsakoff syndrome** (i.e., thiamine deficiency commonly associated with chronic alcohol abuse) should receive thiamine, 100 mg intravenously.

   b. **Dextrose administration.** One ampule of **50% dextrose** can be administered intravenously to empirically treat hypoglycemia, if a fingerstick test for glucose is not readily available.

HOT

Alcoholic patients should receive thiamine (100 mg intravenously) prior to dextrose administration to prevent the development of Wernicke-Korsakoff syndrome.

KEY

---

   c. **Naloxone hydrochloride administration.** Naloxone hydrochloride should be administered if an opiate overdose is suspected. The initial dose is 0.01 mg/kg; higher doses or repeated doses may be required if the patient has respiratory depression or has ingested certain types of synthetic opioids.

B. **If delirium is absent, diagnose the particular type of dementia.**

   1. **Patient history.** Questions should be asked of the informant, as well as of the patient.

      a. **Characterization of the dementing disorder**

         (1) Was the onset sudden or gradual, and how has the disorder progressed?

         (2) What is the nature of the patient's deficits (e.g., memory loss, diminished language skills or other cognitive deficits, personality changes)?

         (3) Does the patient have psychiatric symptoms (e.g., depression, agitation, paranoia, delusions, hallucinations)?

      b. **Past medical history**

         (1) Does the patient have a history of **cardiac, psychiatric, neurologic,** or **oncologic** disease?

(2) What is the patient's **alcohol consumption?**

(3) Is the patient at **risk for HIV?**

(4) Has the patient experienced **head trauma** recently?

c. **Family history.** What is the patient's family history?

d. **Medication history.** Is the patient taking any prescription or over-the-counter drugs?

e. **Social situation.** What is the patient's **home environment** like? A disordered living space or the collapse of previously acceptable hygiene and grooming habits is suggestive of dementia and may indicate a need for a caretaker.

2. **Physical examination.** The goals of the physical examination are to evaluate the extent of the dementia and to assess any comorbid conditions that may increase the patient's disability. Special attention should be paid to the following areas:

a. **General examination,** paying particular attention to signs of thyroid disease (see Chapter 76 III B and Chapter 77 III B)

b. **Cardiovascular examination**

c. **Functional examination,** including assessment of hearing, vision, and risk of falling

d. **Neurologic examination,** including focality, gait, vibration and position sense, and extrapyramidal signs

e. **Mental status examination,** including a brief quantitative screen, such as the **Mini Mental State Examination** (Table 65-1), and assessment of the patient's level of consciousness and affect

3. **Laboratory and imaging studies**

a. **General studies.** All patients should receive the tests used to rule out "reversible dementia" (see IV A 2 a).

b. **Specific studies** may be warranted, as **dictated by the history and physical examination findings.**

(1) **Neuroimaging studies** may be appropriate if the patient has focal signs or symptoms, seizures, gait abnormalities, or a subacute or sudden change in mental status.

(a) **CT** is the least expensive modality.

(b) **MRI** is particularly helpful in HIV-positive patients and patients suspected of having a posterior fossa lesion.

(c) **Positron emission tomography (PET)** and

TABLE 65-1. Mini Mental State Examination

Maximum Score Score

Orientation

(5) __   Ask the patient for the date. Then ask specifically for the parts omitted (e.g., "Can you also tell me what season it is?) Award 1 point for each correct answer.

____ ____ ____ ____ ____
year season date day month

(5) __   Ask the patient in turn, "Can you tell me the name of this: floor? hospital? town? county? state?" Award 1 point for each correct answer.

____ ____ ____ ____ ____
state county town hospital floor

Registration

(3) __   Ask the patient if you may test his memory. Then say the names of 3 unrelated objects, clearly and slowly, allowing about 1 second between each. After you have named all 3 objects, ask the patient to repeat them. This first repetition determines his score (0–3), but keep repeating the objects until the patient can repeat all 3, up to 6 trials. Award 1 point for each correct answer and record the number of trials. If the patient does not eventually learn all 3 objects, recall cannot be meaningfully tested (see below).

____ ____ ____
                        trial #

Attention and Calculation

(5) __   Ask the patient to begin with 100 and count backwards by increments of 7. Stop after 5 subtractions. Award 1 point for each correct answer.
100 ____ ____ ____ ____ ____
      93   86   79   72   65
If the patient cannot or will not perform this task, ask him to spell the "world" backwards. Award 1 point for each letter named in correct order.

____ ____ ____ ____ ____
d   l   r   o   w

Recall

(3) __   Ask the patient if he can repeat 3 objects you previously asked him to remember. Award 1 point for each.

continued

TABLE 65-1. Mini Mental State Examination

Maximum Score Score

Language

Max	Score	
(2)	—	Show the patient a watch and ask him what it is. Repeat for a pencil. Award 1 point for each correct answer.
(1)	—	Ask the patient to repeat the sentence after you: "No ifs, ands or buts." Award 1 point for the correct answer.
(3)	—	Give the patient a blank sheet of paper and ask him to follow a 3 stage command: "Take this paper in your right hand, fold it in half, and place it on the floor." Award 1 point for each part correctly executed.
(1)	—	Ask the patient to read the following statement and do what it says. Award 1 point if the patient performs the action correctly.

CLOSE YOUR EYES.

(1)	—	Ask the patient to write a sentence for you. Do not dictate a sentence. The sentence must contain a subject and a verb, but grammar and punctuation are not necessary. Award 1 point if the patient performs the action correctly.

(1)	—	Ask the patient to copy the following design. Each figure must have 5 sides and 2 of the angles must intersect. Award 1 point if the patient performs the action correctly.

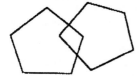

Total Score:____

Assess the patient's level of consciousness along a continuum:

alert   drowsy   stuporous   comatose

Patient: _____   **Unit#:** _____
Examiner: _____   **Date:** _____

Modified with permission from Folsteinn MF, Folsteim SE, McHugh PR: "Mini-mental state." A practical method for grading the cognitive state of patients for the clinician. *J Psychiatr Res* 12(3) :189–198, 1975.

single photon emission computed tomography (SPECT). These modalities, which are used primarily for research, determine disease-specific regional blood flow and glucose metabolism.

(2) **Neuropsychological studies** are especially useful when the patient presents a diagnostic dilemma (e.g., when it is necessary to differentiate depression from dementia).

(3) An **erythrocyte sedimentation rate (ESR)** can help evaluate malignancy or an inflammatory disorder (e.g., vasculitis) as the cause of the patient's dementia.

(4) An **electroencephalogram (EEG)** is rarely indicated, but may help diagnose Creutzfeldt-Jakob disease.

(5) A **lumbar puncture** can be used to rule out infection (including neurosyphilis), malignancy, and vasculitis.

(6) A **brain biopsy** is rarely needed, but may be indicated if imaging studies suggest a tumor, vasculitis, or progressive multifocal leukodystrophy (PML).

 TREATMENT of dementia is directed at optimizing the patient's quality of life and functional status.

A. **General strategies**

1. **Optimize the patient's ability to remain independent.** Measures should be taken to maximize the patient's ability to hear, see, and move independently.

2. **Avoid exacerbating agents.** The use of centrally acting drugs, including over-the-counter preparations, should be minimized.

3. **Educate the patient and his family.** Caregivers should be educated about behavioral management (see V B), environmental manipulation, safety issues, and the importance of respite. Regardless of the cause of the dementia, patients and their families should be referred to the Alzheimer's Association [http://www.alz.org; (800) 272–3900], a national organization with local chapters that can provide support, education, and referrals (e.g., for daycare programs).

4. **Consider the future.** It is important for the provider to accurately assess the patient's ability to manage fi-

nances, drive, cook, get help in an emergency, and ambulate independently in the community, and make recommendations as appropriate.

    a. Discuss and document the patient's wishes for the future use of hospitals, feeding tubes, and nursing homes.

    b. Encourage the patient to establish a Durable Power of Attorney for Health Care.

    c. If the patient is likely to wander, consider a Medic Alert bracelet.

B. Management of behavioral disturbances is largely non-pharmacologic. Medications should be used only if the patient has clear psychotic symptoms or is endangering herself or others.

    1. Nonpharmacologic management. Providing an outlet (e.g., a safe place to pace or wander, regular activity) is often more effective than medication in managing behavioral disturbances.

        a. Identify precipitants. Logging the frequency, timing, and severity of behavioral disturbances can help caregivers identify precipitants. Common precipitants include:

            (1) Delirium

            (2) Depression

            (3) Physical stress (e.g., pain caused by urinary retention or fecal impaction)

            (4) Touch (which the patient may perceive as intrusive)

            (5) Inadequate attention

            (6) Sundowning (i.e., a decline in mental function in the evening)

        b. Teach caregivers how to interact with the patient. Caregiver expectations may need to be lowered.

            (1) A **nondemanding, calm, slow approach** to the patient is best.

            (2) **"Talking the patient through"** (i.e., providing reassurance and explanations of actions and events; orienting the patient to reality) is an important aspect of caring for patients with dementia.

            (3) Patients respond best to **instructions** that are given **using short, concrete phrases,** with the **emphasis on nouns** rather than adjectives.

        c. Minimize the patient's stress.

            (1) Simplify the patient's living environment.

(a) Play quiet or soothing music.

(b) Ensure a direct path to the bathroom, kitchen, and bedroom.

(c) Provide easy mechanics (e.g., door handles instead of doorknobs) and good lighting.

(2) **Structure the patient's day.** Setting schedules for sleeping, eating, engaging in activities, and exercising can minimize stress. Overstimulation, as well as understimulation, should be avoided.

d. **Consider light therapy.** Light therapy, which "resets" melatonin secretion, may be indicated for patients with sleep-wake cycle disturbances.

2. **Pharmacologic management** (Table 65-2)

a. **Antipsychotic agents** may be appropriate if the patient exhibits agitation as a result of psychotic ideation. An agent should be selected on the basis of its side effect profile. There is increasing evidence that the newer drugs (e.g., risperidone, olanzapine) have fewer side effects than the older drugs (e.g., haloperidol) and are at least as effective.

b. **Antidepressant agents.** In many patients with possible dementia, it is difficult to definitely exclude depression as a cause of the mental decline. Often, a trial with an antidepressant is indicated.

(1) **Trazodone** may be the best choice for a patient with prominent sleep disturbance.

(2) **Selective serotonin reuptake inhibitors (SSRIs),** such as **sertraline** and **paroxetine,** have a relatively safe side effect profile and are good choices for treating depression in elderly patients. (Often, a reduced dose is required.)

c. **Mood stabilizers** are most appropriate for patients with labile mood, unpredictable or impulsive aggressive behavior, or mania-like behavior.

d. **Antianxiety agents**

(1) **Benzodiazepines** are indicated for the short-term relief of anxiety, fear, or tension. An agent with a short half-life (e.g., **lorazepam)** should be selected.

(2) **Buspirone** is appropriate for a patient with prominent anxiety and mild depression.

C. **Pharmacologic treatment of Alzheimer's disease.** Several agents are marketed for the treatment of Alzheimer's disease. The patient's cognitive abilities, behavior, and func-

TABLE 65-2. Pharmacological Management of Behavioral Disturbances in Patients with Dementia

Drug	Dosage	Side Effects
Antipsychotic agents		
Haloperidol	0.5 mg twice daily (one dose given at bedtime), to a maximum dose of 1–3 mg/day	High potency side effects (e.g., dystonia, akinesia, dyskinesia)
Risperidone	0.25 twice daily, to a maximum dose of 0.5–4 mg/day	Orthostatic hypotension, parkinsonism
Olanzapine	2.5–15 mg daily	Stomach pain, nausea, dizziness, xerostomia, constipation
Antidepressant agents		
Trazodone	Initial dose is 25 mg at bedtime, but if necessary, two doses may be given daily, up to a maximum dose of 150 mg/day	Daytime sedation*, priapism (rare)
Sertraline	Initial dose is 25 mg/day; increase dose every 1–2 weeks to a maximum dose of 50–150 mg/day	Gastrointestinal and central nervous system (CNS) effects
Paroxetine	Initial dose is 5 mg/day; increase dose every 1–2 weeks to a maximum dose of 20–40 mg/day	Gastrointestinal and CNS effects

continued

TABLE 65-2. Pharmacological Management of Behavioral Disturbances in Patients with Dementia

Drug	Dosage	Side Effects
Mood Stabilizers		
Gabapentin	Initial dose 100 mg at bedtime; depending on sedation and effect, the dosage can be increased in 300-mg increments every 2–5 days to a maximum dose of 1200 mg three times daily	Drowsiness, dizziness, nausea
Valproic acid	Initial dose is 125 mg twice daily; maximum dose is 3000 mg/day	Hepatotoxicity, bone marrow suppression, pancreatitis, thrombocytopenia (follow drug levels)
Carbamazepine	200 mg twice daily	Bone marrow suppression (follow drug levels)
Antianxiety agents		
Lorazepam	0.5 mg as needed every 6–8 hours, up to a maximum dose of 6 mg/day	Falls, sedation, paradoxical agitation
Buspirone	Initial dose is 5 mg twice daily; 40–60 mg daily are often needed	Slow onset of action; may be associated with dizziness and fatigue; drug is often ineffective

*If the patient experiences daytime sedation, increase the bedtime dose and decrease the morning dose.

tional status should be assessed every 1–3 months after initiating therapy.

1. **Donepezil** (5 mg daily for 2–6 weeks, then 10 mg daily if tolerated) is probably the most efficacious agent for the treatment of Alzheimer's disease. Therapy with donepezil may also help moderate behavioral disturbances.

   a. One third of patients improve with dosages of 5 mg, and one half improve when the dosage is increased to 10 mg; however, more gastrointestinal and central nervous system (CNS) side effects are seen with the higher dosage.

   b. Therapy is ongoing.

2. **Tacrine** (10 mg four times daily, increasing to 40 mg four times daily) is associated with more side effects than donepezil, and the dosing is more frequent. Baseline liver function should be assessed; after initiating therapy with tacrine, evaluation of liver function at regular intervals is required.

3. **Gingko biloba** (40 mg three times daily) is not subject to Food and Drug Administration (FDA) review, and therefore, the purity and dose cannot be controlled. However, as many as one third of patients showed improvement after taking EGb 761, a ginkgo biloba extract that has been approved for use in Germany.

4. **Vitamin E.** One large study showed that 1000 IU of vitamin E twice daily increased patient survival and delayed the need for institutionalization, but the study's methodology was poor.

5. **Estrogen** and **nonsteroidal anti-inflammatory drugs (NSAIDs)** may help prevent the development of Alzheimer's disease, but results from prospective trials are not yet available.

VI FOLLOW-UP AND REFERRAL

A. **Follow-up.** Patients should be seen every 3–6 months to ensure optimal management of comorbidities, to monitor patient (and caregiver) well-being, and to evaluate the efficacy of pharmacologic therapy.

B. **Referral.** Most patients with dementia can be managed by primary care physicians. However, if the presentation is atypical or the diagnosis or management of the disease is difficult, patients can be referred to a neurologist, geriatrician, or geriatric psychiatrist.

References
Borson S, Raskin MA: Clinical features and pharmacologic treatment of behavioral symptoms of Alzheimer's disease. *Neurology* 48(Suppl 6):S17-S24, 1997.
Small GW, Rabins PV, Barry PP, et al: Diagnosis and treatment of Alzheimer disease and related disorders. *JAMA* 278(16):1363–1371, 1997.

66. Polyneuropathy

I **INTRODUCTION.** There are three types of **peripheral neuropathies:** polyneuropathy, mononeuritis multiplex, and mononeuropathy. Of these three, polyneuropathy is the most common and poses the greatest difficulty in differential diagnosis; therefore, it is the focus of this chapter.

A. **Polyneuropathy** is characterized by **symmetrical abnormalities** of **sensation, motor strength,** or **both.**

B. **Mononeuritis multiplex** is characterized by **asymmetric abnormalities** in more than one nerve trunk. The abnormalities occur either simultaneously or over days to years.

C. **Mononeuropathy** is characterized by a **focal abnormality** of a single nerve (e.g., carpal tunnel syndrome) and usually results from local nerve compression or stretch.

II **CLINICAL MANIFESTATIONS OF POLYNEUROPATHY**

A. **Sensory abnormalities** in the feet are usually the first symptom of a polyneuropathy.

1. **Hypesthesia** (decreased sensation), **anesthesia** (absent sensation), **paresthesia** ("pins and needles" sensation without any stimuli), **dysesthesia** (burning sensation with or without stimuli), and **hyperpathia** (exaggerated pain perception) may all be noted. Initially, subjective complaints may not be accompanied by objective findings.

2. Later, a **pansensory loss in the feet** may occur and progress centrally. Finger involvement often occurs once the shins are affected; eventually, the classic **"stocking-glove" pattern** may be seen.

B. **Motor abnormalities** may also occur. The extensors are usually more involved than the flexors (i.e., **weakness of dorsiflexion of the toes** is a common finding). A **diminished ankle reflex** is often seen early in the course of the disease, and a **diminished knee reflex** and **foot drop** are seen as the disease progresses.

III **CAUSES OF POLYNEUROPATHY.** The differential diagnosis is long, and can be remembered using the mnemonic, "DANG THERAPIST."

Causes of Polyneuropathy ("DANG THERAPIST")

Diabetes (and other metabolic disorders)
Alcohol abuse
Nutritional deficiency (e.g., vitamin B_{12}, thiamine, pyridoxine, folate)
Guillain-Barré syndrome and other idiopathic causes

Tumor-related (i.e., paraneoplastic syndrome)
Hereditary disorders (e.g., Charcot-Marie-Tooth disease)
Endocrine disorders (e.g., hypothyroidism, acromegaly)
Renal disease (i.e., uremia)
Amyloidosis
Porphyria or **P**olycythemia
Infections and **I**mmune-mediated disorders (e.g., AIDS, leprosy, Lyme disease, syphilis, vasculitis)
Sarcoidosis
Toxins and drugs (e.g., alcohol, heavy metals, pesticides)

IV APPROACH TO THE PATIENT. Many of the disorders that can cause polyneuropathies are potentially life-threatening if not appropriately diagnosed and treated. Because the differential is extensive and the cause of the polyneuropathy may not be obvious, evaluation of the patient needs to be tailored to the situation. If the diagnosis is not initially apparent, a four-step process may be used to cover most of the possibilities.

A. Take a thorough patient history.
   1. Be sure to ask about **recent events** that may provide a clue to the diagnosis. Specifically, inquire about recent **viral illnesses** (which may suggest Guillain-Barré syndrome), the presence of **similar symptoms in family members or co-workers** (which may suggest a toxic exposure), and **systemic symptoms** (e.g., weight loss, which may raise suspicion for an occult malignancy or a chronic infection).
   2. Obtain a **medication history.** Some drugs that may be responsible for a polyneuropathy include **phenytoin, isoniazid, hydralazine, dapsone, amiodarone, metro-**

nidazole, nitrofurantoin, vincristine, colchicine, anti-retroviral medications, and high doses of pyridoxine.
3. Inquire about toxic exposures. The most common toxins include heavy metals (e.g., arsenic, thallium, lead, mercury), industrial agents, and pesticides (e.g., organophosphates); diphtheria toxin should also be considered but is quite rare.

HOT

KEY

Remember, common things are common. If diabetes or ure-mia is present or the patient is a longtime alcoholic, you may not need to look any further.

B. **Assess the time course.** Only a few disorders commonly result in an **acute polyneuropathy** (i.e., one that occurs over a few days). Furthermore, unlike subacute or chronic polyneuropathies, acute disorders usually produce predictable patterns on **electrodiagnostic evaluation** (i.e., **electromyography, nerve conduction studies**).
   1. **Acute axonal polyneuropathies** are characterized by relatively **preserved nerve conduction** and are usually caused by **porphyria** or **intoxications** (e.g., arsenic).
   2. **Acute demyelinating polyneuropathies** display a **marked decrease in nerve conduction. Guillain-Barré syndrome** is the most common type of acute demyelinating polyneuropathy, although **diphtheria toxin** and **toxic berry (buckthorn) ingestion** occasionally produce the same clinical picture.
C. **Perform appropriate laboratory studies** if the diagnosis is not evident. Review the list of possible causes and obtain the laboratory tests that will help you shorten the list. Tests that may be requested include:
   1. Complete blood count (CBC)
   2. Erythrocyte sedimentation rate (ESR)
   3. Renal panel with electrolytes
   4. Fasting glucose and glycosylated hemoglobin levels
   5. Vitamin B_{12} level
   6. Thyroid function tests
   7. Liver function tests
   8. Venereal Disease Research Laboratory (VDRL) test
   9. Serum and urine protein electrophoresis
D. **Consider occult disorders.** The simple laboratory tests outlined in IV C may not rule out some of the more occult

processes (e.g., tumor, vasculitis, sarcoidosis), but they may provide evidence for or against a possible diagnosis (e.g., a normal ESR makes vasculitis less likely). The following tests may be useful in certain clinical settings:

1. **Antinuclear antibody (ANA), rheumatoid factor (RF),** and **serum cryoglobulin assessments** may be used in the evaluation of a suspected vasculitis.
2. **Imaging studies**
   a. **Chest radiographs** may show evidence of sarcoidosis or an occult tumor.
   b. A **computed tomography (CT) scan** may be obtained if an intra-abdominal malignancy is suspected.
3. **Urinary heavy metal** and **porphobilinogen levels** can be used to evaluate the possibility of toxic metal exposures and acute intermittent porphyria, respectively.
4. **Lyme titers** are only useful in the appropriate clinical setting because they lack specificity.
5. **Cerebrospinal fluid (CSF) evaluation**
   a. Findings include high protein levels and a normal cell count in patients with Guillain-Barré syndrome or chronic inflammatory demyelinating polyneuropathy (CIDP).
   b. In patients with AIDS and cytomegalovirus (CMV) polyradiculopathy, findings include pleocytosis, high protein levels, and low glucose levels.
6. **Electrodiagnostic studies** may be performed (if they have not been already) to help categorize whether there is primarily axonal degeneration or demyelination. These studies may be especially helpful in diagnosing CIDP.
7. **Sural nerve biopsy.** The ankle is the easiest place to obtain a cutaneous nerve biopsy.
   a. Nerve biopsy is of low yield in patients with polyneuropathies, but should be considered for patients with suspected **mononeuritis multiplex** because a vasculitis may be more likely. The yield of biopsy is also increased in patients with suspected **vasculitis, amyloidosis, sarcoidosis,** or **leprosy,** and in those with **palpably thickened nerves.**
   b. Because **heredofamilial disorders** often present at an early age and have a characteristic

histopathology, a sural nerve biopsy should also be considered for **children.**

V TREATMENT

A. **Relief of neuropathic pain** is usually not easily accomplished. Regimens for the treatment of neuropathic pain are discussed in Chapter 3 IV D 1 and Table 3-4.

B. **Definitive therapies.** Treatment is generally aimed at the underlying disorder (e.g., treating the infection, removing the toxic exposure, replacing the nutritional deficiency). Other specific therapies are as follows:

1. **Diabetic polyneuropathy** is usually progressive. Optimal glucose control has been shown to reduce the development and progression of neuropathy.

2. **Neuropathy associated with renal disease.** Control of uremia with dialysis may slow the progression of the neuropathy.

3. **Guillain-Barré syndrome.** Approximately 85% of patients recover completely or have only mild residual defects. The mortality rate is approximately 3%–4%.

   a. Most patients require hospitalization for observation and **supportive care** (e.g., intubation for respiratory failure).

   b. **Plasmapheresis** is beneficial (especially within the first 2 weeks of illness).

   c. **Steroids** are not usually effective.

4. **CIDP** may be treated with **steroids, immunosuppressants,** or **plasmapheresis**.

5. **Isoniazid overdose** can be treated with **intravenous pyridoxine** (1 gram for each gram of isoniazid ingested).

6. **Acute intermittent porphyria**

   a. **Acute treatment.** Intravenous **glucose** and **hematin** may be needed for acute attacks.

   b. **Chronic treatment** entails **avoiding precipitating factors** (e.g., sulfa drugs) and adhering to a **high-carbohydrate diet.**

VI FOLLOW-UP AND REFERRAL

A. **Referral**

1. Patients with rapidly progressive disorders (e.g., Guillain-Barré syndrome) require admission to a hospital and urgent consultation with a neurologist.

    2. Referral to a neurologist is also indicated if a specific diagnosis cannot be established after a thorough history, physical examination and laboratory evaluation.

B. Follow-up. Patients with an established diagnosis (e.g., vitamin B_{12} deficiency) and stable symptoms may be seen every 1–2 months to evaluate the response to therapy.

References

Barohn BJ: Approach to peripheral neuropathy and neuronopathy. *Semin Neurol* 18(1):7–18, 1998.

Chalk CH: Acquired peripheral neuropathy. *Neurol Clin* 15(3):501–528, 1997.

67. Carpal Tunnel Syndrome

I INTRODUCTION

A. Carpal tunnel syndrome—the most common **entrapment neuropathy**—is caused by compression of the **median nerve,** which arises from the C6-T1 nerve roots and innervates the flexor muscles of the wrist and fingers. Carpal tunnel syndrome occurs when the median nerve is compressed within the carpal tunnel.

B. Carpal tunnel syndrome affects 0.1% of the population in the United States. Middle-aged women and those with a history of repetitive use of the hands are most often affected.

II CLINICAL MANIFESTATIONS OF CARPAL TUNNEL SYNDROME

A. Pain, paresthesias, or **both** in the distribution of the median nerve (i.e., the thumb, index finger, and middle finger) is the initial complaint. **Aching pain** may radiate proximally into the forearm, shoulder, neck, and chest, or distally into the other fingers of the hand.

    1. The pain is classically **worse at night** and **exacerbated by hand movement.**

    2. **Tinel's sign** and **Phalen's sign** may be positive (each has an approximate sensitivity of 50% and an approximate specificity of 80%).

        a. **Tinel's sign** is positive when percussion (or touching) the volar area of the wrist produces tingling or pain.

        b. **Phalen's sign** is considered positive if pain or paresthesia occur when the patient flexes both wrists to 90° with the dorsal areas of the hands in apposition for 1 minute (reverse praying position).

B. Sensory loss and **weakness** or **atrophy of the affected hand muscles** (especially the abductor pollicis brevis) may be present.

III CAUSES OF CARPAL TUNNEL SYNDROME.
Carpal tunnel syndrome is most often **idiopathic;** however, it can also occur secondary to several disorders. An easy way to remember the causes of secondary carpal tunnel syndrome is with the mnemonic, "WRIST PAIN."

Secondary Causes of Carpal Tunnel Syndrome ("WRIST PAIN")

Work-related
Rheumatoid arthritis
Infiltrative disorders (e.g., amyloidosis)
Sarcoidosis
Thyroid dysfunction (i.e., hypothyroidism) and other endocrine disorders (e.g., diabetes mellitus)

Pregnancy
Acromegaly
Inflammatory tenosynovitis (caused by Reiter's syndrome, gout, soft tissue infection, disseminated gonococcal infection)
Neoplasm (primarily leukemia)

IV **DIFFERENTIAL DIAGNOSIS.** Conditions that may be confused with carpal tunnel syndrome include:

A. C6 or C7 cervical radiculopathy
B. Brachial plexus neuropathy (caused by thoracic outlet syndrome)
C. Median nerve compression in the forearm or arm
D. Mononeuritis multiplex
E. Cervical cord abnormalities, such as syringomyelia or demyelinating disease
F. Angina pectoris, if the pain is left-sided

V **APPROACH TO THE PATIENT**

A. **Establish the diagnosis.** The diagnosis is usually made on the basis of the **history** and **physical examination.** If the diagnosis is unclear, **nerve conduction studies** can be helpful; however, false-negative results may occur in early, mild cases.

B. **Determine the underlying cause.** Once carpal tunnel syndrome is diagnosed, secondary causes should be considered. Laboratory and imaging studies should only be ordered if the patient has signs or symptoms suggesting an underlying disease. The following studies may provide useful information, depending on the clinical situation:

1. Erythrocyte sedimentation rate (ESR)
2. Rheumatoid factor
3. Complete blood count (CBC)
4. Fasting blood glucose level
5. Thyroid-stimulating hormone (TSH) level
6. Uric acid level
7. Hemoglobin A_{1c} level
8. Urine pregnancy test
9. Protein electrophoresis
10. Chest radiograph

VI TREATMENT

A. **Conservative measures** should be tried first.
  1. **Hand rest.** Resting the hand and modifying repetitive motion activities (e.g., by lowering the keyboard, adjusting the chair height or position, and increasing hand rest time during the workday) may alleviate symptoms.
  2. **Splinting.** A wrist splint should be worn, especially at night.
  3. **Anti-inflammatory medications** (e.g., ibuprofen, 400–600 mg three times daily as needed) can provide symptomatic relief.
  4. **Steroid injections.** Injection of steroids into the carpal tunnel should only be performed by physicians experienced with the procedure.
B. **Surgical decompression**. A minority of patients require surgery. Most patients improve after surgery; however, the prognosis is worse for those with thenar atrophy.

VII FOLLOW-UP AND REFERRAL

A. **Follow-up.** Patients who are being managed conservatively should see the physician frequently (e.g., monthly), so that the physician can assess the patient's symptoms and the progression of weakness or atrophy. Surgery should be recommended before thenar atrophy occurs.
B. **Referral.** Consultation with a neurologist is recommended if the diagnosis is unclear.

References
Katz RT: Carpal tunnel syndrome: a practical review. *Am Fam Physician* 49(6):1371–1379, 1385–1386, 1994.
Kulick RG: Carpal tunnel syndrome. *Orthop Clin North Am* 27(2):345–354, 1996.

68. Facial Nerve Palsy

I INTRODUCTION

A. The **facial nerve (cranial nerve VII)** innervates the facial muscles and the muscles of the eyelids. In addition, the facial nerve is involved in dampening sound (via the stapedius muscle) and in taste sensation.

B. It is important to distinguish upper motor neuron disease, a central nervous system (CNS) disorder, from lower motor neuron disease (i.e. facial palsy). The following characteristics distinguish upper motor neuron disease from facial palsy:

1. Voluntary movements of the upper face are preserved because the upper forehead muscles are innervated by both facial nerves.

2. Emotional movements of the mouth (e.g., laughing, crying) are curiously unaffected.

3. Neurologic examination often reveals abnormalities in other cranial nerves or in other nerve groups.

II DIFFERENTIAL DIAGNOSIS

A. **Bell's palsy (idiopathic facial palsy),** the most common cause of facial paresis, is a **unilateral lower motor neuron palsy** that occurs abruptly and is thought to be caused by inflammation involving the facial nerve, either in the facial canal or near the stylomastoid canal.

1. **Epidemiology.** Bell's palsy affects men and women equally, with a peak incidence at age 30 years.

2. **Clinical manifestations**

a. **Symptoms.** The cardinal symptom is **facial paresis.** Other symptoms are not universal, but include **pain around the ear, increased or decreased tearing, facial numbness, hyperacusis,** and **altered taste.**

b. **Signs** include a **less prominent nasolabial fold** and **weakness of the eyebrow, eyelid,** and **mouth muscles** on the affected side.

HOT

KEY

Features that predict a less than complete recovery for patients with Bell's palsy include age greater than 40 years, hyperacusis, and severe initial pain or paralysis.

B. **Infection.** Many infections can lead to facial nerve palsy; the following are the most common:
   1. **Infectious mononucleosis (Epstein-Barr virus infection).** Painful mononeuropathies (including facial nerve palsy) are one manifestation of nervous system involvement in infectious mononucleosis.
   2. **Ramsay Hunt syndrome (herpes zoster virus infection).** Facial paresis results from involvement of the geniculate ganglion by a herpes zoster virus infection; usually, vesicles can be seen in the auricle or external auditory canal.
   3. **Lyme disease**. A small proportion of patients with Lyme disease develop facial palsies within months of the tick bite.

HOT

KEY

Suspect Lyme disease in patients with bilateral facial nerve palsy.

C. **Trauma.** Fracture of the facial bones occasionally affects the facial nerve.
D. **Neoplasia.** Cancer of the ear or parotid gland can lead to facial nerve palsy.
E. **Demyelinating disorders**
   1. **Multiple sclerosis** should be considered in patients with other neurologic symptoms or signs; the key to making the diagnosis is involvement of different parts of the nervous system at different points in time.
   2. **Guillain-Barré syndrome.** Although weakness usually begins in the legs before involving the upper trunk and face, the **Miller Fisher variant** of Guillain-Barré syndrome may begin in the face.

F. Heerfordt's syndrome is parotid enlargement, fever, anterior uveitis, and facial palsy in patients with sarcoidosis.

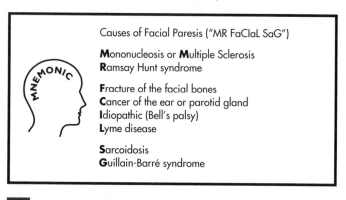

Causes of Facial Paresis ("MR FaClaL SaG")

Mononucleosis or **M**ultiple Sclerosis
Ramsay Hunt syndrome

Fracture of the facial bones
Cancer of the ear or parotid gland
Idiopathic (Bell's palsy)
Lyme disease

Sarcoidosis
Guillain-Barré syndrome

III TREATMENT

A. Bell's palsy (idiopathic facial palsy). As many as 50% of patients recover fully within 8 weeks; 90% are ultimately satisfied with their recovery.

1. **Reassurance** is important; many patients believe that they have had a stroke.
2. **Artificial tears** (2 drops four times daily) and the application of a **lubricating ointment** to the affected eye at night are essential if the patient cannot close her eye. Patients complaining of eye discomfort should be evaluated for corneal pathology.
3. **Oral corticosteroids** should be considered for patients with severe initial facial pain or paralysis who present within 5 days of the onset of symptoms. One common regimen is oral prednisone, 40 mg twice daily for 5 days to start. The dose is then tapered by 10 mg each day over the next week.

B. Secondary facial palsy. Therapy focuses on supportive care and is aimed at the underlying disorder.

IV FOLLOW-UP AND REFERRAL. Referral to an otolaryngologist or neurologist should be considered if a space-occupying lesion is suspected or the diagnosis is unclear.

References
Blaustein BH, Gurwood A: Differential diagnosis in facial nerve palsy: a clinical review. *J Am Optom Assoc* 68(11):715–724, 1997.
Hashisaki GT: Medical management of Bell's palsy. *Compr Ther* 23(11):715–718, 1997.

PART X

Hematology and Oncology

Hematology and Oncology

69. Anemia

INTRODUCTION. Anemia is **a manifestation of disease,** not a disease in and of itself.

A. Definition. Anemia is defined as **a decrease in the volume of red blood cells (RBCs) as reflected by the hematocrit.**

B. Normal values
1. In **men,** a hematocrit of less than 40% is considered anemic.
2. In **women,** a hematocrit of less than 37% is considered anemic.

C. Clinical manifestations of anemia. Patients with anemia may be asymptomatic, or they may complain of **fatigue, dyspnea on exertion,** or **exertional angina.** Signs and symptoms of the underlying disorder may also be present.

D. Classification. Anemia is classified as **microcytic, normocytic,** or **macrocytic** using the **mean corpuscular volume (MCV)** as a basis for the classification.
1. The **normal MCV** is **80–100 μm^3.**
2. If more than one disorder is present, the MCV may be an average of the different populations of RBCs, producing a normal MCV. In mixed disorders, the **red cell distribution width (RDW)** will be increased.

II MICROCYTIC ANEMIA (MCV < 80 μm^3)

A. Causes of microcytic anemia
1. **Iron deficiency** is the most common cause of microcytic anemia and is important to diagnose because it may be indicative of an underlying gastrointestinal malignancy.
2. **Thalassemias** are hereditary disorders characterized by a reduction in the synthesis of α or β globin chains.
3. **Anemia of chronic disease (ACD)** is associated with inflammatory diseases (e.g., rheumatoid arthritis, serious infection, carcinoma).
4. **Sideroblastic anemias** are a heterogenous group of disorders that have in common various defects in the porphyrin pathway. Causes of sideroblastic anemia include:
   a. **Inherited disorders**
   b. **Drugs** and **toxins** (e.g., **L**ead, **I**soniazid, **E**thanol — **LIE**)

c. **Malignancy** (e.g., leukemia, lymphoma, myelofibrosis, multiple myeloma, solid tumor)
d. **Collagen vascular disease** (e.g., rheumatoid arthritis)

HOT

Although sideroblastic anemias often lead to microcytic anemia, they can also be a cause of normocytic or macrocytic anemia.

KEY

B. **Approach to the patient.** It is important to differentiate iron deficiency from the other causes of microcytic anemia.
   1. **Iron deficiency versus thalassemia**
      a. Iron deficiency may be distinguished from thalassemia using the **thalassemia index** [i.e., **the MCV divided by the RBC count**]. A thalassemia index of **less than 13 suggests thalassemia;** one greater than 13 suggests iron deficiency.
      b. An abnormal **hemoglobin electrophoresis** is also useful in diagnosing a thalassemia.
   2. **Iron deficiency versus ACD**
      a. **Determine the probability that a patient has iron deficiency.** The pretest probability is based on clinical factors. By estimating the pretest probability and using likelihood ratios for a given ferritin level (Table 69-1) , you can estimate the posttest probability (see Chapter 1 III C 3).
      b. **Laboratory studies**
         (1) Serum ferritin. This test is useful in all patients, except perhaps those with liver disease. Obtaining the serum ferritin level is most useful when the pretest probability is between 20% and 80%.
            (a) If the serum ferritin is less than 15 μg/L, it practically guarantees that the patient has iron deficiency.
            (b) Similarly, a value greater than 100 μg/L essentially rules out the diagnosis.
         (2) **Serum transferrin** is occasionally helpful because it is usually elevated in iron deficiency and decreased in ACD.
      c. **Bone marrow biopsy** remains the gold standard

TABLE 69-1. Serum Ferritin Values and Corresponding Likelihood Ratios

Serum Ferritin (μg/L)	Likelihood Ratio
>100	0.1
25–100	Not helpful
15–24	10
<15	50

Based on data from: Guyatt GH, Oxman AD, Ali M, et al: Laboratory diagnosis of iron-deficiency anemia: an overview. *J Gen Inter Med* 7(2):145–153, 1992.

for diagnosing iron deficiency, and is the usual method of diagnosing sideroblastic anemia.

HOT

KEY

If iron deficiency is diagnosed in an older patient or young man, endoscopy of the upper and lower gastrointestinal tract needs to be performed because of the possibility of an underlying gastrointestinal malignancy.

III MACROCYTIC ANEMIA (MCV >100 μm³)

A. **Megaloblastic anemia** is caused by defects in DNA synthesis, which lead to hematologic abnormalities. Causes of megaloblastic anemia include:
   1. **Vitamin B_{12} (cobalamin) deficiency**
      a. **Causes** of vitamin B_{12} deficiency include **pernicious anemia, gastrectomy, blind loop syndrome, pancreatic insufficiency,** and **surgical resection** or **Crohn's disease** of the distal ileum. Dietary deficiency of vitamin B_{12} is rarely a cause because the body usually has stores of vitamin B_{12} sufficient to last for 3–5 years after vitamin B_{12} intake stops.
      b. **Clinical manifestations** of vitamin B_{12} deficiency may include gastrointestinal disturbances (e.g., anorexia, diarrhea, glossitis) and a neurologic syndrome consisting of paresthesias, imbalance, and occasionally, dementia.

HOT

KEY

Approximately 10% of patients with vitamin B_{12} deficiency will not be anemic; therefore, vitamin B_{12} levels should be checked in patients with suspected vitamin B_{12} deficiency regardless of the hematocrit.

    2. **Folate deficiency**
        a. **Causes.** Folate deficiency is almost always the result of **inadequate dietary intake**—body stores of folate last only 3–5 months after intake ceases. Other rare causes of folate deficiency include **tropical sprue, chronic hemolytic anemia, pregnancy,** and **dialysis.**
        b. **Clinical manifestations.** Gastrointestinal complaints may occur as with vitamin B_{12} deficiency; however, neurologic sequelae do not.
    3. **Drugs** (e.g., **methotrexate, azathioprine**) can be associated with megaloblastic anemia.

HOT

KEY

Practically all patients taking zidovudine (for the treatment of HIV) have an elevated MCV; therefore, this finding can aid in gauging compliance with medications.

    4. **Miscellaneous causes** of megaloblastic anemia include **Lesch-Nyhan syndrome** and **thiamine-responsive** or **pyridoxine-responsive anemias.**

HOT

KEY

The finding of hypersegmented polymorphonuclear neutrophils (PMNs) on the peripheral blood smear strongly suggests megaloblastic anemia.

    B. **Chronic liver disease** causes a macrocytosis as a result of ineffective erythropoiesis and acute blood loss.
    C. **Reticulocytosis.** Because reticulocytes are much larger than normal RBCs, patients with reticulocytosis can have

MCV readings that are increased. However, an MCV greater than 110 μm^3 is usually not caused by reticulocytosis alone.

D. Alcoholism produces erythrocyte membrane abnormalities, leading to macrocytic anemia.

E. Hypothyroidism causes macrocytic anemia via an unclear mechanism.

HOT

Macrocytosis + neurologic symptoms = vitamin B_{12} deficiency, alcoholism, or hypothyroidism.

KEY

F. Myelodysplasia. There are five myelodysplastic syndromes that are characterized by ineffective hematopoiesis:
1. **Refractory anemia**
2. **Refractory anemia with ringed sideroblasts**
3. **Refractory anemia with excess blasts**
4. **Refractory anemia with excess blasts in transformation**
5. **Chronic myelomonocytic leukemia**

 NORMOCYTIC ANEMIA. An **absolute reticulocyte count** is the initial test to order in a patient with normocytic anemia, because the absolute reticulocyte count allows the anemia to be classified as **proliferative** or **hypoproliferative** (Figure 69-1).

A. Proliferative normocytic anemia is characterized by erythrocyte loss.
1. **Hemolysis.** Clues that hemolysis is present may include **elevated lactate dehydrogenase (LDH)** and increased **total bilirubin levels.** If hemolysis is a concern, the **peripheral smear** must be examined. Based on the morphology of the erythrocytes (e.g., schistocytes, sickle cells) the cause of the hemolytic anemia may be determined. **Microangiopathic hemolytic anemia (MAHA),** an important causes of hemolysis, is characterized by intravascular shearing of RBCs, which leads to schistocyte formation. A few of the important causes of MAHA are listed here.
   a. **Disseminated intravascular coagulation (DIC).** In acute DIC, the major concern is bleeding, whereas in chronic DIC, thrombosis is more of a problem.

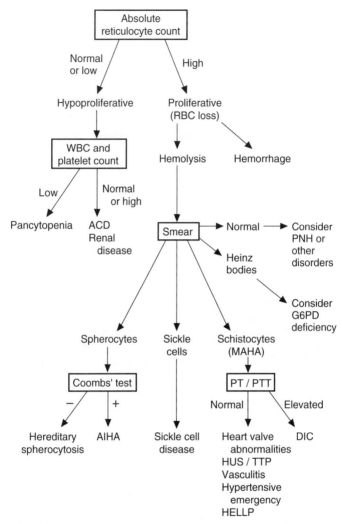

FIGURE 69-1. Determining the cause of normocytic anemia. *ACD* = anemia of chronic disease; *AIHA* = autoimmune hemolytic anemia; *DIC* = disseminated intravascular coagulation; *G6PD* = glucose-6-phosphate dehydrogenase; *HELLP* = hemolysis, elevated liver enzymes, and low platelet count syndrome; *HTN* = hypertension; *HUS/TTP* = hemolytic-uremic syndrome/thrombotic thrombocytopenic purpura; *MAHA* = microangiopathic hemolytic anemia; *PNH* = paroxysmal nocturnal hemoglobinuria; *PT* = prothrombin time; *PTT* = partial thromboplastin time; *RBC* = red blood cell; *WBC* = white blood cell. (Modified with permission from Saint S, Frances C: *Saint-Frances Guide to Inpatient Medicine.* Baltimore, Williams & Wilkins, 1997, p 321.)

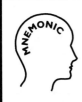

Causes of DIC ("MOIST")

Malignancy
Obstetric complications
Infection
Shock
Trauma

   b. **Hemolytic-uremic syndrome/thrombotic throm-
       bocytopenic purpura (HUS/TTP).** The triad of
       HUS is hemolysis, uremia, and thrombocytope-
       nia. TTP is hemolytic-uremic syndrome accompa-
       nied by fever and neurologic changes. In general,
       if uremia is the prominent disorder, the disease is
       referred to as HUS. If the central nervous system
       (CNS) manifestations are more significant, then
       TTP is the appropriate term.

HOT

An LDH level less than 1000 U/L makes HUS/TTP very unlikely.

KEY

   2. **Hemorrhage.** If hemorrhage is suspected, the source
       of the blood loss must be determined (e.g., the gas-
       trointestinal tract).
 B. **Hypoproliferative normocytic anemia.** Anemia accom-
     panied by **low white blood cell (WBC)** and **platelet
     counts** indicates pancytopenia. A hypoproliferative
     normocytic anemia accompanied by normal or high
     WBC and platelet counts usually indicates ACD or re-
     nal disease.

V TREATMENT

 A. **Symptomatic therapy.** Patients who have acute symp-
     toms because of their anemia require **blood transfusions**
     (and perhaps hospitalization).

HOT

KEY

One unit of packed RBCs increases the hematocrit by approximately 3%. In patients with coronary artery disease (CAD), it is usually advisable to keep the hematocrit above 30%.

   B. Iron deficiency is best treated with **ferrous sulfate** (325 mg orally, 3 times daily). The hematocrit returns halfway to normal after about 4 weeks of therapy and should be completely normal after 8 weeks. Seeing the patient after 4 weeks of therapy is advisable to monitor compliance and recheck the hematocrit.

HOT

KEY

Determining the underlying cause of iron deficiency (i.e., excluding gastrointestinal malignancy in patients older than 40 years) is of the utmost importance.

   C. Vitamin B$_{12}$ deficiency as a result of **pernicious anemia** is treated with **intramuscular vitamin B$_{12}$** (100 μg daily for the first week, weekly for the next 3 weeks, and then monthly for life).
      1. Patients usually feel better within a few days of therapy, and the hematocrit should return to normal in 2 months.
      2. Patients should be seen every 2–4 weeks initially.

HOT

KEY

Neurologic symptoms may be reversible if therapy is initiated within 6 months of symptom onset.

   D. Folate deficiency is treated with **folic acid** (1 mg orally daily). As with therapy for vitamin B$_{12}$ deficiency, therapy for folate deficiency usually results in rapid improvement in symptoms, followed by a return to the normal hematocrit within 2 months.

HOT KEY

In patients with concomitant vitamin B_{12} and folic acid deficiencies, large doses of folic acid may produce an increase in the hematocrit but will allow the neurologic damage caused by the vitamin B_{12} deficiency to progress.

E. **Sickle cell disease (SCD)**
1. Although specific therapy for SCD is not available, **hydroxyurea** (500–700 mg/day) may reduce the frequency of painful crises and should be considered for those with very frequent painful crises. (The long-term safety of the drug remains a concern.)
2. Patients should be given **oral folate** (1 mg daily).
3. **Transfusions should be avoided.**

F. **Autoimmune hemolytic anemia. Prednisone** (1 mg/kg/day in divided doses) is usually the initial therapy for this disorder. **Transfusion, intravenous immunoglobulin therapy,** and **splenectomy** may be necessary, but only after consultation with a hematologist.

VI FOLLOW-UP AND REFERRAL

A. Referral to a **hematologist** is advised if the cause of the anemia remains unclear after initial evaluation, or if bone marrow biopsy is being contemplated.

B. Consultation with a **gastroenterologist** is necessary if endoscopy is required to rule out a gastrointestinal cause of blood loss.

References
Charache S: Mechanism of action of hydroxyurea in the management of sickle cell anemia in adults. *Semin Hematol* 34(3 Suppl 3):15–21, 1997.
Fireman Z, Kopelman Y, Sternberg A: Endoscopic evaluation of iron deficiency anemia and follow-up in patients older than age 50. *J Clin Gastroenterol* 26(1):7–10, 1998.
Toh BH, van Driel IR, Gleeson PA: Pernicious anemia. *N Engl J Med* 337(20):1441–1448, 1997.

70. Polycythemia

I **INTRODUCTION.** Polycythemia [i.e., an **abnormal increase in the red blood cell (RBC) mass]** may be a secondary, physiologic response to another disorder (e.g., chronic hypoxia), or it may herald a primary, more malignant disorder (e.g., polycythemia vera or an erythropoietin-secreting tumor). A **hematocrit greater than 54% in men** or **51% in women** indicates polycythemia, and requires further evaluation.

A. **Absolute polycythemia** is characterized by an increase in RBC mass.

B. **Relative polycythemia** is characterized by a decrease in plasma volume.

II **CLINICAL MANIFESTATIONS OF POLYCYTHEMIA**

A. Patients are **often asymptomatic if the hematocrit is lower than 60%.**

B. Higher hematocrits may be associated with **vaso-occlusive episodes** resulting in **headaches, blurry vision, dizziness, strokes, cardiac ischemia,** and **peripheral thromboses.** A **"ruddy" cyanosis** may be found on physical examination.

C. **Polycythemia vera,** a myeloproliferative disorder characterized by prominent proliferation of the RBC line, may present with **pruritus** and **peptic ulcers** in addition to the symptoms described in II B, due to increased histamine levels from a larger number of circulating basophils. Both **thrombosis** and **bleeding** may occur as a result of abnormal platelet function, and **splenomegaly** is common.

III **CAUSES OF POLYCYTHEMIA**

A. **Absolute polycythemia.** There are five common causes of absolute polycythemia. Remember, "Hypoxia Can Cause Polycythemia Every Time."

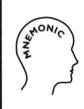

Causes of Absolute Polycythemia ("Hypoxia Can Cause Polycythemia Every Time")

Hypoxia (chronic)
Carboxyhemoglobinemia
Cushing's syndrome or **C**orticosteroids
Polycythemia vera
Erythropoietin-secreting **T**umors

1. **Hypoxia.** Chronic hypoxia, as a result of cardiopulmonary disease or high altitude, can lead to polycythemia.

2. **Carboxyhemoglobinemia** or **methemoglobinemia.** Carboxyhemoglobin, methemoglobin, and other high-affinity variants cause a leftward shift of the hemoglobin dissociation curve, decreased oxygen delivery to the tissues, and a compensatory polycythemia. Smoking is a common cause of carboxyhemoglobinemia.

3. **Cushing's syndrome or corticosteroid therapy.** Corticosteroids have an erythropoietic effect, which can lead to polycythemia.

4. **Polycythemia vera** causes polycythemia by clonal proliferation of stem cells independent of erythropoietin.

5. **Erythropoietin-secreting tumors** are primarily renal, cerebellar, or hepatic.

B. **Relative polycythemia.** There are two main causes of relative polycythemia.

1. **Dehydration** (e.g., from vomiting, diarrhea, excessive perspiration, or diuretics) can deplete plasma volume, leading to a relative polycythemia.

2. **Stress erythrocytosis (Gaisböck's disease)** actually results from contraction of the plasma volume, and is therefore a misnomer. This benign disorder is seen most often in hypertensive, obese men.

IV APPROACH TO THE PATIENT

A. **Rule out hypoxia and carboxyhemoglobinemia.** These are common, relatively easy-to-evaluate causes of polycythemia. If abnormalities significant enough to result in the polycythemia are found, the need for additional work-up may be eliminated. An **arterial blood gas with carboxyhemoglobin level** is necessary for all patients who smoke, and is more accurate than oxygen saturation measurements. The methemoglobin level can also be checked if clinical suspicion warrants doing so.

B. Look at the patient's hematocrit.

1. A **hematocrit greater than 60% in men** or **55% in women** essentially rules out steroid excess, which usually causes a mild polycythemia, and usually reduces the list of possible diagnoses to either polycythemia vera (more common) or an erythropoietin-secreting tumor (less common).

    a. **Polycythemia vera.** The following criteria help to diagnose polycythemia vera.

       (1) **Polycythemia associated with splenomegaly, thrombocytosis,** and a **normal oxygen saturation** is diagnostic for polycythemia vera.

       (2) An **increased leukocyte alkaline phosphatase (LAP) score, concomitant iron-deficiency anemia,** and/or an **increased vitamin B$_{12}$ level** offer additional evidence for polycythemia vera.

       (3) A **decreased erythropoietin level** is also useful (almost all patients with polycythemia vera have a level less than 20 mU/ml).

       (4) A **marrow erythroid progenitor cell culture** shows independent growth with polycythemia vera, but not with secondary polycythemia. However, this test is usually not routinely available.

    b. **Erythropoietin-secreting tumors.** In patients without a definitive diagnosis, the possibility of an erythropoietin-secreting tumor should be considered.

       (1) An **abdominal computed tomography (CT)** scan may help rule out renal pathology (including cancer) and hepatic malignancies.

       (2) **Brain imaging** [preferably a magnetic resonance imaging (MRI) scan] may be performed if there is any clinical suspicion of a cerebellar lesion.

2. A **hematocrit less than 60% in men** or **55% in women** suggests mild polycythemia, which is more common with secondary polycythemia. An **RBC mass study** should be ordered to rule out **decreased plasma volume,** which is responsible for the polycythemia in approximately 50% of cases.

V **TREATMENT.** Definitive therapy is aimed at the underlying disorder. Stress erythrocytosis requires no treatment. Supportive measures include the following.

A. Oxygen therapy is useful in patients with an arterial oxygen tension (Pao_2) lower than 60 mm Hg.

B. Smoking cessation is encouraged (especially in patients with carboxyhemoglobinemia).

C. Hydration is recommended for patients with evidence of dehydration.

D. Phlebotomy lowers the hematocrit, reducing blood viscosity, preventing thromboembolic complications, and improving oxygen delivery.

    1. Phlebotomy is the **treatment of choice for polycythemia vera** and has been shown to dramatically prolong survival. Patients with a hematocrit greater than 60% should have 500 ml of blood removed every 2–3 days until a hematocrit lower than 55% is obtained.

        a. The target hematocrit is in the mid to low 40s.

        b. The timing of phlebotomy and the amount of blood drawn in order to achieve this goal vary among patients. Smaller blood draws (e.g., 250 ml) may be required in elderly patients.

    2. Because the risk of thrombotic complications increases dramatically when the hematocrit is greater than 55%, phlebotomy is also recommended for other causes of polycythemia when the hematocrit remains elevated despite correction of the underlying disorder. Patients gradually become iron deficient with repeated phlebotomy, which results in decreased production of red blood cells. **Iron supplementation should therefore be avoided** because it causes phlebotomy requirements to increase, over time.

E. Aspirin. The use of anti-platelet agents in the treatment of polycythemia is controversial, but aspirin and other anti-platelet agents may be indicated for patients with thrombotic complications.

F. Allopurinol (300 mg daily in patients with normal renal function) is often indicated for patients who have hyperuricemia and gout, which often accompany the increased cell turnover that is characteristic of polycythemia vera.

G. Histamine-2 (H_2 blockers (e.g., ranitidine, 300 mg daily) may be useful for patients with polycythemia vera who have pruritus.

H. Hydroxyurea is sometimes used as a myelosuppressive agent for patients with polycythemia vera.

VI FOLLOW-UP AND REFERRAL

A. A hematologist can help guide specific anti-platelet and myelosuppressive therapy; all patients with polycythemia vera should be managed in consultation with a hematologist.

B. Patients with marked polycythemia must be seen for phlebotomy every 1–3 days until the hematocrit is lowered to less than 55%; the target hematocrit can then be reached with weekly blood draws. Regular monitoring of the hematocrit (at least monthly) and phlebotomy are essential in order to prevent life-threatening complications.

References

Messinezy M, Pearson TC: ABC of clinical haematology: polycythemia, primary (essential) thrombocythaemia and myelofibrosis. *BMJ* 314(7080):587–590, 1997.

Tatarsky I, Sharon R: Management of polycythemia vera with hydroxyurea. *Semin Hematol* 34(1):24–28, 1997.

71. Thrombocytopenia and Thrombocytosis

I **INTRODUCTION.** Thrombocytopenia and thrombocytosis are common disorders that may be discovered during an evaluation for bleeding or clotting disorders, or noted as a response to another illness.

   A. **Thrombocytopenia** is defined as a **platelet count less than 150,000 cells/μl.**

   B. **Thrombocytosis** is defined as a **platelet count greater than 450,000 cells/μl.**

II. **THROMBOCYTOPENIA**

   A. **Clinical manifestations.** Signs and symptoms are related to the degree of thrombocytopenia (in the absence of concomitant disorders of coagulation or platelet dysfunction).

      1. **Platelet count of 50,000–150,000 cells/μl.** Clinical manifestations are usually absent.

      2. **Platelet count of 20,000–50,000 cells/μl.** Patients may report **easy bruisability,** but spontaneous bleeding is usually not seen.

      3. **Platelet count less than 20,000 cells/μl.** Patients are at increased risk for **spontaneous bleeding** (e.g., **petechiae, gastrointestinal bleeding).**

   B. **Causes of thrombocytopenia.** It is easiest to remember the causes of thrombocytopenia if you classify them according to the underlying mechanism: decreased production, splenic sequestration, or increased destruction (Figure 71-1) .

      1. **Decreased production.** Because diseases of the bone marrow are involved, there is often a decrease in other cell lines as well. The causes of decreased platelet production are almost identical to those of pancytopenia ("PANCYTO"), with the exception of consumption ("C").

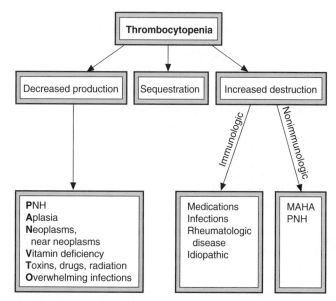

FIGURE 71-1. Causes of thrombocytopenia. *MAHA* = microangiopathic hemolytic anemia; *PNH* = paroxysmal nocturnal hematuria. (Reprinted with permission from Saint S, Frances C: *Saint-Frances Guide to Inpatient Medicine.* Baltimore, Williams & Wilkins, 1997, p 310.)

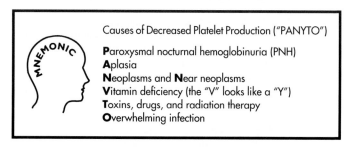

Causes of Decreased Platelet Production ("PANYTO")

Paroxysmal nocturnal hemoglobinuria (PNH)
Aplasia
Neoplasms and **N**ear neoplasms
Vitamin deficiency (the "V" looks like a "Y")
Toxins, drugs, and radiation therapy
Overwhelming infection

a. **PNH** is more commonly associated with increased destruction, but may also be associated with a production defect.

b. **Aplasia. Aplastic anemia** usually causes pancytopenia but occasionally can result in isolated thrombocytopenia.

c. **Neoplasms** and **near neoplasms** include **leukemia, metastatic malignancies,** and **myelodysplasia.**

    d. **Vitamin deficiencies,** including **vitamin B$_{12}$** and **folate deficiency,** are rare causes of isolated thrombocytopenia.

    e. **Toxins, drugs,** and **radiation therapy. Heparin, ethanol, thiazide diuretics, estrogens,** and **chemotherapeutic agents** can lead to decreased platelet production.

    f. **Overwhelming infections,** including sepsis, tuberculosis, fungal infection, and HIV disease, can cause thrombocytopenia as a result of decreased platelet production.

2. **Increased splenic sequestration** can result from **hypersplenism** of any cause, leading to thrombocytopenia.

3. **Increased destruction** is probably the most common cause of isolated thrombocytopenia. Disorders that cause increased destruction of platelets can be classified as nonimmunologic or immunologic.

    a. **Nonimmunologic** causes of platelet destruction include the following.

        (1) **Microangiopathic hemolytic anemia (MAHA)** may cause platelet destruction as a result of shearing in small vessels (see also Chapter 69 IV A 1 b). MAHA is often seen in the setting of disseminated intravascular coagulation (DIC) or hemolytic-uremic syndrome/thrombotic thrombocytopenic purpura (HUS/TTP).

        (2) **PNH** causes defects in all cell lines, which predisposes cells to complement-mediated lysis. Therefore, PNH is a rare cause of isolated thrombocytopenia.

    b. **Immunologic** causes of platelet destruction include:

        (1) **Drugs** (e.g., heparin)

        (2) **Infections**

        (3) **Rheumatologic disease**

        (4) **Idiopathic thrombocytopenic purpura (ITP).** An acute form of ITP that is usually related to a viral illness and resolves spontaneously over 3–6 months may be seen in children. In adults, ITP usually follows a chronic course.

C. **Approach to the patient**

1. **Exclude pseudothrombocytopenia.** Pseudothrombocytopenia is an artifact of platelet clumping in the test tube in EDTA-anticoagulated blood. Clumps of platelets in the peripheral blood smear may alert you to the problem. Sending a heparinized specimen corrects the clumping and confirms your suspicion.

2. Try to determine the cause of the thrombocytopenia.

   a. Patient history. Pay particular attention to the patient's medications. Risk factors for HIV or a history of substance abuse (e.g., alcohol) also deserve attention. A review of systems and asking about "B symptoms" (i.e., fevers, night sweats, and weight loss) may help reveal an occult malignancy.

   b. Physical examination. A complete physical examination is always necessary.

     (1) Splenomegaly suggests sequestration.

     (2) Lymphadenopathy suggests an underlying malignancy or chronic infection.

   c. Laboratory studies

     (1) Peripheral blood smear. A peripheral blood smear is often helpful.

       (a) Large platelets. This finding implies increased destruction and early release of platelets from the bone marrow. Large platelets on the peripheral blood smear are a classic finding in ITP.

       (b) Schistocytes. The finding of fragmented red blood cells (RBCs) implies MAHA.

       (c) Leukoerythroblastosis

         (i) The finding of **early (nucleated) RBCs** and **early white blood cells (WBCs)** [e.g., **bands, metamyelocytes, and myelocytes**] on a peripheral smear implies marrow invasion by malignancy, fibrosis, or infection.

         (ii) Teardrop cells (i.e., RBCs shaped like teardrops as a result of being squeezed out of the bone marrow) may be seen in a leukoerythroblastic smear.

       (d) Megaloblasts imply vitamin B_{12} or folate deficiency.

       (e) Neutrophils with bilobed nuclei (i.e., the Pelger-Huët anomaly) are seen in patients with myelodysplasia.

     (2) The **prothrombin time (PT),** the **partial thromboplastin time (PTT),** and the **lactate dehydrogenase (LDH) level** may be used to evaluate the possibility of MAHA. **Blood urea nitrogen (BUN)** and **creatinine levels** should be obtained when HUS/TTP is a consideration.

(3) **Serologic studies.** Antinuclear antibody (ANA), HIV, and other specific viral serologies are useful for evaluating the possibility of immunologic destruction associated with a rheumatologic disorder [e.g., systemic lupus erythematosus (SLE)] or infection (e.g., HIV).

   (a) An HIV test is especially necessary in patients with HIV risk factors.

   (b) Epstein-Barr virus, cytomegalovirus (CMV), hepatitis virus, and toxoplasmosis serologies are most useful when the patient has systemic symptoms or lymphadenopathy or splenomegaly on examination.

(4) **Vitamin B_{12} and folate levels** and **tests for PNH** are sometimes performed, but are usually not helpful because these disorders are rarely associated with isolated thrombocytopenia.

(5) **Antiplatelet antibody testing** is not necessary to make the diagnosis of ITP, and is therefore usually not performed.

d. **Bone marrow biopsy** is performed in many patients with thrombocytopenia. Pertinent findings on bone marrow biopsy include the following.

(1) **Decreased megakaryocytes** are diagnostic of one of the production problems. Evidence of the specific cause of the decreased production may also be found (e.g., malignancy, infection).

(2) **Increased megakaryocytes** are found when increased destruction or sequestration is the mechanism of thrombocytopenia. Increased megakaryocytes on bone marrow biopsy without other identifiable causes of increased destruction or sequestration is usually diagnostic for ITP.

(3) **Evidence for myelodysplasia** (e.g., hypercellularity, megaloblastic features, nuclear budding, multinucleated erythroblasts) can also be seen on bone marrow biopsy.

HOT **KEY** If the cause of the patient's thrombocytopenia is readily identifiable (e.g., thiazide diuretic therapy), a trial of removing the possible inciting agent may be both diagnostic and therapeutic, and obviate the need for a bone marrow biopsy.

D. Treatment
   1. General treatment
      a. Discontinue medications that may cause thrombocytopenia. Usually, the platelet count returns to normal in 7–10 days.

HOT **KEY** Heparin-induced thrombocytopenia and thrombosis (HITT) is a disorder where immune-mediated thrombocytopenia and, paradoxically, systemic thrombosis coexist. Increasing the heparin dose in patients with HITT is contraindicated; the only therapy is heparin withdrawal.

---

   b. Platelet transfusions
      (1) Contraindications
         (a) Platelet transfusions are not indicated for patients with platelet counts greater than 20,000 cells/μl and no evidence of bleeding.
         (b) In general, patients with TTP should not receive platelet tranfusions because transfusions may exacerbate the TTP.
      (2) Indications. Platelet transfusions are indicated in the following situations:
         (a) Prior to surgery. The platelet count is usually maintained above 50,000 cells/μl when surgery is to be performed, although in patients with ITP, this may be both impossible and unnecessary. When neurosurgery is to be performed, the platelet count is usually maintained above 90,000 cells/μl in an attempt to normalize the bleeding time.
         (b) In a patient with active bleeding
            (i) Severe bleeding. The platelet count is always maintained above 50,000 cells/μl and is sometimes increased to 90,000–100,000 cells/μl.
            (ii) Mild bleeding or **petechiae.** The platelet count should be maintained above 20,000 cells/μl.
         (c) To prevent spontaneous bleeding. The platelet count is usually kept above 10,000–20,000 cells/μl, depending on physician preference.

HOT

KEY

Unnecessary platelet transfusions should be avoided because they may induce immune resistance; if this complication occurs, human leukocyte antigen (HLA)-matched platelets can be administered.

2. **Treatment of ITP**
   a. **Observation** is often appropriate for patients with platelet counts greater than 20,000 cells/µl and no evidence of bleeding.
   b. **Pharmacologic therapy**
      (1) **Steroids** (e.g., prednisone, 1–2 mg/kg/day) benefit approximately two thirds of patients, leading to an increase in platelet count in approximately 3 weeks. Counts often fall again when steroids are tapered.
      (2) **Intravenous gammaglobulin** often increases the platelet count faster than steroids; it is therefore useful for actively bleeding patients and those with extremely low counts in the "window" before steroids take effect.
      (3) **Immunosuppressive agents** can be used for patients with ITP associated with SLE or other connective tissue disorders.
      (4) **Danazol** (600 mg/day) is sometimes useful for patients with refractory ITP.
      (5) **Zidovudine** may be useful for patients with HIV-associated ITP.
   c. **Splenectomy** is indicated when steroid therapy fails or relapse occurs following a steroid taper.
E. **Follow-up and referral.** Consultation with a hematologist is indicated when the cause of the thrombocytopenia cannot be identified despite a thorough evaluation, or when the thrombocytopenia is severe, prolonged, or complicated by bleeding or abnormal clotting.

III THROMBOCYTOSIS

A. **Clinical manifestations**
   1. **Primary thrombocytosis.** If the thrombocytosis is caused by a myeloproliferative disorder, the platelets are frequently abnormal and the patient may be prone to both bleeding and clotting events.
   2. **Secondary (reactive) thrombocytosis.** If the thrombo-

cytosis is secondary to another disorder, even patients with extremely high platelet counts (e.g., greater than 1,000,000 cells/μl) are usually asymptomatic.

B. Causes of thrombocytosis

1. **Primary thrombocytosis** is caused by **myeloproliferative disorders,** which increase the platelet count through clonal proliferation of the stem cells. The four myeloproliferative disorders are:

   a. **Essential thrombocytosis,** characterized by prominent proliferation of platelets

   b. **Chronic myelogenous leukemia (CML),** characterized by prominent proliferation of the WBC line

   c. **Polycythemia vera,** characterized by prominent proliferation of the RBC line

   d. **Myelofibrosis,** characterized by prominent proliferation of fibroblasts

2. **Secondary thrombocytosis** is more common than primary thrombocytosis. Causes include:

   a. **Malignancies**

   b. **Infections**

   c. **Connective tissue disorders**

   d. **Iron deficiency anemia**

   e. **Splenectomy**

C. Approach to the patient

1. **Patient history**

   a. A history of **gastrointestinal bleeding** may imply iron deficiency.

   b. **Fevers, night sweats,** or **weight loss** may implicate malignancy or chronic infection (e.g., tuberculosis). A complete review of systems should be performed to help identify the presence of an occult malignancy or infection.

   c. A history of recent **splenectomy** may provide a simple explanation for the thrombocytosis.

2. **Physical examination.** Perform a thorough physical examination, including pelvic and rectal examinations. Pay special attention to the spleen and lymph nodes because enlargement may signal malignancy or infection.

3. **Laboratory studies** can further narrow the differential diagnosis.

   a. **Serum ferritin level.** The serum ferritin level helps to evaluate the possibility of iron deficiency anemia and is especially important in patients with a history of gastrointestinal bleeding, guaiac-positive stools, or a low mean corpuscular volume (MCV).

   b. **Hematocrit** and **WBC count.** The hematocrit and WBC count are often elevated in patients with myeloproliferative disorders, although essential thrombocytosis may result in an isolated elevation of the platelet count.

   c. **Other tests** may be performed if a reactive thrombocytosis is suspected [e.g., a purified protein derivative (PPD) test for possible tuberculosis, a computed tomography (CT) scan for suspected intra-abdominal malignancy].

D. Treatment

   1. **Primary thrombocytosis. Hydroxyurea** should be considered for patients with marked thrombocytosis (i.e., a platelet count greater than 700,000 cells/μl), or if symptomatic thromboses occur.

   2. **Secondary thrombocytosis.** Most patients with reactive thrombocytosis do not require treatment to lower the platelet count. The platelet count usually returns to normal following treatment of the underlying disorder.

E. Follow-up and referral

   1. A hematologist can provide recommendations concerning long-term therapy for patients with thrombocytosis that is caused by a myeloproliferative disorder.

   2. Most other cases of thrombocytosis respond to treatment of the underlying disorder, and platelet counts should be followed every 1–4 weeks until they return to normal. Patients with persistent abnormalities require referral.

References

Murphy S, Peterson P, Iland H, Laszlo J: Experience of the polycythemia vera study group with essential thrombocythemia: a final report on diagnostic criteria, survival, and leukemic transition by treatment. *Semin Hematol* 34(1):29–39, 1997.

Rutherford CJ, Frenkel EP: Thrombocytopenia: issues in diagnosis and therapy. *Med Clin North Am* 78(3):555–575, 1994.

72. Leukocytosis

I INTRODUCTION

A. The **circulating pool of white blood cells** (WBCs, leukocytes) consists of:
   1. **Neutrophils**
   2. **Lymphocytes**
   3. **Monocytes**
   4. **Eosinophils**
   5. **Basophils**

B. **Definitions**
   1. **Leukocytosis.** In leukocytosis, the total WBC count **exceeds 11,000 cells/mm^3 (11 x 10^9/L).**
   2. **Leukemoid reaction.** A leukemoid reaction is said to occur when the leukocyte count **exceeds 30,000 cells/mm^3** and there is no evidence of immature WBCs or nucleated red blood cells (RBCs) on the peripheral smear. This process reflects a healthy bone marrow that is reacting to some type of stress (e.g., trauma, inflammation, infection, malignancy).
   3. **Leukoerythroblastosis.** This term is used when there is evidence of immature WBCs or nucleated RBCs on the peripheral smear, regardless of the total WBC count. Leukoerythroblastosis usually implies bone marrow infiltration (e.g., from tumor).

C. Because each cell type can be increased in response to various stimuli, determining the predominant cell type in patients with leukocytosis may offer some insight into the cause.

II TYPES OF LEUKOCYTOSIS

A. **Neutrophilia** is defined as a neutrophil count that **exceeds 7500 cells/mm^3.**
   1. **Causes of neutrophilia.** Neutrophilia can be caused by many of the major disease categories listed in Chapter 1 II B 2 (Table 72-1).
   2. **Approach to the patient**
      a. When evaluating patients with neutrophilia, the most important initial consideration should be **infection**.
      b. If this and other benign disorders are excluded, a search for **malignancy** (which may necessitate a bone marrow biopsy) is usually warranted.

TABLE 72-1. Common Causes of Neutrophilia

Category of Disease	Specific Causes
Hematologic	Hemolytic anemia, splenectomy
Pregnancy-related	Pregnancy-induced neutrophilia
Drugs/toxins	Corticosteroids, lithium, mercury, ethylene glycol
Metabolic/endocrine	Hyperthyroidism, ketoacidosis
Inflammatory	Rheumatoid arthritis, vasculitis, gout
Infectious	Bacteria, viruses, fungi, parasites
Neoplastic	Myeloproliferative disorders, myelodysplastic syndromes, gastrointestinal or renal malignancy, melanoma, Hodgkin's disease
Trauma	Insect bites, jellyfish stings, crush injuries, electric shock

HOT

KEY

Acutely infected or injured patients have elevated levels of endogenous glucocorticoids, which, in turn, lead to low levels of eosinophils and basophils. The presence of eosinophils and basophils in acutely ill patients with neutrophilia indicates concomitant adrenal insufficiency, a granulocyte-macrophage colony-stimulating factor (GM-CSF)—secreting tumor, or a hematologic malignancy.

B. Lymphocytosis is defined as a lymphocyte count that **exceeds 5000 cells/mm ^{3}.**
   1. Causes of lymphocytosis. The severity of the lymphocytosis is usually indicative of the cause (Table 72-2).
   2. Approach to the patient. Look for leukoerythroblastosis on the peripheral smear.
      a. If **leukoerythroblastosis** is **present, malignancy** is likely and bone marrow biopsy is necessary.
      b. If **leukoerythroblastosis** is **not present, infection** is likely. A bone marrow biopsy is necessary if the diagnosis remains unclear.
C. Monocytosis is defined as a monocyte count that **exceeds 500 cells/mm³.** Monocytes play an important role in

TABLE 72-2. Common Causes of Lymphocytosis

Type of Lymphocytosis	Specific Causes
Mild to moderate (5000–15,000/mm^3)	Viral illness (mononucleosis, hepatitis) Secondary to other infections (e.g., tuberculosis, toxoplasmosis, syphilis) Malignancy (e.g., Hodgkin's disease, early CLL)
Severe (>15,000/mm^3)	Mononucleosis Hepatitis Pertussis Late CLL ALL

ALL = acute lymphocytic leukemia; CLL = chronic lymphocytic leukemia.

killing obligate intracellular parasites and are associated with granulomatous inflammation.

1. **Causes of monocytosis** are given in Table 72-3.
2. **Approach to the patient.** If the levels of monocytes are extremely high, a hematologic malignancy should be suspected.

D. **Eosinophilia.** Eosinophils normally dwell in the tissues. The normal range of eosinophils in the blood is 0–450 cells/mm^3 (0%–4%); eosinophilia is defined as an eosinophil count that exceeds 450 cells/mm^3. Counts are highest in the morning and fall during the day, as glucocorticoid levels increase. Causes of eosinophilia include the following.

1. **Pulmonary disease.** Many primary lung disorders can lead to eosinophilia, including **Löffler's syndrome, hypersensitivity pneumonitis,** and **eosinophilic pneumonia.**
2. **Helminthic infections**. Eosinophils play a major role in defending the host against multicellular, helminthic parasites. Examples of helminthic infections include:
   a. **Filariasis**
   b. **Ascariasis**
   c. **Schistosomiasis**
   d. **Trichinosis**
   e. ***Strongyloides* infection**

TABLE 72-3. Common Causes of Monocytosis

Category of Disease	Specific Cause
Infectious	Tuberculosis, endocarditis, brucellosis, syphilis, fungal or protozoal infections, listeriosis
Neoplastic	Hodgkin's disease, leukemia, carcinoma
Inflammatory	Inflammatory bowel disease, sarcoidosis

HOT **KEY**

Disseminated *Strongyloides* infection sometimes does not cause eosinophilia because of the superimposed bacterial infection that may accompany parasitic dissemination.

3. **Other infections** may also be associated with eosinophilia.
   a. **Allergic bronchopulmonary aspergillosis**

HOT **KEY**

Invasive aspergillosis does not cause eosinophilia.

   b. **Coccidioidomycosis**
   c. **Tuberculosis,** especially chronic tuberculosis
4. **Contaminated L-tryptophan** can cause eosinophilia-myalgia syndrome.
5. **Immunologic disorders,** such as vasculitis (especially Churg-Strauss syndrome), severe rheumatoid arthritis, and eosinophilic fasciitis, can cause eosinophilia.
6. **Addison's disease (corticosteroid deficiency)** can be associated with eosinophilia.
7. **Cutaneous disorders** associated with eosinophilia include **bullous pemphigoid, scabies,** and **eosinophilic cellulitis.**

8. **Allergic disorders.** Eosinophils induce the release of allergic mediators by mast cells and basophils. Therefore, eosinophilia is often seen in **asthma, allergic rhinitis, atopic dermatitis, drug reactions, acute urticaria,** and other allergic disorders.
9. **Neoplasms.** Solid tumors of epithelial origin, mucus-secreting tumors, lymphoma, and leukemia can lead to eosinophilia.

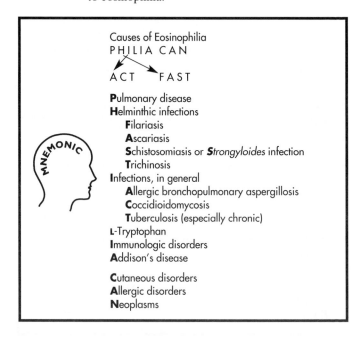

Causes of Eosinophilia
PHILIA CAN
ACT   FAST

Pulmonary disease
Helminthic infections
  Filariasis
  Ascariasis
  Schistosomiasis or **S**trongyloides infection
  Trichinosis
Infections, in general
  Allergic bronchopulmonary aspergillosis
  Coccidioidomycosis
  Tuberculosis (especially chronic)
L-Tryptophan
Immunologic disorders
Addison's disease

Cutaneous disorders
Allergic disorders
Neoplasms

III ▮ FOLLOW-UP AND REFERRAL

A. **Follow-up.** During the process of evaluation, the patient should be seen every 2–4 weeks. More frequent visits may be necessary if the patient is moderately to severely symptomatic.
B. **Referral.** A referral to a hematologist can be helpful when the diagnosis remains unclear after a preliminary evaluation. Referral to a hematologist is necessary when a hematologic malignancy or bone marrow biopsy is being contemplated.

References
Rothenberg ME: Eosinophilia. *N Engl J Med* 338(22):1592–1600, 1998.
Reding MT, Hibbs JR, Morrison VA, et al: Diagnosis and outcome of 100 consecutive patients with extreme granulocytic leukocytosis. *Am J Med* 104(1):12–16, 1998.

73. Bleeding Disorders

I **INTRODUCTION.** A predisposition to bleeding can result from **problems with platelets** (either number or function) or **problems with coagulation** (factor deficiency or factor inhibitors).

II **CLINICAL MANIFESTATIONS OF BLEEDING DISORDERS**
A. **Inherited problems. Recurrent bleeding since childhood** or a **family history of bleeding** implies an inherited coagulation factor deficiency or an inherited problem with platelet function.
B. **Platelet problems** usually cause **mucocutaneous petechiae** or **ecchymoses.**
C. **Coagulation problems** are suspected in patients with **spontaneous deep bleeding** into hematomas or joints (hemarthroses) or **delayed bleeding** after surgery or trauma.

III **APPROACH TO THE PATIENT.** Figure 73-1 summarizes the general approach to a patient with a bleeding disorder.

A. **Platelet count.** The platelet count must be less than 90,000–100,000 cells/μl to prolong the bleeding time. Therefore, mildly decreased counts are not responsible for clinical bleeding, and a concurrent problem of platelet function or coagulation should be considered.
B. **Prothrombin time (PT)/partial thromboplastin time (PTT).** There are three types of PT/PTT abnormalities: increased PT/normal PTT, increased PT and PTT, and normal PT/increased PTT.
   1. **Increased PT/normal PTT**
      a. **Differential diagnoses**
         (1) Early disseminated intravascular coagulation (DIC)
         (2) Liver disease
         (3) Warfarin therapy
         (4) Vitamin K deficiency
         (5) Factor VII deficiency (rare)
      b. Recommended work-up

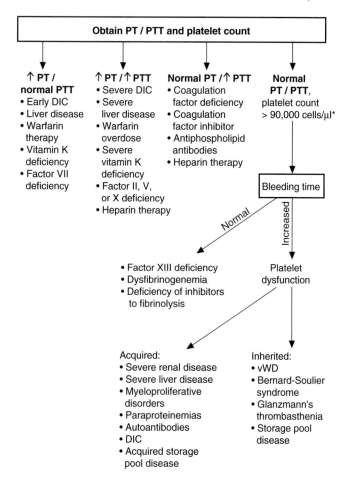

| Obtain PT / PTT and platelet count |

↑ PT / normal PTT
• Early DIC
• Liver disease
• Warfarin therapy
• Vitamin K deficiency
• Factor VII deficiency

↑ PT / ↑ PTT
• Severe DIC
• Severe liver disease
• Warfarin overdose
• Severe vitamin K deficiency
• Factor II, V, or X deficiency
• Heparin therapy

Normal PT / ↑ PTT
• Coagulation factor deficiency
• Coagulation factor inhibitor
• Antiphospholipid antibodies
• Heparin therapy

Normal PT / PTT, platelet count > 90,000 cells/μl*

Bleeding time

Normal — *Increased*

• Factor XIII deficiency
• Dysfibrinogenemia
• Deficiency of inhibitors to fibrinolysis

Platelet dysfunction

Acquired:
• Severe renal disease
• Severe liver disease
• Myeloproliferative disorders
• Paraproteinemias
• Autoantibodies
• DIC
• Acquired storage pool disease

Inherited:
• vWD
• Bernard-Soulier syndrome
• Glanzmann's thrombasthenia
• Storage pool disease

* A platelet count less than 90,000 cells/μl may result in an increased bleeding time and a bleeding disorder. Patients with platelet counts greater than 90,000 cells/μl may still be thrombocytopenic (i.e., a platelet count less than 150,000 cells/μl), but this level of thrombo-cytopenia is usually not the cause of a bleeding disorder; therefore, other causes should be considered.

Figure 73-1. Approach to the patient with a bleeding disorder. *DIC* = disseminated intravascular coagulation; *PT* = prothrombin time; *PTT* = partial thromboplastin time; *vWD* = von Willebrand's disease. (Reprinted with permission from Saint S, Frances C: *Saint-Frances Guide to Inpatient Medicine.* Baltimore, Williams & Wilkins, 1997, p 334.)

      (1) Patient history. Ask about medications (e.g., warfarin) and note factors that may predispose a patient to vitamin K deficiency (e.g., malnutrition, alcoholism, pancreatic insufficiency, recent antibiotic use).

      (2) DIC panel (D-dimers, fibrinogen) and **peripheral smear.** Evidence for DIC may include a low fibrinogen level (< 150 mg/dl), elevated D-dimers, or schistocytes on the peripheral blood smear. Because D-dimers may be elevated in patients with liver or renal disease or with clinical bleeding, and hypofibrinogenemia may occur with severe liver dysfunction, the presence of schistocytes may be the only distinguishing feature for DIC in a patient with concomitant liver failure.

      (3) Liver function tests (bilirubin, albumin, and transaminase levels) are often obtained.

      (4) A **factor VII level** is rarely necessary but can be obtained if the cause of the increased PT is still unknown.

2. Increased PT and PTT

  a. Differential diagnoses. Generally, more severe versions of the same conditions that cause an isolated elevated PT cause an increase in both the PT and PTT.

      (1) DIC

      (2) Severe liver disease

      (3) Warfarin overdose

      (4) Severe vitamin K deficiency

      (5) Factor II, V, or X deficiency (rare)

      (6) Heparin therapy (usually the PT is only mildly increased)

  b. Recommended work-up. The recommended evaluation is the same as that for increased PT/normal PTT, except that on the rare occasion of a completely negative work-up, different factor levels need to be tested.

3. Normal PT/increased PTT

  a. Differential diagnoses. After excluding the obvious cause (i.e., heparin therapy), you only need to consider three possibilities.

      (1) Coagulation factor deficiency

      (2) Coagulation factor inhibitor

      (3) Antiphospholipid antibodies (including lupus anticoagulant and anticardiolipin antibody)

    b. Recommended work-up
       (1) Patient history. If the patient has a history of bleeding, a factor deficiency or a factor inhibitor is likely. If the patient has a history of clotting, an antiphospholipid syndrome is implicated.
       (2) 50:50 mixing study. Only 30% factor activity is needed to have a normal PTT. By mixing the patient's blood with an equal amount of blood with normal coagulation (i.e., blood with a normal PTT), enough factor will be provided to correct any factor deficiency (if that is the problem).
          (a) If the PTT corrects (and stays corrected on later testing) a **factor deficiency** is diagnosed. The most common factor deficiencies are factor VIII (hemophilia A), factor IX (hemophilia B), and factor XI deficiencies (mostly seen in Ashkenazi Jews); therefore, **factor VIII, IX,** and **XI levels should be drawn first.**
          (b) If the PTT does not correct with mixing, an **antiphospholipid antibody** or a **factor inhibitor** is present. **Send laboratory tests for lupus anticoagulant and anticardiolipin antibody.**
          (c) If the PTT initially corrects, but prolongs on later testing, a **factor inhibitor** is probably present (i.e., the added factor has been consumed by the inhibitor). **Factor VIII inhibitor is the most common and should be checked first.**
C. Bleeding time
    1. If the bleeding time is prolonged and the platelet count is more than 90,000 cells/μl, platelet dysfunction is implicated.
       a. Acquired platelet dysfunction
          (1) Differential diagnoses. Acquired platelet disorders are usually systemic.
             (a) Severe renal disease leading to uremia can cause platelet dysfunction.
             (b) Severe liver disease. Factor deficiency as a result of liver disease is a well-known cause of coagulopathy. In addition, liver disease can cause coagulopathy by inducing platelet dysfunction.

(c) **Malignancy.** Multiple myeloma and Waldenstrom's macroglobulinemia (which can cause paraproteinemia) and myeloproliferative disorders can lead to platelet dysfunction.

(d) **Autoantibodies** [from β-lactam antibiotic therapy or idiopathic thrombocytopenic purpura (ITP)] can coat platelets and increase the bleeding time even with a normal platelet count.

(e) **DIC.** The fibrin split products produced in DIC inhibit platelet function.

(f) **Acquired storage pool disease.** Cardiopulmonary bypass surgery or vasculitis can cause platelets to release all of their granules, resulting in dysfunctional platelets.

(g) **Aspirin** irreversibly inhibits platelet function for the life of the platelet (7–10 days); other nonsteroidal anti-inflammatory drugs (NSAIDs) reversibly inhibit platelet function and the effect is more transient.

HOT

The bleeding time may be mildly prolonged with aspirin or NSAIDs, but will only become abnormally prolonged if an underlying cause of platelet dysfunction is present.

KEY

---

(2) **Recommended work-up**

(a) **Patient history.** A medication history (including all over-the-counter drugs) should always be obtained. Immune-mediated platelet dysfunction may be suspected with the use of certain medications, a history of ITP, or with mild thrombocytopenia accompanied by obvious platelet dysfunction (prolonged bleeding time).

(b) A **complete blood count (CBC) with differential** will help evaluate the possibility of a myeloproliferative disorder.

(c) A **DIC panel** can help evaluate the possibility of DIC.

(d) **Liver function tests** and **blood urea nitro-**

gen **(BUN)** and **creatine levels** help exclude liver and renal disease, respectively.

(e) **Protein electrophoresis** may be used to detect a paraproteinemia.

b. **Inherited platelet dysfunction.** Normally, platelets first adhere to the endothelium during injury, and then they aggregate by binding fibrinogen.

(1) **Differential diagnoses.** The first two disorders involve problems with platelet adherence, and the second two involve problems with platelet aggregation.

(a) **von Willebrand's disease (vWD).** von Willebrand's factor (vWF) is made by megakaryocytes and endothelial cells, and circulates in the plasma in multimers of varying size bound to factor VIII (which vWF stabilizes). vWF binds to the glycoprotein Ib receptor on platelets, and helps platelets adhere to the endothelium.

(i) In **type I vWD** (80% of cases), there is a decreased quantity of vWF.

(ii) In **type III vWD,** there is a complete absence of vWF.

(iii) In **type II vWD,** there is a qualitative decrease in vWF activity.

In **type IIa vWD,** the qualitative defect results from a decrease in the large multimers of vWF, the active forms in platelet adhesion.

In **type IIb vWD,** there is also a decrease in the large multimers of vWF; however, the decrease is caused by abnormal vWF adherence to platelets.

(b) **Bernard-Soulier syndrome** results from a loss in the platelet receptor for vWF (glycoprotein Ib).

(c) **Glanzmann's thrombasthenia** results from the loss of the IIa-IIIb glycoprotein platelet receptor, which leads to decreased fibrinogen binding and, therefore, defective platelet aggregation.

(d) **Storage pool disease** is caused by the defective release of platelet granules [especially adenosine diphosphate (ADP)], which results in decreased platelet aggregation.

(2) Recommended work-up

(a) Patient history. Obtaining the family history is important. vWD is an autosomal dominant disorder, while Bernard-Soulier syndrome and Glanzmann's thrombasthenia are autosomal recessive.

(b) vWD panel. Screen for vWD first because vWD is the most common inherited disorder of platelet function. A vWD panel includes the following tests.

(i) Ristocetin cofactor activity test. The patient's plasma is mixed with normal platelets and ristocetin. Ristocetin should cause plasma vWF to bind to the platelet surface (via the glycoprotein Ib receptor), resulting in platelet aggregation. Lack of aggregation implies vWD.

(ii) The **factor VIII antigen level** is another way of assessing the vWF level.

(iii) Factor VIII activity may be decreased with a decrease in vWF level, resulting in a prolonged PTT.

HOT Type I vWD often causes a parallel decrease in all parts of the panel, while type III vWD demonstrates no activity in any part of the panel. In type II vWD, there will be decreased ristocetin cofactor activity out of proportion to the decreased **KEY** factor VIII antigen level.

(c) Ristocetin aggregation test. The patient's plasma and platelets are mixed with ristocetin. **Bernard-Soulier syndrome** is diagnosed by a normal vWD panel, but an abnormal ristocetin aggregation test.

(d) Platelet aggregometry is used to diagnose **Glanzmann's thrombasthenia** and **storage pool diseases.**

2. **If the bleeding time is not prolonged** in a patient with a **normal PT/PTT** and **platelet count,** but there is still clinical suspicion of a bleeding diathesis, **rare disorders that involve a defect in cross-linking of fibrin** should be considered. These disorders include:

a. Dysfibrinogenemia

   b. Factor XIII ("fibrin-stabilizing factor") deficiency

   c. Deficiency of inhibitors to fibrinolysis (i.e., plasminogen activator inhibitor or α_2 plasmin inhibitor)

IV TREATMENT

A. Platelet problems

  1. Quantitative problems. Patients may require platelet transfusions (see Chapter 71 II D 1 b).

  2. Qualitative problems are usually only treated when the patient is bleeding or surgery is planned. The use of aspirin and NSAIDs should be avoided.

    a. Desmopressin (DDAVP), 0.3 μg/kg per day, works presumably by increasing the release of stored vWF from endothelial cells. This drug can be used as prophylaxis prior to surgery or for treatment during an episode of bleeding in patients with mild type I vWD or other disorders of platelet dysfunction (e.g., uremia).

     (1) Stores of vWF are depleted in 2–3 days, so desmopressin is usually only effective as short-term treatment.

     (2) Desmopressin is ineffective in type III vWD. In type IIb vWD, large multimers of vWF are already stuck to platelets, and exposure to desmopressin can trigger paradoxical thromboses and thrombocytopenia (from splenic removal). Therefore, the use of desmopressin should be avoided in patients with these subtypes.

    b. Cryoprecipitate and **platelet transfusions** may be necessary for patients who have been hospitalized as a result of refractory bleeding.

    c. Specific therapies may include dialysis for uremia, myelosuppression for myeloproliferative disorders, or steroids for immune disorders.

B. Coagulation problems

  1. Vitamin K (10 mg subcutaneously, daily for 3 days) should be administered routinely in case vitamin K deficiency has a primary or contributing role in the patient's disorder.

  2. Warfarin. If the PT is higher than desired, the **warfarin dose** is usually **decreased** or **withheld,** and the PT is rechecked daily. Low doses of vitamin K (e.g., 1 mg intravenously or orally) can be administered to gradually lower the PT in patients with marked PT elevations. Remember, there is approximately a 3-day lag between the changes in warfarin dose and the changes in the PT. If you have withheld the warfarin, do not wait until the PT is in the appropriate range to resume therapy because the PT will continue to drop. Therapy is best resumed when the PT is slightly higher than desired.

3. **Factor replacement**
   a. **Factor deficiencies.** Hemophilia A and B are treated with **factor VIII** and **IX concentrates** respectively; other factor deficiencies are replaced with **fresh frozen plasma.**
   b. **Factor inhibitors.** Aggressive factor replacement (to "overwhelm" the inhibitor) can be tried. Activated factor IX can be used for patients with factor VIII inhibitors, thereby bypassing the point in the coagulation pathway where factor VIII is needed.
4. **Plasmapheresis** can be used to remove factor inhibitors.
5. **Steroids** and **other immunosuppressants** (e.g., **cyclophosphamide)** are used for chronic therapy in patients with factor inhibitor disorders.
6. **Fresh frozen plasma** and **cryoprecipitate** may be helpful for hospitalized patients with bleeding.

References

Cohen AJ, Kessler CM: Treatment of inherited coagulation disorders. *Am J Med* 99(6):675–682, 1995.

74. Lymphadenopathy

LYMPHADENOPATHY

A. Introduction

1. In lymphadenopathy, the lymph nodes are enlarged or have an abnormal consistency. Lymphadenopathy can be regional (i.e., affecting only one group or a few contiguous groups of nodes) or generalized. Lymphadenopathy usually signals the presence of regional or systemic disease and therefore warrants medical evaluation.

2. Lymphadenopathy must not be confused with lymphangitis or lymphadenitis.

    a. **Lymphangitis** is inflammation of the lymphatics. Generally, red streaks that pass from a wound toward the draining lymph node are seen in lymphangitis.

    b. **Lymphadenitis,** a subtype of lymphadenopathy, is inflammation of the lymph node. The affected node is red, enlarged, and tender.

HOT

Both lymphangitis and lymphadenitis are classically caused by streptococcal or staphylococcal infection.

KEY

B. Causes of lymphadenopathy. There are numerous causes of lymphadenopathy; fortunately, four factors help guide the work-up and narrow the differential.

1. **Location of the lymphadenopathy**

    a. **Generalized lymphadenopathy.** If the lymphadenopathy involves more than two separate sites, the most likely causes can be remembered with the mnemonic, "SHE HAS CUTE LAN (lymphadenopathy)."

Causes of Generalized Lymphadenopathy ("SHE HAS CUTE LAN")

Syphilis
Hepatitis
Epstein-Barr virus

Histoplasmosis
AIDS/HIV
Serum sickness

Cytomegalovirus (CMV)
Unusual drugs (e.g., hydantoin derivatives, antithyroid medications, antileprosy medications, isoniazid)
Toxoplasmosis
Erythrophagocytic lymphohistiocytosis

Leishmaniasis
Arthritis (rheumatoid)
Neoplasm (i.e., leukemia, lymphoma)

    b. **Localized lymphadenopathy.** Causes of localized lymphadenopathy are given in Table 74-1.
2. **HIV status of the patient.** HIV status must always be considered whenever a patient has lymphadenopathy, whether it is regional or generalized. Typically, in patients with HIV, the lymphadenopathy is generalized and occurs early in the course of the HIV infection. The lymphadenopathy can be caused either by the HIV itself or by other systemic diseases that are common in HIV-infected patients.
3. **Clinical scenario**
    a. **Patient age.** Lymphadenopathy in patients younger than 30 years is most often benign and caused by an infection, whereas in patients older than 30 years, malignancy becomes a much more worrisome possibility.

HOT KEY As many as 50% of patients younger than 50 years have palpable cervical lymphadenopathy. Significant cervical, axillary, or inguinal lymphadenopathy in patients older than 60 years usually represents a serious underlying disorder.

TABLE 74-1. Causes of Localized Lymphadenopathy

Location of Lymphadenopathy	Potential Causes
Cervical nodes	Head or neck malignancy or infection Mononucleosis Tuberculosis Lymphoma
Supraclavicular nodes	Lung or gastrointestinal malignancy Lymphoma
Axillary nodes	Hand or arm infection or trauma (including bites) Cat-scratch disease Lymphoma Brucellosis Breast cancer
Epitrochlear nodes	Unilateral: hand infections, lymphoma, tularemia Bilateral: sarcoidosis, syphilis
Inguinal nodes	Leg or foot infections Pelvic malignancy Lymphoma Sexually transmitted diseases (STDs)
Hilar or mediastinal nodes	Sarcoidosis Tuberculosis Lymphoma Fungal infection Lung cancer
Abdominal nodes	Lymphoma Tuberculosis *Mycobacterium avium-intracellulare* infection Metastatic malignancy

      b. Associated findings

        (1) Symptoms of **fever, chills, night sweats,** and **weight loss** (constitutional or "B" symptoms) usually imply a serious systemic infection or malignancy.

        (2) Symptoms or signs of a **local infection** (e.g., pharyngitis, conjunctivitis, otitis, skin infection) or **trauma** usually imply an infectious cause.

        (3) **Exposures** (e.g., cigarette smoke, cats) should also be ascertained.

    4. **Characteristics of the node on palpation.** The physical attributes of the affected lymph nodes may assist in narrowing the differential diagnosis, although physical examination findings can be misleading. The following correlations tend to be true:

      a. **Infections,** which are associated with rapid growth of the node and capsular stretching. tend to cause **tender nodes.** In addition, the nodes tend to be **asymmetric** and the skin that covers them tends to be **erythematous.**

      b. **Lymphoma** classically leads to **large, firm, rubbery, non-tender nodes.**

      c. **Metastatic cancer** usually results in **very firm ("rock hard") non-tender nodes** that are **immobile** (i.e., fixed to the underlying tissue).

C. Approach to the patient

    1. **Ensure that the lymph nodes are truly abnormal.** Certain lymph nodes [e.g., the submandibular nodes (in young adults) and the inguinal nodes] are commonly palpable. The submandibular and inguinal nodes should measure less than 1 and 2 centimeters, respectively.

    2. **Generate a differential diagnosis** based on the location of the lymphadenopathy, the HIV status of the patient, the clinical scenario, and the physical attributes of the node. The differential will help you determine which laboratory and imaging studies to order initially [e.g., complete blood count (CBC), peripheral blood smear, monospot test, hepatitis serologies, serum lactate dehydrogenase (LDH) level, sedimentation rate, Venereal Disease Research Laboratory (VDRL) test, chest radiograph].

    3. **Perform fine needle aspiration or an excisional biopsy of the node if lymphoma or metastatic malignancy is likely.** Fine needle aspiration is good for diagnosing metastatic malignancies (and infections), but not for lymphomas. If lymphoma is a strong possibility, excisional biopsy is usually required to evaluate the lymph node architecture.

4. **Consider a period of observation if the most likely diagnosis is infection.** In those with a likely bacterial cause (e.g., *Streptococcus, Staphylococcus*), a trial of antibiotics is appropriate (e.g., 250–500 mg of cephalexin orally, 4 times daily for 7–10 days). If there is no evidence of resolution after 2–3 weeks, fine needle aspiration, an excisional biopsy, or both is usually required.

D. Treatment depends on the underlying cause.

E. Follow-up and referral

1. **Follow-up.** It is important to follow patients every 1–2 weeks until a diagnosis is made or the lymphadenopathy resolves.

   a. Lymphadenopathy as a result of infection or inflammation resolves within 3 weeks in most patients.

   b. Follow-up is essential for patients with lymphadenopathy of unclear etiology, because a small but significant percentage of these patients develop lymphoma within 1 year.

2. **Referral.** If the patient has lymphoma or another malignancy, prompt referral to a hematologist-oncologist is necessary.

II **LYMPHOMA** is a malignant disorder of the lymphoreticular system. When patients first notice lymphadenopathy, they are usually most concerned about lymphoma. It is important for primary care providers to have an overview of lymphoma in order to counsel their patients appropriately.

A. Introduction. Lymphoma is classified as belonging to one of two groups. Distinguishing the two is important because the treatment and prognosis depend on which type of lymphoma a patient has.

1. The classification is based on the histologic presence or absence of multinucleated giant cells (Reed-Sternberg cells).

   a. **Hodgkin's disease.** Reed-Sternberg cells are present.

   b. **Non-Hodgkin's lymphoma (NHL).** Reed-Sternberg cells are absent.

2. Hodgkin's disease and NHL are compared in Table 74-2.

B. Hodgkin's disease

    1. Epidemiology

        a. Incidence. Fewer than 10,000 cases of Hodgkin's disease are diagnosed in the United States each year.

        b. Patient profile

            (1) Hodgkin's disease has a **bimodal age distribution.** Patients are most often between the ages of 20 and 25 years or older than 55 years.

            (2) Men are affected more often than women.

TABLE 74.2. Comparison of Hodgkin's Disease and Non-Hodgkin's Lymphoma (NHL)

	Hodgkin's Disease	NHL
Cause	Unknown; viral cause suspected	Unknown, although Burkitt's lymphoma is associated with Epstein-Barr virus infection
Malignant cell line	Unclear	B cell: 90% T cell: 10%
Site of origin	Nodal	Extranodal (in as many as 40% of cases)
Spread	Contiguous	Non-contiguous
Mediastinal involvement	Common	Rare
Bone marrow involvement	Rare	Very common in low-grade NHL; unusual in high-grade NHL
Systemic or "B" symptoms	Very common	Seen in fewer than 50% of patients
Best prognostic indicator	Stage*	Grade*

*"Stage" refers to the extent of spread of the tumor, while "grade" refers to the degree of differentiation (i.e., histopathology).

(3) Whites are affected more often than African-Americans.

(4) Hodgkin's disease in young adults is often associated with **middle- to upper-class socio-economic status, advanced educational status,** and **small family size.**

2. **Clinical manifestations**
   a. **Painless, superficial lymphadenopathy** (usually involving the cervical or supraclavicular nodes) may be noted on physical examination, or **mediastinal lymphadenopathy** may be seen on a chest radiograph.
   b. **Constitutional ("B") symptoms** (i.e., fever, night sweats, and weight loss) and **severe pruritus** (usually confined to the lower extremities) are common patient complaints.
   c. **Symptoms of spinal cord compression** or **superior vena cava syndrome.** Both of these entities are rare initial presentations of Hodgkin's lymphoma.
   d. **Immunologic dysfunction** may develop simultaneously with the onset of the lymphoma. Immunologic dysfunction is manifested as:
      (1) A loss of cell-mediated immunity (with cutaneous anergy)
      (2) A decrease in the ratio of T helper cells to T suppressor cells
      (3) Leukopenia and an increased susceptibility to infection as the disease progresses

---

HOT

KEY

Some patients with Hodgkin's disease experience pain in the lymphoid tissue following the consumption of alcohol. Some believe that the development of a headache shortly after drinking alcohol may also suggest Hodgkin's disease.

---

3. **Disease progression.** Unlike NHL, Hodgkin's disease progresses in an **orderly** fashion.
   a. Initially, the tumor spreads to the anatomically adjacent lymph tissues.
   b. Hematogenous spread to the liver, bone marrow, and other viscera occurs only in advanced disease.

C. **NHL**
   1. **Epidemiology**

      a. Incidence. The incidence of NHL is four times that of Hodgkin's disease. The HIV epidemic has lead to an increase in the incidence of NHL over the last several years.

      b. Patient profile

        (1) The **median age** at the time of diagnosis is **50 years.**

        (2) Men are affected more often than women.

        (3) Whites are affected more often than African-Americans.

        (4) NHL is more common in **immunocompromised patients** (e.g., those with AIDS, congenital immunodeficiencies, or autoimmune disease; those undergoing immunosuppressive therapy).

2. Clinical manifestations. The presentation depends on the site and subtype of tumor. Common complaints include:

    a. Asymptomatic superficial lymphadenopathy

    b. Constitutional ("B") symptoms (much less common than in Hodgkin's disease and with less prognostic significance)

    c. Abdominal complaints (e.g., fullness, discomfort)

    d. Bone pain or pathologic fractures

    e. Symptoms related to pancytopenia

    f. Acute emergencies (e.g., superior vena cava syndrome, spinal cord compression, airway compression)

3. Disease progression. Unlike Hodgkin's disease, the spread of tumor in NHL is **not contiguous.**

D. Treatment. Both types of lymphoma are treatable and frequently curable; patients should be referred to a hematologist-oncologist for therapy.

References

Smith DL: Cat-scratch disease and related clinical syndromes. *Am Fam Physician* 55(5):1783–1789, 1793–1794, 1997.

Baroni CD, Uccini S: The lymphadenopathy of HIV infection. *Am J Clin Pathol* 99(4):397–401, 1993.

Skarin AT, Dorfman DM: Non-Hodgkin's lymphomas: current classification and management. *CA Cancer J Clin* 47(6):351–372, 1997.

PART XI

Endocrinology

75. Diabetes Mellitus

I. INTRODUCTION

A. Diabetes mellitus (DM) affects approximately 5%–6% of the United States population (approximately **15 million Americans**). The disease is the leading cause of adult blindness, end-stage renal disease, and nontraumatic amputation, and it is a major risk factor for coronary artery disease (CAD) and stroke.

B. There are two forms of DM.

1. **Type I DM [insulin-dependent DM (IDDM)].** Approximately 10% of patients with DM have type I DM, which usually presents in childhood or early adulthood. The disorder is caused by autoimmune destruction of the insulin-secreting beta cells in the pancreas. Patients develop an absolute deficiency of insulin and require daily injections to prevent severe hyperglycemia and diabetic ketoacidosis.

2. **Type II DM [non-insulin-dependent DM (NIDDM)].** Most diabetic patients (90%) have this form of DM, which is more common in obese adults. Hyperglycemia in these patients is attributable to a combination of factors: impaired pancreatic insulin secretion, insulin resistance in the peripheral tissues, and increased hepatic glucose production.

II. CLINICAL MANIFESTATIONS.
Many patients are asymptomatic at the time of diagnosis, however, the following may be seen:

A. **Polyuria, polydipsia,** and **polyphagia (the 3 "P"s).** Hyperglycemia leads to glycosuria, which is responsible for this classic triad of symptoms.

B. **Weight change, fatigue, blurred vision,** and **vaginitis** or **balanitis** are also commonly reported.

C. **Diabetic ketoacidosis** (seen in patients with type I DM) or **nonketotic hyperosmolar coma** (seen in patients with type II DM). Some patients with undiagnosed DM present with these serious conditions.

III. APPROACH TO THE PATIENT (Figure 75-1)

A. **Blood glucose levels.** In patients who present with symptoms suggestive of DM, the diagnosis can be established

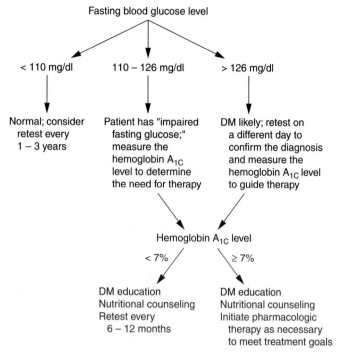

Fasting blood glucose level

< 110 mg/dl   110 – 126 mg/dl   > 126 mg/dl

Normal; consider retest every 1 – 3 years

Patient has "impaired fasting glucose;" measure the hemoglobin A_{1C} level to determine the need for therapy

DM likely; retest on a different day to confirm the diagnosis and measure the hemoglobin A_{1C} level to guide therapy

Hemoglobin A_{1C} level

< 7%   ≥ 7%

DM education
Nutritional counseling
Retest every
  6 – 12 months

DM education
Nutritional counseling
Initiate pharmacologic
  therapy as necessary
  to meet treatment goals

Figure 75-1. Approach to the patient with signs and symptoms of diabetes mellitus (*DM*).

with **laboratory testing.** Diagnosis is based on finding **persistent hyperglycemia,** a characteristic of both forms of DM. DM can be diagnosed when the patient meets either one of the following two criteria on two separate days.

1. A **random blood glucose level** greater than or equal to 200 mg/dl is consistent with DM in a patient with classic symptoms of DM.

2. A **fasting blood glucose level** (i.e., one taken 8 or more hours after eating) greater than 126 mg/dl is also consistent with DM.

HOT ▶ **KEY** Patients who do not meet the definition of DM but who have abnormal laboratory test results (i.e., a fasting blood glucose level of 110–126 mg/dl) have **"impaired fasting glucose."** These patients are at high risk for developing DM, and should be screened annually.

B. Hemoglobin A$_{1c}$ level. Although this test is not used for the diagnosis of DM, it is excellent for monitoring control of DM and response to therapy. The hemoglobin A$_{1c}$ level indicates the amount of glucose attached to hemoglobin in red blood cells (RBCs). Higher hemoglobin A$_{1c}$ levels occur with higher blood glucose levels over time; therefore, the hemoglobin A$_{1c}$ level reflects the average degree of glucose control over 2–4 months.

IV TREATMENT

A. General considerations

1. **Goal of therapy.** The goals of therapy are to **minimize symptoms** and **prevent complications.**

2. **Team approach.** DM is best managed when the patient and the doctor share the responsibility for patient care. All new patients should be enrolled in a DM education program that addresses diet, exercise, monitoring of blood glucose levels, warning signs, and the importance of establishing emergency contacts.

3. **Intensity of therapy.** In patients with type I DM who undergo intensive insulin therapy, the risk of developing complications from DM (e.g., retinopathy, nephropathy, neuropathy) is decreased by 50%–75%. However, intensive treatment is associated with an increased incidence of hypoglycemia. Therefore, the decision to initiate intensive treatment depends on the patient's risk profile and preferences.

   a. Patients who are poorly compliant, have problems with repeated episodes of hypoglycemia, or have complicating medical problems may not be appropriate candidates for intensive treatment.

   b. Table 75-1 shows target fasting blood glucose and hemoglobin A$_{1c}$ levels. The values in Table 75-1 can be used to help guide the intensity of therapy, as desired by the primary care provider and the patient.

HOT **KEY** Intensive insulin therapy should only be attempted by providers who have experience with this technique. Patients are likely to have a higher incidence of hypoglycemia and may require more training and more frequent contact and follow-up.

TABLE 75-1. Target Fasting Blood Glucose and Hemoglobin A_{1c} Levels

	Patients at Risk for Hypoglycemia*	Ideal†	Normal‡
Fasting blood glucose level (mg/dl)	80–150	80–120	60–110
Hemoglobin A_{1c} level (%)	< 8	< 7	< 6

*In patients with complicating medical problems, higher fasting blood glucose and hemoglobin A_{1c} levels may be appropriate to avoid the risk of hypoglycemia.
† In patients with diabetes mellitus (DM).
‡ In patients without DM.

B. Type II DM
1. **Weight loss** and **exercise** have been shown to reduce and even correct insulin resistance in patients with type II DM. Patients who can lose weight may be able to reduce their reliance on medications and potentially cure the disease.
2. **Oral medications**. Patients with type II DM who are unable to adequately lower their hemoglobin A_{1c} levels or who remain symptomatic despite diet and exercise should be started on oral medication.
   a. **Biguanides** are believed to decrease hepatic glucose production and increase peripheral tissue sensitivity to insulin. The only biguanide available in the United States is **metformin**.
      (1) **Dose.** The starting dose is 500 mg or 850 mg daily, taken with a meal. The dose can be increased gradually as necessary every 2 weeks (to a maximum dose of 850 mg three times daily).
      (2) **Side effects.** Lactic acidosis is the major concern. Gastrointestinal side effects (e.g., diarrhea, bleeding, nausea) are common, but usually diminish over time and are less common with gradual dose increases.
      (3) **Contraindications.** Metformin therapy should

be avoided under any of the following circumstances:

(a) Decreased renal function (i.e., a serum creatinine level greater than 1.4 in women or 1.5 in men)

(b) Acute or chronic liver disease

(c) Significant alcohol use

(d) Studies using iodinated intravenous contrast agents

(e) Acute illness, such as sepsis, myocardial infarction, congestive heart failure (CHF), shock, or hypoxia

(4) **Monitoring**. Periodic serum creatinine levels should be obtained for all patients.

b. **Sulfonylureas** (Table 75-2) act by increasing pancreatic insulin release.

(1) The first-generation agents (e.g., tolbutamide) have the shortest half-lives.

(2) The second generation agents (e.g., glyburide, glipizide) have longer half-lives, increasing the risk of hypoglycemia (especially in patients who skip meals).

HOT **KEY**

All of the sulfonylureas can cause hypoglycemia, so monitor the patient's blood glucose level daily while advancing the dose.

---

c. **Acarbose** is taken with each meal and delays the breakdown of ingested complex carbohydrates, decreasing postprandial glucose concentrations. Because it does not cause hypoglycemia, acarbose therapy combined with diet and exercise may be a reasonable first choice for patients with mild to moderate hyperglycemia.

d. **Troglitazone** acts by increasing insulin sensitivity in muscle and fat. Because of its potentially serious side effects, this agent should only be used when treatment goals cannot be reached using the other oral agents.

(1) Because troglitazone has been associated with fatal hepatitis, patients with alanine amino-

TABLE 75-2. Characteristics of Selected Sulfonylureas

Agent	Starting Dose	Maximum Dose	Half-Life (Hours)
First generation			
Tolbutamide	500 mg daily	1000 mg three times daily	6–12
Second generation			
Glipizide	2.5–5 mg daily	20 mg twice daily*	12–24
Glyburide	1.25–2.5 mg daily	20 mg daily	16–24

*Must be administered twice daily if the total dose is greater that 15 mg/day.

transferase (ALT) levels greater than 1.5 times normal are not candidates for troglitazone therapy.

   (2) Patients receiving troglitazone therapy should have their ALT levels measured monthly for 8 months, then every 2 months for the remainder of the first year of therapy, and then periodically at the discretion of the provider.

   (a) If the ALT levels are two or more times the upper limit of normal, the frequency of monitoring should be increased to every 2 weeks.

   (b) If the ALT levels exceed three times the upper limit of normal, troglitazone therapy should be terminated.

3. **Insulin therapy.** Insulin should be used cautiously in patients with type II DM because it promotes weight gain, and because hyperinsulinemia may promote CAD.

   a. **Always try diet and exercise first, then oral agents.**

   b. If the patient's DM is still not controlled, consider continuing the oral agents and adding a once-daily injection of NPH insulin at bedtime. In order to simplify therapy, some providers prefer to discontinue all oral therapy for DM and rely only on insulin. Titrate the dose to control the fasting (morning) glucose level. If more insulin is required, use the four-step approach described in IV C 3.

HOT

KEY

When patients with type II DM require insulin, they usually require much higher doses than those required by patients with type I DM.

C. **Type I DM.** These patients require **insulin therapy.**

1. **Insulin preparations** (Table 75-3). Insulin preparations vary in the time to maximum effect and duration of action; therefore, the clinical situation dictates the choice of insulin.

2. **Approximating initial insulin requirements.** There are many strategies for achieving the best blood glucose profile in patients with DM who are taking insulin. Here is one effective, simple strategy that uses only NPH and regular insulin:

TABLE 75-3. Characteristics of Commonly Used Subcutaneous Insulin Preparations

Type*	Class	Onset of Action	Time to Maximum Effect (hours)	Duration (hours)
Regular	Short-acting	15–30 minutes	3	10–12
NPH	Intermediate-acting	30–60 minutes	4–6	14–24
Lente	Intermediate-acting	30–60 minutes	10	21–26
Ultralente	Long-acting	1–3 hours	10–14	24–36

*Mixtures of NPH and regular insulin are also available in 70%/30% and 50%/50% combinations.

    a. Calculate the total daily insulin dose based on the patient's weight.

      (1) Newly diagnosed type I DM. These patients often have a "holiday" period during which only small doses of insulin are required (e.g., 0.3 units/kg/day).

      (2) Established type I DM. These patients require approximately 0.5 units/kg/day.

    b. Divide the dose (Figure 75-2). Give two thirds of the total daily dose 30 minutes before breakfast and one third 30 minutes before the evening meal.

      (1) The morning dose should be two thirds NPH insulin and one third regular insulin.

      (2) The evening dose should be one half NPH insulin and one half regular insulin.

3. Monitoring therapy. A simple way to monitor therapy is to use a step-wise approach based on the four times of the day when the blood glucose level is measured (Figure 75-3).

    a. NPH, an intermediate-acting insulin, can be thought of as the patient's basal insulin; therefore, the NPH dose should be adjusted first. In general, the **morning** and **pre-evening meal blood glucose levels** reflect the action of NPH; these levels are targeted in steps 1 and 2.

    b. Regular insulin, a short-acting insulin, is used for "fine-tuning" and targets the **pre-lunch** and **bedtime blood glucose levels** (steps 3 and 4).

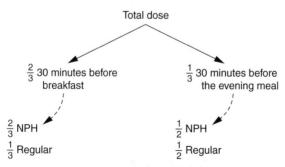

Figure 75-2. One simple strategy for using insulin therapy to achieve a normal plasma glucose profile in a patient with diabetes.

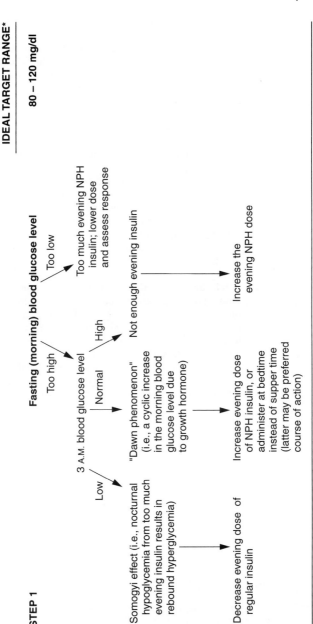

IDEAL TARGET RANGE*

80 – 120 mg/dl

STEP 1

Fasting (morning) blood glucose level

Too low → Too much evening NPH insulin; lower dose and assess response

Too high → 3 A.M. blood glucose level

High → Not enough evening insulin → Increase the evening NPH dose

Normal → "Dawn phenomenon" (i.e., a cyclic increase in the morning blood glucose level due to growth hormone) → Increase evening dose of NPH insulin, or administer at bedtime instead of supper time (latter may be preferred course of action)

Low → Somogyi effect (i.e., nocturnal hypoglycemia from too much evening insulin results in rebound hyperglycemia) → Decrease evening dose of regular insulin

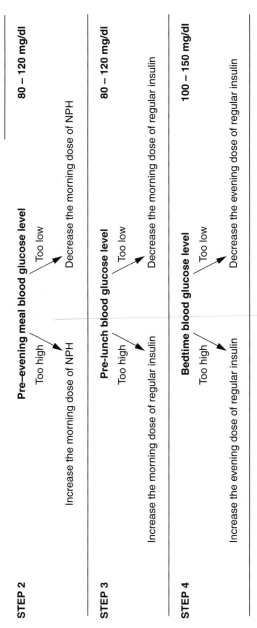

IDEAL TARGET RANGE*

STEP 2

Pre–evening meal blood glucose level 80 – 120 mg/dl

Too high → Increase the morning dose of NPH

Too low → Decrease the morning dose of NPH

STEP 3

Pre-lunch blood glucose level 80 – 120 mg/dl

Too high → Increase the morning dose of regular insulin

Too low → Decrease the morning dose of regular insulin

STEP 4

Bedtime blood glucose level 100 – 150 mg/dl

Too high → Increase the evening dose of regular insulin

Too low → Decrease the evening dose of regular insulin

* *Higher blood glucose levels may be acceptable in patients at risk for hypoglycemia.*

Figure 75-3. A step-wise approach to monitoring insulin therapy. Once the fasting (morning) blood glucose level is within the target range, move on to the pre-evening meal blood glucose level, the pre-lunch blood glucose level, and the bedtime blood glucose level. A pattern of hypoglycemia requires immediate attention.

FOLLOW-UP AND REFERRAL. Patients with DM require ongoing monitoring (Table 75-4). The frequency of visits varies, depending on the need for medication adjustments, the presence of other illnesses, and the patient's understanding of his DM. The goal at each follow-up visit is to maximize the effectiveness of treatment and prevent the progression of complications.

A. **Monitoring for complications.** The patient should be evaluated for symptoms and signs of all major long-term complications at each follow-up visit.
1. The **patient history** should be reviewed and a **physical examination** should be performed at each visit.
   a. **Neuropathy.** The skin, particularly that of the feet, should be examined for signs of neuropathy. Patients with evidence of skin breakdown or loss of sensation to light touch should be seen by a podiatrist.
   b. **Cardiovascular** and **peripheral vascular disease.** Signs and symptoms suggestive of vascular disease should be sought at each visit. Providers must try to reduce the diabetic patient's already high risk of CAD by identifying and treating other known risk factors (e.g., hypertension, hypercholesterolemia, smoking).

HOT

KEY

Because angiotensin-converting enzyme (ACE) inhibitors are known to protect against diabetic nephropathy, this class of drugs is considered the first choice for patients with DM and hypertension.

---

2. **Retinopathy.** An annual **ophthalmology examination** is necessary to monitor for retinopathy.
3. **Nephropathy.** An annual **timed overnight 10-hour urine collection** (or **spot urine,** if available) should be used to assess for microalbuminuria, an early sign of diabetic nephropathy.

HOT

 A urine dipstick for protein can be normal in patients with significant microalbuminuria.

KEY

TABLE 75-4. Areas To Address During Follow-Up Visits with Patients with Diabetes

Patient history
- ☐ Symptoms of hypo- or hyperglycemia
- ☐ Results of home monitoring
- ☐ Symptoms of complications of diabetes mellitus (e.g., visual changes, chest pain, shortness of breath, neuropathy)
- ☐ Medication history, including any adjustments in insulin therapy
- ☐ Lifestyle issues (e.g., smoking, exercise, diet, psychosocial concerns)

Physical examination
- ☐ Evaluation of vital signs (i.e., weight and blood pressure)
- ☐ Fundoscopic examination
- ☐ Cardiovascular examination
- ☐ Examination of the skin and feet

Laboratory studies
- ☐ Hemoglobin A_{1c} level (biannually)
- ☐ HDL and LDL levels (annually if normal, more often if patient is being treated for hypercholesterolemia)
- ☐ Urinalysis
- ☐ Urinary microalbumin level on a spot urine or timed overnight 10-hour urine collection (annually, unless the patient is on treatment)
- ☐ Creatinine level in patients with nephropathy (annually)
- ☐ Consider a baseline EKG

Referrals
- ☐ Ophthalmologist for an annual eye examination
- ☐ Podiatrist (as needed)

EKG = electrocardiogram; HDL = high-density lipoprotein; LDL = low-density lipoprotein.

B. **Patient education**
   1. The **importance of diet** and **exercise** should always be stressed because weight loss can improve glucose tolerance in overweight patients with DM.
   2. **Psychosocial** and **lifestyle issues** should also be addressed, especially in patients with a new diagnosis or in those who have had a deterioration in their clinical condition.

HOT

KEY

To reduce risk to the fetus, women with DM who wish to have children should consult with an endocrinologist before becoming pregnant. Contraception must therefore be discussed with all women with DM who are of reproductive age.

References

Intensive blood-glucose control with sulphonylureas or insulin compared with conventional treatment and risk of complications in patients with type 2 diabetes (UKPDS33). UK Prospective Diabetes Study (UKPDS) Group. *Lancet* 352(9131): 837–853, 1998.

The effect of intensive treatment of diabetes mellitus on the development and progression of long-term complications in insulin-dependent diabetes mellitus. The Diabetes Control and Complications Trial Research Group. *N Engl J Med* 329(14):977–986, 1993.

Lewis EJ, Hunsicker LG, Bain RP, et al: The effect of angiotensin-converting-enzyme inhibition on diabetic nephropathy. *N Engl J Med* 329(20):1456–1462, 1993.

76. Hypothyroidism

I INTRODUCTION

A. Hypothyroidism is the clinical state in which the availability of thyroid hormone is diminished.

    1. Primary hypothyroidism (99% of cases) refers to thyroid gland failure.

    2. Secondary (central) hypothyroidism (1% of cases) is caused by a disorder of the pituitary gland, hypothalamus, or hypothalamic-pituitary portal circulation.

B. Hypothyroidism is five to seven times **more common in women** than in men. The condition is seen in as many as 10% of women older than 50 years.

II CAUSES OF HYPOTHYROIDISM

are summarized in Table 76-1. **Chronic autoimmune thyroiditis (Hashimoto's disease)** is the most common cause of hypothyroidism.

HOT KEY

Hashimoto's disease is often associated with other autoimmune conditions, including primary adrenal insufficiency, type I diabetes mellitus (DM), pernicious anemia, and Sjögren's syndrome.

III CLINICAL MANIFESTATIONS OF HYPOTHYROIDISM.

The disease process, which can be nonspecific and insidious, often mimics the normal aging process. Most of the clinical manifestations of hypothyroidism result from **slowing of metabolic processes,** which is caused by thyroid hormone deficiency.

A. Symptoms include fatigue, generalized weakness, cold intolerance, hair loss, dry skin, myalgias, paresthesias, constipation, menstrual irregularities, weight gain, and cognitive decline.

TABLE 76-1. Causes of Hypothyroidism

Primary hypothyroidism
  Thyroiditis
    Chronic autoimmune thyroiditis (Hashimoto's disease)
    Subacute thyroiditis
    Postpartum thyroiditis
    External irradiation
  Iatrogenic
    Radioiodine ablation (iodine 131 treatment)
    Thyroidectomy
  Infiltrating disorders
    Infection
    Granulomatous disease
    Malignancy
  Drugs
    Antithyroid agents (e.g., methimazole, propylthiouracil)
    Lithium
    Iodide
    Amiodarone
    Cytokines
    Perchlorate
  Iodine deficiency
  Congenital disorders
    Thyroid dysgenesis
    Defects in thyroid hormone synthesis
  Idiopathic
    Thyroid gland atrophy (probably autoimmune)
Secondary hypothyroidism (central)
  TSH deficiency due to pituitary disease
    Postpartum infarction
    Tumor infiltration (e.g., pituitary macroadenoma)
    Granulomatous disease
    Infection
    Irradiation
    Idiopathic
  TRH deficiency due to hypothalamic disease
    Tumor (e.g., craniopharyngioma)
    Irradiation
    Transient occurence in nonthyroidal illness

TRH = thyroid-releasing hormone; TSH = thyroid-stimulating hormone.

HOT

KEY

Hypothyroidism leads to cold intolerance.

B. **Signs** include bradycardia, diastolic hypertension, hoarseness, doughy skin, and mucinous edema (myxedema). The relaxation phase of the skeletal muscle reflexes may be delayed.

HOT

KEY

If hypothyroidism occurs early in life, the patient may experience mental and growth retardation.

 IV **APPROACH TO THE PATIENT.** If hypothyroidism is suspected on the basis of the patient's clinical presentation, **laboratory studies should be ordered.** Typically, the biochemical profile consists of an **increased serum thyroid-stimulating hormone (TSH) level** and **decreased peripheral thyroid hormone** [i.e., **free thyroxine (FT$_4$)** and **free triiodothyronine (FT$_3$)**] **levels.**

A. A **TSH level** is the best test to obtain in the outpatient setting if primary hypothyroidism is suspected. TSH elevation is caused by the loss of negative feedback effects (as a result of low thyroid hormone levels) on pituitary thyrotrophs. A peripheral FT$_4$ level, rather than a serum TSH level, is helpful if pituitary dysfunction (i.e., secondary hypothyroidism) is suspected.

B. A **FT$_4$ level** should be obtained to confirm the diagnosis. If the peripheral FT$_4$ level is normal but the serum TSH level is elevated, then the patient has subclinical hypothyroidism.

HOT KEY

Triiodothyronine (T_3) levels are generally not used to diagnose hypothyroidism because the T_3 value may be transiently decreased by nonthyroidal illness or malnutrition and may not truly represent a hypothyroid state.

C. **Antithyroid antibody** (i.e., **antithyroid peroxidase** or **antithyroglobulin) titers** should be obtained in patients diagnosed with hypothyroidism.
1. If positive, underlying autoimmune thyroid disease is confirmed. Approximately 90% of patients with autoimmune thyroiditis have positive antithyroid antibodies on testing.
2. If negative, then the patient probably has a nonautoimmune thyroiditis and may have a transient hypothyroid state (e.g., subacute thyroiditis).

HOT KEY

The practice of screening for hypothyroidism in asymptomatic patients is controversial, but screening should be considered for women older than 60 years and for patients with hypercholesterolemia, elevated creatinine kinase levels, hyponatremia, hyperprolactinemia, or a family history of thyroid disease.

V TREATMENT

A. **Clinical hypothyroidism.** Treatment is the same for all patients, regardless of the cause of the hypothyroidism.
1. **Levothyroxine (T_4) therapy** (thyroid hormone replacement)*
   a. In **otherwise healthy young adults,** treatment can be initiated at a near-total replacement dose of **75–100 μg daily.** The usual levothyroxine requirement is 1.6 μg/kg/day, but the dose may need to be increased for patients with conditions associated with malabsorption or increased serum levels of thyroid-binding globulin (e.g., pregnancy).

---

*There is little role in the outpatient setting for therapy with mixtures of T_3 and T_4 or T_3 alone (except in preparing a patient for iodine 131 therapy in the setting of a well-differentiated thyroid carcinoma).

HOT

KEY Patients with a history of thyroid carcinoma may be given higher doses of levothyroxine in an attempt to keep the serum TSH level at a lower value. Because TSH can promote thyroid growth and possibly tumor genesis, keeping the TSH level low may decrease the patient's risk of cancer recurrence or growth.

    b. In **elderly patients** or **those with risk factors for heart disease,** it is prudent to initiate treatment at a dose of **25–50 μg daily,** unless the patient is markedly symptomatic. The dose can then be increased in 25 μg increments each month, as tolerated. This approach decreases the risk of precipitating an untoward cardiac event.

HOT

KEY Multivitamins with iron, sucralfate, cholestyramine, fiber, possibly calcium, and other similar substances can interfere with the absorption of levothyroxine. Patients should be advised to take their levothyroxine separate from other medications and preferably on an empty stomach.

  2. Monitoring
    a. Ongoing evaluation of thyroid status. Thyroid hormone requirements may decrease with aging; therefore, the patient's thyroid status should be evaluated at least annually, even when the patient has become euthyroid.
      (1) In patients with **primary hypothyroidism,** a **TSH level** can be used to follow thyroid status. The TSH level should be checked 6–8 weeks after any dosage adjustment.

HOT

KEY It takes approximately 6–8 weeks for the serum TSH level to equilibrate after an adjustment in thyroid hormone dose.

        (2) In patients with **secondary hypothyroidism,** an **FT$_4$ level** (rather than a serum TSH level) should be used to evaluate thyroid status.

    b. Monitoring for adrenal insufficiency. In some instances, initiation of thyroid hormone replacement therapy unmasks underlying adrenal insufficiency secondary to increased metabolism of cortisol. Therefore, signs and symptoms of adrenal insufficiency need to be monitored.

B. Subclinical hypothyroidism. Treatment with levothyroxine should be considered if the patient is only midly symptomatic, but has a TSH level greater than normal, or has a positive antithyroid antibody status.

VI FOLLOW-UP AND REFERRAL

A. Follow-up. Patients should see their primary care physician annually for clinical evaluation, or sooner if they experience a change in clinical status.

B. Referral to an endocrinologist is indicated in the following circumstances:

    1. Thyroid function tests continue to be abnormal, despite what appear to be appropriate changes in dose.

    2. The hypothyroidism is determined to be secondary rather than primary.

References

Lindsay RS, Toft AD: Hypothyroidism. *Lancet* 349(9049):413–4177, 1997.

Weetman AP: Hypothyroidism: screening and subclinical disease. *BMJ* 314(7088): 1175–1178, 1997.

77. Hyperthyroidism

....

▐ I ▌ INTRODUCTION

A. Hyperthyroidism is the clinical state in which the availability of thyroid hormone is increased.

    1. Excessive production of thyroid hormone by the thyroid gland is responsible for most cases of hyperthyroidism.

    2. Ectopic production of thyroid hormone accounts for the diagnosis in a minority of cases.

B. Hyperthyroidism is **more common in women.** The overall incidence of hyperthyroidism is 0.2%–0.4%.

▐ II ▌ CAUSES OF HYPERTHYROIDISM

A. Graves' disease, the most common cause of hyperthyroidism, is an autoimmune process in which an abnormal immunoglobulin (thyroid-stimulating immunoglobulin) stimulates the thyroid gland to produce excess hormone. Graves' disease is most common in women between the ages of 20 and 40 years.

B. Toxic multinodular goiter and **toxic adenoma of the thyroid** result in autonomous thyroid hormone production.

C. Iodine exposure (jodbasedow). Some patients may become overtly hyperthyroid after ingesting or being exposed to iodine (e.g., in contrast agents). The iodine serves as a fuel for thyroid hormone production.

D. Subacute thyroiditis (e.g., as a result of viral infection) and **certain drugs** (e.g., amiodarone) can lead to injury and disruption of the thyroid follicles, causing preformed thyroid hormone to be released into the circulation.

E. Factitious hyperthyroidism may be caused by inappropriate ingestion of thyroid hormone by patients. Inadvertent overdose may have the same effect.

F. Struma ovarii and **hydatiform moles** may be associated with ectopic production of thyroid hormone.

G. Pituitary adenomas can produce thyroid-stimulating hormone (TSH), leading to hyperthyroidism.

H. Pituitary resistance to thyroid hormone with peripheral tissue resistance is a rare cause of clinical hyperthyroidism.

III CLINICAL MANIFESTATIONS OF HYPERTHYROIDISM.
Most of the clinical manifestations of hyperthyroidism result
from the **acceleration of metabolic processes** that is caused
by thyroid hormone excess.

A. Symptoms. Palpitations, tremulousness, irritability or anxiety, heat intolerance, diaphoresis, hyperdefecation, menstrual irregularities, hair loss, increased appetite, and
weight loss are common.

B. Signs include tachycardia, atrial fibrillation, fine tremor,
hyperreflexia, proximal muscle weakness, thyromegaly,
moist skin, and gynecomastia. Patients with Graves' disease may have associated ophthalmopathy (i.e., propto-
sis, lid lag, and conjunctival irritation) and dermopathy
(e.g., pretibial myxedema).

HOT

Elderly patients may have very subtle or no symptoms despite overt biochemical evidence (apathetic hyperthyroidism).

KEY

 IV APPROACH TO THE PATIENT

A. Patient history. Typical symptoms are described in III A.

B. Physical examination

1. A **diffusely but symmetrically enlarged thyroid gland**
    is suggestive of Graves' disease, especially when as-
    sociated with ophthalmopathy or dermopathy.

2. An **irregularly enlarged thyroid gland** is suggestive of
    either a toxic multinodular goiter or a toxic adenoma.

3. A **tender thyroid gland** suggests thyroiditis.

C. Laboratory studies are useful for confirming a clinical diagnosis of hyperthyroidism as well as for determining the
cause.

1. **Confirming the clinical diagnosis.** Typically, the bio-
    chemical profile consists of a **decreased serum TSH
    level** and **increased peripheral thyroid hormone** [i.e.,
    free thyroxine (FT$_4$) and **free triiodothyronine (FT$_3$)**]
    levels.

    a. **Subclinical hyperthyroidism.** Patients have a de-
        creased TSH level but normal FT$_4$ and FT$_3$ levels.

HOT

KEY

Because chronic exposure to excess thyroid hormone may lead to decreased bone density and cardiac abnormalities (e.g., left ventricular hypertrophy, atrial fibrillation), most experts now agree that treating subclinical hyperthyroidism is indicated.

      b. **T$_3$ thyrotoxicosis** is characterized by a low TSH level, a normal FT$_4$ level, and an elevated FT$_3$ level.

      c. **TSH-producing pituitary adenomas** or **thyroid resistance hormone syndrome** may result in increased FT$_4$ and FT$_3$ values but normal or elevated serum TSH levels.

  2. **Determining the underlying cause**

      a. **Thyroid scan.** A radioiodine tracer (i.e., iodine 123) is administered and then the thyroid gland is imaged. The amount and distribution of radioiodine uptake usually pinpoints the cause of the hyperthyroidism (Table 77-1).

TABLE 77-1. Narrowing the Differential Using Thyroid Scan Results

Radioiodine Uptake		Likely Cause of
Amount	Distribution	Hyperthyroidism
Increased	Homogeneous	Graves' disease
Increased	Multiple focal "hot spots"	Toxic multinodular goiter
Increased	One focal "hot spot"	Toxic adenoma
Decreased ("white out")	. . .	Thyroiditis or factitious hyperthyroidism

HOT

KEY

Radioiodine thyroid scans are not useful in patients who have recently been exposed to iodine (e.g., by eating shell-fish or seaweed, having a contrast study with iodine, or us-ing povidone iodine). Thyroid ultrasound may be a useful alternative for these patients, who must wait at least 1 month before having a thyroid scan.

    b. **Antithyroid antibody titers** are positive in the majority of patients with Graves' disease.

    c. **Thyroid-stimulating immunoglobulin levels.** This test is specific for Graves' disease, but not very sensitive and usually not necessary.

    d. **Thyroglobulin levels** are decreased in patients with factitious hyperthyroidism.

    e. **Erythrocyte sedimentation rate (ESR).** The ESR is increased in patients with thyroiditis.

    f. **Alpha subunit levels** are elevated in patients with TSH-producing pituitary adenomas.

HOT

KEY

Laboratory abnormalities seen in many patients with hy-perthyroidism include hypercalcemia and elevated alkaline phosphatase (AP) levels, which are indicative of increased bone turnover.

V   **TREATMENT.** If possible, treatment should be tailored to the cause; however, it is not always possible to determine the cause promptly. Treatment should never be deferred while awaiting the results of a pending study if the patient is mod-erately or severely ill.

    A. Pharmacologic therapy

        1. **Thiourea agents** (e.g., **methimazole, propylthiouracil**) inhibit thyroid hormone synthesis. Propylthiouracil has the theoretical benefit of inhibiting peripheral conversion of T_4 to T_3 (T_3 is the more active form), while methimazole has the advantage of less frequent dosing.

            a. Indications

                (1) Graves' disease. Thiourea agents are the first choice for therapy of Graves' disease because these patients have a reasonable chance of full remission.

HOT

KEY

Patients who take thiourea agents for Graves' disease optimize their chances for full remission if they continue treatment for at least 1 year after becoming euthyroid.

  (2) Toxic multinodular goiter or **toxic adenoma.** Methimazole or propylthiouracil may be used to treat toxic multinodular goiter or toxic adenoma when radioiodine ablation is not desired by the patient.

  b. Doses. Typical starting doses are:
    (1) Propylthiouracil, 300–600 mg daily in two or three divided doses
    (2) Methimazole, 20–40 mg daily in two doses

  c. Side effects most commonly include an allergic reaction (occasionally accompanied by serum sickness) and gastrointestinal distress. Rarely, severe hepatotoxicity or idiosyncratic agranulocytosis occurs; pharmacologic therapy must be discontinued immediately in these patients.

HOT

KEY

If a patient taking a thiourea agent develops a sore throat or a fever, then blood should be drawn immediately for a complete blood count (CBC) to rule out agranulocytosis.

  2. Sodium ipodate, a potent inhibitor of peripheral T_4 conversion, is effective for treating all causes of hyperthyroidism. Sodium ipodate is usually used in combination with other agents.

  a. Because sodium ipodate acts quickly (i.e., within 1–2 days of initiating therapy), it can be used in conjunction with thiourea agents (which take longer to become effective) to treat moderate or severe hyperthyroidism.

  b. Sodium ipodate is particularly useful in the treatment of thyroiditis, because it induces symptomatic improvement while the underlying process resolves itself.

3. **β Blockers** decrease tissue response to catecholamines and, to a lesser degree, decrease peripheral conversion of T_4 to T_3. Therefore, they provide symptomatic relief and are usually used as an adjunct to other treatments.

4. **Steroids** primarily work by decreasing the immune response and, to a lesser degree, by decreasing peripheral conversion of T_4 to T_3.

    a. The use of systemic steroids should be reserved for patients with severe hyperthyroidism (e.g., thyroid storm) or ophthalmopathy. Topical steroids have a role in the local treatment of Graves' dermopathy.

    b. In general, steroid therapy should be avoided in patients with thyroiditis, because although the steroids provide initial relief, the thyroiditis often returns as soon as the steroids are tapered and many patients then require chronic high-dose treatment.

5. **Nonsteroidal anti-inflammatory drugs (NSAIDs)** are used to relieve neck discomfort in patients with thyroiditis.

B. **Radioiodine ablation (iodine 131 treatment)** takes advantage of the thyroid gland's selective uptake of iodine. One dose of iodine 131 can significantly decrease the size and function of the thyroid gland.

    1. **Indications.** Radioiodine ablation is most often used to treat toxic multinodular goiter, toxic adenoma, and Graves' disease.

    2. **Side effects.** The treatment is generally well tolerated. The most common long-term side effect is hypothyroidism.

HOT **KEY** Radioiodine ablation should be used with caution in elderly patients, who may develop a transient post-treatment thyroiditis leading to temporary thyrotoxicosis and possible cardiac complications (e.g., angina, atrial fibrillation).

C. **Surgery** is a last resort. Possible indications include:

    1. Failure of primary treatment

    2. Significant local symptoms as a result of an enlarged thyroid gland

    3. Pregnancy, when the patient's hyperthyroidism can-

not be controlled with medication (radioiodine ablation is contraindicated in pregnant women)

VI FOLLOW-UP AND REFERRAL

A. **Follow-up.** Frequent visits (i.e., every 1–2 months) are necessary during the initial treatment phase. Once the patient is euthyroid, the frequency of visits can be reduced to once every 3–4 months for 1 year after the onset of euthyroidism.

1. Periodic liver function tests are prudent to screen for hepatotoxicity in patients taking thiourea agents.

2. Periodic thyroid function tests are critical to monitor response to treatment.

   a. Because patients who have undergone radioiodine ablation are at increased risk over time for developing hypothyroidism, thyroid function should be checked at least annually in these patients.

   b. Remember that the TSH level may remain suppressed for several months after the patient becomes euthyroid; therefore, measurement of peripheral FT_4 and FT_3 levels may be more helpful.

B. **Referral**

1. Given the complexity of diagnosing and treating hyperthyroidism and the potentially rapid dynamics of the patient's clinical status, you should have a low threshold to refer the patient to an endocrinologist.

2. Patients with significant ophthalmopathy warrant referral to an ophthalmologist, and those with dermopathy warrant evaluation by a dermatologist.

3. Some patients (e.g., pregnant women, patients with very large goiters) may need to be referred to a surgeon for evaluation.

HOT **KEY** Any patient with suspected thyroid storm (characterized by fever, psychosis, nausea, vomiting, and seizures) requires inpatient intensive care and immediate consultation with an endocrinologist.

References

Cooper DS: Antithyroid drugs for the treatment of hyperthyroidism caused by Graves' disease. *Endocrin Metab Clin North Am* 27(1):225–247, 1998.

Gittoes NJ, Franklyn JA: Hyperthyroidism. Current treatment guidelines. *Drugs* 55(4):543–553, 1998.

Lazarus JH: Hyperthyroidism. *Lancet* 349(9048):339–343, 1997.

78. Solitary Thyroid Nodule

I INTRODUCTION

A. Solitary thyroid nodules are common, occurring in 4%–7% of the population of the United States. Improved imaging techniques (e.g., ultrasound) have led to an increase in the number of thyroid nodules that are discovered incidentally.

B. Women are affected four times more often than men.

II DIFFERENTIAL DIAGNOSIS. The following conditions must be ruled out:

A. Benign colloid nodule
B. Benign follicular adenoma
C. Malignancy
D. Cyst
E. Inflammatory condition
F. Developmental abnormality (i.e., thyroglossal duct)

III APPROACH TO THE PATIENT. The goals of evaluation are to determine if the nodule is malignant, assess compression of nearby structures (e.g., the trachea and esophagus), and determine the patient's thyroid functional status.

> **HOT**
>
>
>
> Most solitary thyroid nodules are benign (approximately 5% are malignant).
>
> **KEY**

A. **Patient history.** Patients are typically euthyroid and asymptomatic. Important questions to ask include:

1. Does the patient have **local symptoms** (e.g., dysphagia, difficulty breathing, chronic irritative cough, hoarseness) as a result of compression of adjacent structures?
2. Are there any **symptoms of hyper-** or **hypothyroidism?**
3. Does the patient have a **history of external radiation exposure to the neck region** (e.g., as a result of treatment for cancer, acne, or an enlarged thymus)?

4. Does the patient have a **family history of medullary thyroid carcinoma** or **multiple endocrine neoplasia, type II (MEN-II)?**

B. **Physical examination.** Palpate the neck to assess the size and firmness of the nodule, adherence to surrounding tissue, lymphadenopathy, and tracheal deviation. Be sure to note any tenderness.

HOT **KEY**   Factors that increase the chance of malignancy are age younger than 20 years or older than 60 years; history of head and neck irradiation; male gender; rapidly growing or firm nodule; hoarseness; surrounding lymphadenopathy; and a family history of medullary thyroid carcinoma or MEN-II.

HOT **KEY**   A sudden increase in size, pain, or both in a preexisting nodule is usually caused by an acute hemorrhage and is less concerning for malignancy.

C. **Laboratory studies**
1. A **thyroid-stimulating hormone (TSH) level** should be obtained to evaluate the functional status of the thyroid gland.
2. A **calcitonin level** should be considered, especially if the patient has a family history of medullary thyroid carcinoma or MEN-II.
3. A **serum thyroglobulin level** should be considered. If the nodule turns out to be a well-differentiated thyroid carcinoma, then this measurement may provide insight into the tumor's ability to make thyroglobulin.

D. **Fine needle aspiration biopsy** is the mainstay of evaluation. When performed by an experienced endocrinologist, the false-negative rate is less than 5% and the false-positive rate is approximately 1%.
1. The diagnostic accuracy, convenience, and minimal risk associated with fine needle aspiration biopsy has significantly reduced the role of radioiodine thyroid scanning in the diagnostic work-up of a solitary thyroid nodule.

    2. Four basic results can be seen. These results, which guide further work-up and treatment, are:

      a. **Benign**

      b. **Malignant or suspicious for malignancy**

      c. **Insufficient for diagnosis**

      d. **Follicular neoplasm**

E. **Imaging studies** have little use during the early stages of evaluation because they cannot rule out or confirm a diagnosis of malignancy. However, in certain situations, imaging studies may be indicated.

    1. **Ultrasound** can determine the size and consistency of the nodule. In addition, ultrasound can be used to help guide fine needle aspiration biopsy of a nodule that is difficult to palpate.

    2. **Computed tomography (CT)** and **magnetic resonance imaging (MRI)** may help determine the degree of local compression of neighboring structures.

    3. **Radioiodine thyroid scan**

      a. Radioiodine thyroid scanning is helpful when the TSH level is suppressed, because it can determine if the nodule in question is "hot," possibly obviating the need for fine needle aspiration biopsy.

        (1) "Hot" nodules, often seen in hyperthyroid patients (i.e., those with decreased TSH levels) function autonomously and suppress the uptake of iodine by the surrounding thyroid tissue on a radioiodine scan. **"Hot" nodules are rarely malignant.**

        (2) "Cold" and "warm" nodules may be malignant.

      b. Some advocate thyroid scanning when fine needle aspiration biopsy results reveal a follicular neoplasm. It is believed that if the nodule takes up iodine, then the risk of malignancy is decreased.

IV TREATMENT

A. **Approach to management.** Management primarily depends on the patient's TSH level and results on fine needle aspiration biopsy (Figure 78-1). However, if a nodule is rapidly increasing in size or causing local compressive symptoms, then surgical evaluation is warranted independent of the results of TSH evaluation and fine needle aspiration biopsy.

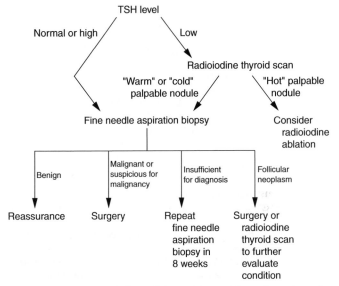

FIGURE 78-1. Approach to managing a patient with a solitary thyroid nodule. *TSH* = thyroid-stimulating hormone.

1. **TSH level**
   a. If the TSH level is **normal** or **high,** then the results of fine needle aspiration biopsy dictate the approach to management (see IV A 2).
   b. If the TSH level is **low,** then a radioiodine thyroid scan may be performed. If the nodule is "hot," then radioiodine ablation should be considered because these nodules are rarely malignant.

2. **Fine needle aspiration biopsy results**
   a. **Benign.** The patient should be reassured and advised that re-evaluation may be necessary if the nodule increases in size or if local symptoms develop.
   b. **Malignant or suspicious for malignancy.** The patient should be referred for surgery unless the diagnosis is primary lymphoma, in which case chemotherapy may be indicated. If the results are suggestive of medullary thyroid carcinoma, then the patient and other family members need to be evaluated for MEN-II.
   c. **Insufficient for diagnosis.** This finding warrants a

repeat fine needle aspiration biopsy. Because inflammatory changes from the previous biopsy can confuse results on subsequent biopsies, adequate time (e.g., 8 weeks) should be allowed between biopsies.

   d. Follicular neoplasm. Cytologic evaluation cannot determine the exact nature of this lesion. Either capsular or vascular invasion is required to diagnose malignancy. Approximately 10%–20% of follicular neoplasms are found to be malignant at surgery. Many physicians recommend surgery given this risk, although some advocate a radioiodine scan to further evaluate the patient's risk of malignancy (see III E 3 b).

B. Treatment modalities

1. **Thyroid hormone administration.** The underlying rationale is that thyroid nodules will shrink in response to doses of thyroid hormone, which suppresses TSH secretion.

   a. Recent prospective studies have demonstrated that fewer than 15% of nodules respond to this therapy. In addition, long-term risks are associated with thyroid hormone suppression (e.g., decreased bone density, tachyarrhythmias).

   b. For these reasons, the role of thyroid hormone suppression in the management of thyroid nodules is limited and should be used only in selective situations and for a limited period of time. A means of objectively documenting change in nodule size (e.g., serial ultrasounds) should be in place.

2. **Near-total thyroidectomy.** Many experts recommend near-total thyroidectomy (without fine needle aspiration biopsy) for patients with a history of neck irradiation and a solitary nodule, due to the high incidence of malignancy in this population (30%–50%).

 FOLLOW-UP AND REFERRAL. Referral to an endocrinologist or surgeon should be considered when it is necessary to perform fine needle aspiration biopsy, or when the TSH level is decreased or results of fine needle aspiration biopsy are inconclusive.

References

Boigon M, Moyer D: Solitary thyroid nodules. Separating benign from malignant conditions. *Postgrad Med* 98(2):73–74, 77–80, 1995.

Hermus AR, Huysmans DA: Treatment of benign nodular thyroid disease. *New Engl J Med* 338(20):1438–1447, 1998.

79. Calcium Disorders

I **INTRODUCTION.** At any given time, 99% of the body's calcium stores is within the skeleton. Of the remaining 1% in the circulation, 40% is bound to albumin, 10% is complexed (citrate, phosphate), and 50% is free (ionized). It is the free (ionized) component that is biologically active and thus of primary clinical importance.

A. The **serum ionized calcium level** is maintained within a relatively narrow range (1.0–1.3 mmol/L), primarily via regulation by parathyroid hormone (PTH) and vitamin D.

B. The **total serum calcium level** is normally 8.4–10.6 mg/dl. Measurements of the total serum calcium level need to be interpreted with caution because they depend on the concentration of other proteins in the serum (e.g., albumin). For every 1 mg decrease in the serum albumin level (normally 4 mg/dl), you must increase the total serum calcium level by 0.8 mg/dl. For example, if the total serum calcium level is 7.5 mg/dl and the serum albumin level is 2 mg/dl, then the corrected total serum calcium level is 9.1 mg/dl (and the patient is normocalcemic). However, this rule is an approximation and loses validity at extremes of albumin levels. Thus, the serum ionized calcium level is the preferred laboratory test for determining calcium status.

II **HYPOCALCEMIA** is a serum ionized calcium level of less than 1 mmol/L.

A. **Clinical manifestations of hypocalcemia.** The severity of signs and symptoms depends on both the degree and the acuity of the hypocalcemia. Patients with chronic hypocalcemia may be asymptomatic, whereas patients who experience a sudden decrease in calcium may have severe symptoms. Because hypocalcemia leads to enhanced excitation of the nervous system and muscle cells, the symptoms and signs primarily involve the neuromuscular and cardiovascular systems.
   1. **Symptoms**
      a. Mild symptoms include **muscle cramps** and **paresthesias of the lips and extremities.**

      b. More severe symptoms include **tetany, stridor,** (as a result of laryngospasm), **seizures,** and **altered mental status.**

  2. **Signs** may include:

      a. **Chvostek's sign** (tapping the facial nerve leads to contraction of the facial muscles)

      b. **Trousseau's sign** (occlusion of the brachial artery with a blood pressure cuff leads to carpal spasm)

      c. **Extrapyramidal signs**

      d. **Hypotension,** signs of **congestive heart failure (CHF),** or **prolongation of the QT interval** or **atrioventricular (AV) block** on an electrocardiogram (EKG)

      e. **Cataract formation** (in patients with chronic hypocalcemia)

B. **Causes of hypocalcemia**

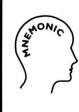

Causes of Hypocalcemia ("HIPOCAL")

Hypoparathyroidism
Infection
Pancreatitis
Overload states
Chronic renal failure
Absorption abnormalities
Loop diuretics and other drugs

  1. **Hypoparathyroidism**

      a. Causes of hypoparathyroidism include **thyroidectomy, autoimmune destruction of the thyroid, DiGeorge syndrome,** and **thyroid damage** (e.g., as a result of irradiation or surgery).

      b. Functional hypoparathyroidism (i.e., decreased secretion of PTH) may occur secondary to **magnesium deficiency.**

  2. **Infection.** As many as 20% of patients with Gram-negative sepsis are hypocalcemic due to acquired defects in the parathyroid-vitamin D axis. This hypocalcemia may cause hypotension that is responsive to calcium replacement.

  3. **Pancreatitis.** A serum calcium level of less than 8 mg/dl is one of Ranson's criteria; the calcium level correlates well with the severity of acute pancreatitis.

  4. **Overload states.** Occasionally, hypocalcemia may

be seen in cases of rapid intravascular volume expansion.

5. **Chronic renal failure.** Vitamin D is metabolized in the normal kidney to 1,25-dihydroxyvitamin D, which promotes intestinal calcium absorption. With renal failure, intestinal calcium absorption decreases and the patient becomes hypocalcemic.

6. **Absorption abnormalities.** Patients with malabsorption of calcium, magnesium, or vitamin D (from any cause) often have hypocalcemia.

7. **Loop diuretics and other drugs.** Unlike thiazide diuretics (which can cause hypercalcemia), furosemide and other loop diuretics lead to enhanced renal excretion of calcium. Other drugs (e.g., foscarnet, citrate, edathamil) or blood transfusions may also lead to hypocalcemia.

C. **Approach to the patient**
   1. Obtain a **serum ionized calcium level** to confirm the clinical diagnosis of hypocalcemia.
   2. Obtain a **concomitant serum magnesium level** to rule out hypomagnesemia, which, if corrected, may correct the hypocalcemia and prevent the need for additional work-up or intervention.
   3. Obtain the following **serum levels:**
      a. **PTH**
      b. **25-Hydroxyvitamin D** and **1,25-dihydroxyvitamin D**
      c. **Phosphate** and **chloride**
      d. **Creatinine**
      e. **Amylase** and **lipase** (if pancreatitis is suspected)
   4. Obtain an **EKG** to evaluate for QT prolongation.

HOT

KEY

Because hypocalcemia can be associated with a generalized polyglandular syndrome, consider evaluation for other endocrine deficiencies (e.g., adrenal insufficiency).

D. **Treatment**
   1. **Severe symptoms.** If the patient has tetany, arrhythmias, or seizures, immediate referral to the emergency department (ED) is indicated.
      a. **Calcium gluconate.** An initial bolus of 1–2 am-

pules (100–200 mg) should be administered intravenously, followed by infusion at a rate of 0.5–1.5 mg/kg/hr.

   b. Magnesium sulfate (2 g over 10 minutes) should be administered to most patients. If the patient is hypomagnesemic, then the magnesium deficiency must be corrected before the serum calcium level will normalize.

2. **Mild symptoms.** If the patient is relatively asymptomatic, then oral administration of elemental calcium and vitamin D is usually all that is required. In order to minimize hypercalciuria, which can lead to nephrolithiasis or nephrocalcinosis, the doses of calcium and vitamin D should be titrated to keep the serum ionized calcium level in the low-normal to mid-normal range.

   a. Elemental calcium. The dose is usually 2–4 g in two or three divided doses, each 1 day.

   b. Vitamin D. Because of its relatively short half life, greater potency, and greater availability, **calcitriol** (1,25-dihydroxyvitamin D) is used most commonly. The dose ranges from 0.25–0.5 μg, administered twice daily.

HOT

Patients with hypoparathyroidism usually require larger doses of calcium and vitamin D.

KEY

E. Follow-up and referral
   1. **Follow-up**
      a. The **serum ionized calcium level** should be measured **every 6 months** once levels have been established in the normal range.
      b. Consider obtaining a **24-hour urine collection annually** to ensure that the patient is not developing hypercalciuria (defined as > 400 mg calcium/24 hours).
   2. **Referral** to an endocrinologist should be made when patients have fluctuating serum calcium levels, inordinate calcium or vitamin D requirements, or concomitant endocrine dysfunction.

HYPERCALCEMIA is a serum ionized calcium level of more than 1.30 mmol/L.

A. Clinical manifestations of hypercalcemia. As with hypocalcemia, both the degree and acuity of the hypercalcemia influence the severity of the patient's signs and symptoms.

 1. **Symptoms** are usually nonspecific and tend to occur when the serum calcium level exceeds 12 mg/dl. "**Abdominal MOAN, psychiatric GROAN, kidney STONE,** and **urination ZONE** (i.e., the bathroom)" is an easy way to remember the common symptoms of hypercalcemia.

  a. **Gastrointestinal** symptoms include constipation, nausea, vomiting, and anorexia.

  b. **Central nervous system (CNS)** symptoms include confusion, depression, lethargy, and weakness. Symptoms can progress to coma and death.

  c. **Renal** complications include nephrolithiasis, polyuria and polydipsia as a result of decreased concentrating ability of the kidney, and renal failure.

 2. **Signs** of hypercalcemia include hypertension, hypotonia, decreased deep tendon reflexes, and a shortened QT interval on the EKG.

B. Causes of hypercalcemia. In 80%–90% of cases, hypercalcemia is caused either by malignancy or hyperparathyroidism. In the hospital setting, malignancy is the more common cause, while in the ambulatory setting, hyperparathyroidism predominates.

Causes of Hypercalcemia ("My Favorite MISHAP")

Medications (e.g., lithium, thiazide diuretics)
Familial hypocalciuric hypercalcemia (FHH)

Malignancy
Intoxication (vitamin D or A overdose) or **I**mmobilization
Sarcoidosis (and other granulomatous diseases)
Hyperparathyroidism or **H**yperthyroidism
Addison's disease or milk-**A**lkali syndrome
Paget's disease or **P**heochromocytoma

1. **Medications**
   a. **Lithium.** Chronic exposure to lithium can alter the set point for PTH secretion, resulting in a hyperparathyroid state.
   b. **Thiazide diuretics** result in increased renal reabsorption of calcium.
2. **FHH** is a benign autosomal dominant disorder characterized by hypercalcemia, hypocalciuria, and occasional hypermagnesemia. A defect in the calcium sensors in the kidneys and the parathyroid glands results in altered set points for renal calcium reabsorption and PTH secretion, respectively.
3. **Malignancy.** Several mechanisms can be responsible for the hypercalcemia of malignancy.
   a. Some tumors (e.g., breast, lung, renal cell) produce PTH-related peptide. (This is the most common underlying mechanism).
   b. Other malignancies (e.g., multiple myeloma, possibly some lymphomas) produce osteoclast-activating factors, which stimulate osteoclastic bone resorption.
   c. Hypercalcemia can result from local osteolysis (seen with extensive bone involvement).
4. **Intoxication.** Some patients take large amounts of vitamin D for unclear reasons. Vitamin A intoxication can also occur, but is much less common than vitamin D intoxication.
5. **Immobilization** is a diagnosis of exclusion. Hypercalcemia (as a result of increased bone resorption) may be seen in patients who have been immobilized for a significant amount of time.
6. **Sarcoidosis** and **other granulomatous diseases** (e.g., tuberculosis, berylliosis, lymphoma). Hypercalcemia results from increased conversion of 25-hydroxyvitamin D to 1,25-hydroxyvitamin D within macrophages.
7. **Hyperparathyroidism**
   a. Primary hyperparathyroidism caused by a solitary adenoma accounts for more than 80% of cases of hyperparathyroidism.
   b. Four-gland hyperplasia (10% of cases), multiple adenomas (fewer than 5% of cases), carcinoma (fewer than 5% of cases), and multiple endocrine neoplasia, type I or type II (MEN-I, MEN-II) can also cause hyperparathyroidism.
8. **Hyperthyroidism.** Hypercalcemia occurs in 15%–20%

of hyperthyroid patients and is most likely related to increased osteoclastic bone resorption.

9. **Addison's disease.** The mechanism by which adrenal insufficiency induces hypercalcemia is unclear and may be multifactorial. One contributing aspect may be significant volume depletion and resultant hemoconcentration.

10. **Milk-alkali syndrome.** Hypercalcemia occurs secondary to excess calcium carbonate ingestion (often seen in patients with peptic ulcer disease or chronic renal insufficiency who are treated with oral calcium).

11. **Paget's disease,** a nonmetabolic bone disease of unknown cause, is characterized by excessive bone destruction and unorganized repair, which leads to skeletal deformities (e.g., kyphosis, bowing of the tibias, enlargement of the skull with occasional deafness). Hypercalcemia usually occurs in the setting of prolonged immobilization.

12. **Pheochromocytoma.** In some cases, parathyroid hormone-related peptide (PTHrP) may be released, but the mechanism of hypercalcemia is not entirely clear.

C. **Approach to the patient.** As with hypocalcemia, a **serum ionized calcium level** should be obtained to confirm the clinical diagnosis. Once it is determined that hypercalcemia is present, an effort should be made to determine its cause.

1. **Patient history.** Causes such as calcium, vitamin D, or vitamin A ingestion and thiazide diuretic use can usually be ruled out on the basis of the history.

2. **Laboratory studies** may be helpful.

a. Obtain the **serum PTH, alkaline phosphatase (AP), phosphate,** and **chloride levels** to evaluate for **hyperparathyroidism,** which is characterized by elevated serum PTH, chloride, and AP levels and a low phosphate level.

HOT KEY The serum PTH level is often slightly increased in patients with FHH, which can lead to a mistaken diagnosis of hyperparathyroidism. A "normal" PTH level in the setting of hypercalcemia is inappropriate and either represents hyperparathyroidism or FHH.

HOT

KEY

The serum AP level is usually elevated in patients with Paget's disease.

    b. A **24-hour urine collection** to evaluate calcium and creatinine clearance is helpful because if calcium excretion is low ($<$ 50 mg/24 hours), then FHH is a strong possibility. The creatinine clearance also helps determine if there is any renal impairment.

    c. **Serum PTHrP level.** If the serum PTHrP level is elevated, then a thorough work-up to locate an occult malignancy must be undertaken.

    d. **Serum vitamin D level**

        (1) The **25-hydroxyvitamin D level** screens for increased vitamin D intake and rare hematologic malignancies.

        (2) The **1,25 hydroxyvitamin D level** screens for granulomatous processes.

    e. **Thyroid function tests** should be performed to rule out hyperthyroidism.

    f. **Serum protein electrophoresis** is indicated to evaluate for multiple myeloma.

    g. A **morning serum cortisol level** or an **adrenocorticotropic hormone (ACTH) stimulation test** should be performed to rule out adrenal insufficiency if clinical suspicion warrants.

D. **Treatment** focuses on lowering the serum calcium level and treating the underlying cause of hypercalcemia.

    1. **Acute therapy.** Patients with altered mental status, a serum calcium level greater than 13 mg/dl, or unstable medical problems (e.g., acute pancreatitis) must be hospitalized for aggressive treatment of hypercalcemia.

        a. **Hydration with normal saline** (1–2 L initially, followed by infusion at a rate of 250 ml/hour as tolerated by the patient's volume status) usually initiates calciuresis.

        b. **Loop diuretics** (e.g., furosemide, 20–40 mg every 2 hours) should be given once the patient is euvolemic. If these agents are given while the patient is hypovolemic, they may exacerbate the hypercalcemia.

    c. Bisphosphonates also decrease the serum calcium level, independent of the cause of the hypercalcemia. **Pamidronate** given as a constant infusion of 60–90 mg over 24 hours (or 2–4 hours, if the patient is an outpatient) is effective.

        (1) Pamidronate's onset of action is at least 24–48 hours after administration, so repeat doses should not be prematurely administered.

        (2) The effects of pamidronate may last several weeks.

    d. Calcitonin (4 IU/kg administered intramuscularly or subcutaneously) also may be used to decrease the serum calcium level to a modest degree.

        (1) Due to tachyphylaxis, the effects are usually not long lasting.

        (2) Calcitonin can be effective for relieving acute pain associated with osteoporotic compression fractures (seen in patients with hyperparathyroidism).

    e. Steroids, which inhibit conversion of 25-hydroxyvitamin D to 1,25 hydroxyvitamin D, may be especially useful in treating hypercalcemia associated with granulomatous diseases.

    f. Oral phosphates (250–500 mg four times daily) decrease calcium levels through binding. Their role is limited by the possibility of soft tissue deposits and diarrhea.

    g. Other measures. In patients with resistant hypercalcemia, agents such as **gallium** and **mithramycin** can be considered, but these drugs are very toxic. As a last resort, either **peritoneal dialysis** or **hemodialysis** can be performed.

  2. Definitive therapy. When the calcium is lowered to a reasonable level and the patient's symptoms have improved, treatment should focus on the underlying cause.

HOT

KEY

Patients with FHH are treated conservatively (i.e., by ensuring adequate oral hydration and avoiding excessive calcium, excessive vitamin D, and thiazide diuretics).

E. Follow-up and referral

   1. Follow-up depends on the underlying cause. For example, in cases of treated malignancies or parathyroid hyperplasia, periodic measurements of serum calcium are useful because hypercalcemia may herald recurrence of disease.

   2. Referral should be sought in the following circumstances:

      a. When acute hypercalcemia is refractory to conventional treatment

      b. When the underlying cause is best treated by a specialist

      c. When it is unclear whether surgery is the appropriate therapy for hyperparathyroidism

      d. When MEN-I or MEN-II is suspected

References

Barri YM, Knochel JP: Hypercalcemia and electrolyte disturbances in malignancy. *Hematol Onc Clin North Am* 10(4):775–790, 1996.

Bushinsky DA, Monk RD: Calcium. *Lancet* 352(9124):306–311, 1998.

Reber PM, Heath H 3rd: Hypocalcemic emergencies. *Med Clin North Am* 79(1):93–106, 1995.

Rude RK: Hypocalcemia and hypoparathyroidism. *Curr Ther Endocrinol Metab* 6:546–551, 1997.

80. Osteoporosis

I INTRODUCTION

A. Definition. In osteoporosis, bone reabsorption exceeds bone formation, resulting in a low bone mass and an increased propensity for fractures. The World Health Organization (WHO) has developed a classification scheme showing the correlation between bone mass and bone mineral density (BMD) [Table 80-1].

B. Epidemiology

1. It is estimated that more than one half of all women and approximately one third of all men will experience at least one osteoporotic fracture at some point during their lifetimes.

2. In women, the mortality rate associated with osteoporotic fractures is greater then the mortality rates associated with breast and ovarian cancer combined; more than 20% of women with osteoporosis who experience a hip fracture die within 1 year.

C. Risk factors. As we age, osteoblast activity tends to diminish in respect to osteoclast activity, resulting in a net loss of bone mass; therefore, **aging** is the primary risk factor for the development of osteoporosis. Other risk factors are summarized in Table 80-2.

HOT

Osteoporosis and its complications can be prevented.

KEY

II APPROACH TO THE PATIENT

A. Screening

1. **Bone densitometry.** Osteoporotic fracture risk is directly correlated with bone mass, as measured using bone densitometry (Table 80-3).

   a. Method. Bone densitometry is a noninvasive method of measuring bone mass that has been shown to be accurate, safe, and predictive of fracture risk. The most common and accurate method

TABLE 80-1. Correlation Between Bone Mass and Bone Mineral Density (BMD)

Classification	BMD*
Normal	< 1
Osteopenia	1–2.5
Osteoporosis	> 2.5
Severe osteoporosis	> 2.5 + one or more fractures related to osteoporosis

*Standard deviations below the young adult mean.

TABLE 80-2. Risk Factors for the Development of Osteoporosis

Unmodifiable risk factors
  Age
  White race
  First-degree relative with a nontramatic fracture
Modifiable risk factors
  Immobility
  Low calcium or vitamin D intake
  Alcohol use
  Tobacco use
  Caffeine use
  Certain therapeutic drug use (e.g., corticosteroids, heparin, anticonvulsant agents, aluminum-containing antacids)
  Hypogonadal states (most commonly seen in postmenopausal women)
  Comordid conditions (e.g., chronic renal failure, cirrhosis, Cushing's disease, hyperthyroidism, hyperarathyrodism, and Paget's disease)

in widespread use is **dual-energy x-ray absorptiometry (DEXA).**

   b. Indications. High-risk patients should be screened using bone densitometry. Examples of high-risk patients include:

   (1) Women who experience early menopause (i.e.,

TABLE 80.3. Correlation of Bone Mineral Density (BMD) and Ostereoporotic Fracture Risk	
BMD (g/cm^2)*	Fracture Risk (within 4 years)
< 0.6	90%
0.6–0.8	20%
> 0.8	5%

*As measured using bone densitometry.

before the age of 45 years) or who have undergone bilateral oophorectomy prior to a normal menopause

(2) Premenopausal women with amenorrhea or oligomenorrhea

(3) Women who did not receive hormone replacement therapy (HRT) for at least 5 years after menopause

(4) Patients currently undergoing or about to undergo glucocorticosteroid therapy for longer than 3 months

(5) Patients with primary hyperparathyroidism or hyperthyroidism

(6) Patients with a strong family history of osteoporosis

(7) Men with hypogonadism

(8) Patients with vertebral fractures or radiologic evidence of osteopenia

(9) Women considering HRT, when information about bone density is considered essential to decision making

2. **Laboratory studies.** Currently, there are no generally accepted biochemical markers predictive for osteoporosis.

B. **Assessment of patients with suspected osteoporosis**

1. **Laboratory studies** can help rule out secondary causes of osteoporosis (see Table 80-2).

a. **General studies.** The following studies may be ordered for patients when concern for osteoporosis exists:

(1) **Complete blood count (CBC)**

(2) **Creatinine level**
(3) **Alkaline phosphatase (AP) level**
(4) **Calcium and phosphate levels**
(5) **Thyroid-stimulating hormone (TSH) level**
  b. **Specific studies.** When clinical suspicion warrants, a **serum protein electrophoresis** (to evaluate for multiple myeloma) and either a **24-hour urine cortisol test** or **dexamethasone suppression test** (to evaluate for glucocorticoid excess) should be ordered.
2. **Plain film radiography** can be essential for the proper diagnosis of fractures and should be obtained whenever clinical suspicion warrants (e.g., after a fall).

III TREATMENT AND PREVENTION

A. **Lifestyle modifications.** Patients with osteoporosis must take measures to **minimize** their **risk of falling** (e.g., by improving home lighting, wearing proper footwear, and removing hazards such as throw rugs from their homes).
B. **Nutritional therapy**
  1. **Calcium** is an essential component of bone; adequate calcium intake should be ensured throughout life.
    a. Men and premenopausal women require at least 1000 mg/day of calcium.
    b. Postmenopausal women need at least 1500 mg/day of calcium.
  2. **Vitamin D** increases calcium absorption in the gastrointestinal tract; deficiency may lead to secondary hyperparathyroidism, which in turn can cause osteoporosis. Vitamin D deficiency can be a problem among elderly patients because many of these patients have limited sun exposure.
    a. All adults older than 50 years require 200–400 IU/day of vitamin D.
    b. Patients older than 65 years or with documented osteoporosis require 400–800 IU/day of vitamin D.
C. **Pharmacologic therapy**
  1. **Estrogen** markedly slows the progression of age-

HOT

A tablet containing both vitamin D and calcium is available and may improve patient compliance.

KEY

related bone loss and is the **mainstay of osteoporosis prevention** and **treatment in postmenopausal women.** HRT should be discussed with all women at the time of menopause (Figure 80-1).

  a. Contraindications

    (1) Absolute contraindications include breast cancer, unexplained vaginal bleeding, active liver disease, and active vascular thrombosis.

    (2) Relative contraindications include migraines, familial hypertriglyceridemia, fibroids, endometriosis, uterine cancer, gallbladder disease, chronic hepatic disease, a strong family history of breast cancer, or a history of thromboembolism.

  b. Dosages

    (1) The minimum daily dose of estrogen that has been shown to be effective in preventing osteoporosis can be obtained in the following ways:

      (a) Estrogen (equine or **estrone sulfate),** 0.625 mg/day

      (b) Oral estradiol, 1–2 mg/day

      (c) Transdermal estradiol, 50–100 μg/day

    (2) In women who have not had a hysterectomy, progesterone should be given with the estrogen to prevent endometrial hyperplasia and carcinoma. Common combinations include:

      (a) Daily estrogen plus progestin (5–10 mg/day) on days 1 through 10 or 14 of each calendar month

      (b) Daily estrogen plus continuous daily progestin (i.e., 2.5 mg progestin combined with 0.625 mg estrogen)

      (c) Cyclic estrogen and progestin with a pill-free interval (i.e., estrogen, 0.625 mg/day on days 1–25 and progestin, 10 mg/day on days 14–25)

HOT **KEY**   Cyclic progestin therapy may be associated with monthly withdrawal bleeding. Daily progestin therapy is usually not associated with withdrawal bleeding and therefore may be associated with a higher patient compliance rate.

---

  2. Bisphosphonates act by binding to mineralized bone surfaces, thus inhibiting osteoclastic activity.

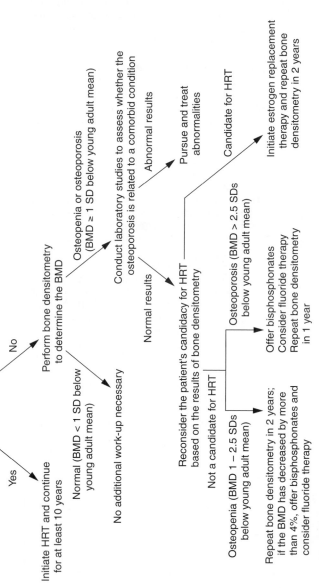

FIGURE 80-1. Hormone replacement therapy (*HRT*) should be discussed with all women at the time of menopause. If the patient is an eligible candidate for HRT and agrees to continue therapy for at least 10 years, then no additional work-up for osteoporosis is necessary, because the patient is already receiving the definitive therapy. If the patient has any relative contraindications to estrogen replacement therapy, then bone densitometry can be used to weigh the risks against the possible benefits. *BMD* = bone mineral density; *SD* = standard deviation.

a. **Indications.** The role of the bisphosphonates in the treatment of osteoporosis is not yet clearly defined, but these drugs have been shown to increase bone mass and prevent fractures (especially in patients who are not taking estrogen). The best application for bisphosphonates may be for patients who are unable or unwilling to take HRT and yet have either low bone mass or risk factors for the development of osteoporosis.

b. **Administration.** The recommended duration of therapy with any of the bisphosphonates is 3–7 years. Bone densitometry should be performed every 2–3 years to assess efficacy.

   (1) **Etidronate** (400 mg/day for 14 days every 3 months) must be used cyclically.

   (2) **Alendronate** (10 mg, taken with a full glass of water at least 30 minutes before breakfast) can be taken daily.

3. **Calcitonin.** In limited studies, calcitonin has been shown to prevent bone loss (but not fractures) in patients with osteoporosis.

   a. **Indications**

      (1) Calcitonin is currently considered primarily for patients who cannot tolerate estrogen or bisphosphonates, or who prove refractory to their effects.

      (2) Calcitonin (50–100 IU/day) has been shown to be effective in treating pain secondary to osteoporotic fractures.

   b. **Administration.** Calcitonin is available as a nasal preparation as well as an injectable.

4. **Fluoride** has been shown to increase bone mass and reduce fractures when given in a cyclic fashion.

   a. **Indications.** Fluoride should be considered for osteoporotic patients who cannot or will not take estrogen, alendronate, or calcitonin, or who have suffered a fracture despite use of other medications.

   b. **Administration.** Slow-release fluoride (25 mg, twice daily) is given for 12 months, followed by a 2-month pill-free interval.

References

Clinical Practice Guidelines for the Diagnosis and Management of Osteoporosis. Scientific Advisory Board, Osteoporosis Association of Canada. *CMAJ* 155(8): 1113–1129, 1996.

Deal CL: Osteoporosis: prevention, diagnosis, and management. *Am J Med* 102(1A): 35S–39S, 1997.

PART XII

Infectious Diseases

81. Sexually Transmitted Diseases

I **INTRODUCTION.** More than 12 million cases of sexually transmitted diseases (STDs) are reported in the United States each year. Many STDs can lead to chronic debilitating conditions, or even death.

HOT KEY

All STDs are preventable. Patients should be counseled about the risk of acquiring HIV and other STDs, and safe sex practices should be emphasized. HIV and syphilis testing should be offered to all patients, and an attempt should be made to identify and treat sex partners of patients with STDs.

II **DIFFERENTIAL DIAGNOSIS.** Most STDs belong to one of the nine categories listed in Table 81-1.

III **GENITAL ULCER DISEASE.** In the United States, genital ulcers are most often caused by genital herpes, chancroid, or syphilis. Clinical examination is usually not enough to differentiate one entity from another; therefore all patients with ulcers should be evaluated using the approach shown in Figure 81-1.

HOT KEY

All patients with a genital ulcer should have a serologic test for syphilis.

A. **Genital herpes** is caused by **herpes simplex virus (HSV).**
1. **Clinical manifestations**
   a. **Initial episode.** After an incubation period of 3–20 days, small vesicles appear and then rupture, forming ulcers. **Ulcers** may be the presenting lesion. **Fever, myalgia,** and **malaise** may accompany the first episode, which can be severe and usually lasts about 12 days.

TABLE 81-1. Differential Diagnosis of Sexually Transmitted Diseases (STDs)

Genital ulcer disease
Genital warts
Urethritis
Cervicitis
Pelvic inflammatory disease (PID)
Vaginal infections
Epididymitis
Hepatitis
HIV

---

    b. Recurrent episodes. Most patients experience recurrent outbreaks after primary infection takes place; the frequency and severity of these outbreaks varies widely. Most recurrences last 5–10 days and decrease in severity over time.

HOT

KEY

Asymptomatic shedding of the virus can occur between outbreaks; therefore, transmission of the disease is possible even in the absence of visible ulcers or vesicles.

---

  2. Approach to the patient. The diagnosis can be established via culture or antigen testing of a swab from the ulcer.

  3. Treatment is with **acyclovir, valacyclovir,** or **famciclovir.**

    a. Primary episode. Acyclovir (400 mg orally three times daily for 10 days or 200 mg orally five times daily for 10 days) shortens the healing time by as many as 5 days, but has no effect on the frequency or severity of recurrences. Valacyclovir (1000 mg orally twice daily for 10 days) or famciclovir (250 mg three times daily for 10 days) may also be used.

    b. Recurrent episodes

      (1) Acute treatment. Acyclovir (in the same dose

Examine the patient
Send VDRL or RPR test in all cases
Discuss safe sex practice and offer HIV testing

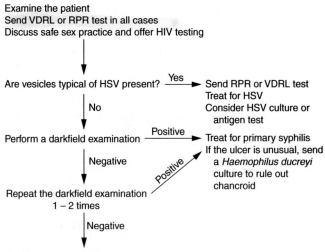

Are vesicles typical of HSV present? —Yes→ Send RPR or VDRL test
Treat for HSV
Consider HSV culture or
antigen test

No

Perform a darkfield examination —Positive→ Treat for primary syphilis
If the ulcer is unusual, send
a *Haemophilus ducreyi*
culture to rule out
chancroid

Negative

Positive

Repeat the darkfield examination
1 – 2 times

Negative

Send a:
- Culture for *Haemophilus ducreyi* to rule out chancroid
- Culture or antigen test for HSV
- Direct fluorescent antibody test for *Treponema pallidum*
- RPR or VDRL test

Treat for the most likely diagnosis*
Arrange a follow-up visit to review test results in 1 week

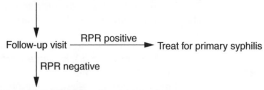

Follow-up visit —RPR positive→ Treat for primary syphilis

RPR negative

Treat for chancroid or HSV (based on test results)
Repeat RPR or VDRL at this visit if the ulcer is still present
Repeat RPR or VDRL again in 6 weeks regardless

* If the patient is pregnant or unlikely to return for follow-up, or if the testing
capability is not great, treat for syphilis. Consider treating for chancroid as
well if there is a high prevalence of chancroid in the community.

FIGURE 81-1. Approach to the patient with a genital ulcer. *HSV* =
herpes simplex virus; *RPR* = rapid plasma reagin.

as for treatment of a primary episode, for 5 days), valacyclovir (500 mg orally twice daily for 5 days), or famciclovir (125 mg orally twice daily for 5 days) may decrease the length of the outbreak by 1–2 days, if initiated during the prodrome or first 2 days of the episode.

(2) **Suppressive therapy** is appropriate if the patient is experiencing frequent (more than 6 per year) or severe outbreaks, or if the outbreaks cause significant emotional distress.

(a) Acyclovir (400 mg orally twice daily) can decrease the rate of recurrence by more than 75%.

(b) Valacyclovir (500–1000 mg orally once daily) or famciclovir (250 mg orally twice daily) may also be effective.

4. **Follow-up and referral**

   a. The patient should be seen 1 week after the initial visit to ensure that proper healing is taking place, and then every 6–12 months thereafter to monitor long-term therapy and to educate the patient about the natural history of HSV infection.

   b. Patients should be counseled to abstain from sex during outbreaks and to use condoms at all times because transmission is possible even when active lesions are not present.

B. **Chancroid** is caused by *Haemophilus ducreyi.*

   1. **Clinical manifestations.** *H. ducreyi* has a short incubation period (i.e., 4–7 days).

      a. Patients usually present with at least one **painful, nonindurated ulcer with irregular borders;** multiple ulcers are common.

      b. **Buboes** (i.e., tender inguinal lymph nodes that may rupture) are seen in approximately 50% of patients.

   2. **Approach to the patient.** Diagnosis is difficult. Culturing requires selective media and temperature control and has a sensitivity of only 80%. A probable diagnosis can be made if:

      a. The lesions do not have the typical appearance of genital herpes and testing for HSV is negative, **and**

      b. There is no evidence of syphilis on darkfield examination or the syphilis serology is negative at 1 and 6 weeks

3. **Treatment.** Large or fluctuant buboes should be incised and drained to promote better healing, and antibiotic therapy with any one of the following regimens should be initiated:

   a. **Ceftriaxone,** 250 mg intramuscularly, administered once

   b. **Azithromycin,** 1 g orally, administered once

   c. **Erythromycin,** 500 mg orally four times daily for 7 days

   d. **Ciprofloxacin,** 500 mg orally twice daily for 7 days

4. **Follow-up and referral**

   a. The patient should be seen within 3–7 days to ensure that the ulcers are healing and the adenopathy is improving.

   b. All sexual contacts within the past 10 days should be treated.

C. **Syphilis** is caused by ***Treponema pallidum.***

1. **Clinical manifestations.** Untreated syphilis may progress through five stages (Figure 81-2).

   a. **Primary syphilis.** Approximately 50% of patients develop a **solitary, painless ulcer with a clean, indurated base** within 3–4 weeks of contracting the disease. The ulcer may be genital, perianal, or oral.

   b. **Secondary syphilis** develops 4–10 weeks after exposure in all untreated patients. Secondary syphilis is often characterized by a **diffuse maculopapular skin rash** (which also involves the palms and soles), **fever, lymphadenopathy,** and **condylomata lata** (i.e., papular lesions in the in-

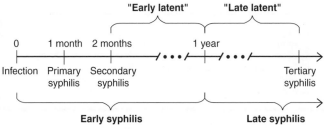

FIGURE 81-2. Natural history of syphilis. The first year of untreated infection is called early (infectious) syphilis and includes primary, secondary, and early latent syphilis. After the first year, untreated patients have late syphilis, which may be latent or have tertiary manifestations.

tertriginous areas that produce a greyish exudate). Some patients with secondary syphilis develop **early neurosyphilis,** which presents as a basilar meningitis.

  c. Early latent phase. This is the term used to describe the remainder of the first year of untreated infection, after all of the manifestations of secondary syphilis have resolved. Approximately 25% of these patients will have a relapse with symptoms of secondary syphilis.

  d. Late latent phase. This is the asymptomatic stage that follows the first year of infection and precedes the development of tertiary syphilis. This phase may last for months or for the rest of the patient's life.

  e. Tertiary syphilis develops in approximately one third of untreated patients and is characterized by a variety of disorders:

    (1) Gummas are benign infiltrative tumors.

    (2) Ophthalmologic problems may include iritis, chorioretinitis, and optic atrophy.

    (3) Cardiovascular complications include aortitis, aortic regurgitation, or aneurysms.

    (4) Neurologic disorders. Patients may be asymptomatic, exhibiting only a positive cerebrospinal fluid (CSF) serology, or they may present with severe signs, including those of meningitis, meningovascular syphilis, dementia, psychosis, generalized paresis, or tabes dorsalis (a syndrome characterized by impaired proprioception and deep tendon reflexes, and Argyll Robertson pupils).

HOT

Although neurosyphilis is usually a form of tertiary syphilis, it can occur during early syphilis.

KEY

---

  2. Approach to the patient
    a. Serologic tests
      (1) Nontreponemal antibody tests include the **Venereal Disease Research Laboratory**

         (VDRL) test and the **rapid plasma reagin (RPR) test.**

         (a) These tests measure antibodies to lipoidal antigens, which increase with treponemal activity but may also increase in other diseases (e.g., connective tissue disorders, chronic infections).

         (b) Both tests are usually positive 1–3 weeks after the appearance of an ulcer (i.e., 4–6 weeks after infection occurs).

      (2) Treponemal antibody tests, such as the **fluorescent treponemal antibody, absorbed (FTA-ABS) test,** measure antibodies to *T. pallidum* antigens. These tests, which are more specific than the nontreponemal antibody tests, are usually used as confirmatory tests. Treponemal antibody tests are usually positive in all stages of syphilis.

  b. Evaluation at various stages

    (1) Primary syphilis

      (a) Darkfield examination or **direct fluorescent antibody tests** of the ulcer exudate may establish the diagnosis.

      (b) Serologic tests become positive 4–6 weeks after infection and are therefore not yet positive in 30%–40% of patients with primary syphilis.

    (2) Secondary syphilis. The diagnosis can be established on the basis of clinical examination and positive serologic tests.

    (3) Latent syphilis is usually only identified by a positive blood test. All patients with latent disease of unknown duration should be considered to have late latent syphilis and treated accordingly. The difficulty is determining if the patient with latent syphilis has neurologic involvement and requires more intensive treatment. **Lumbar puncture** and **CSF analysis** should be performed in patients who meet any of the criteria in Table 81-2.

    (4) Tertiary syphilis

      (a) Neurosyphilis. The diagnosis can be made by a positive CSF VDRL test result. A negative result does not rule out the diagnosis; a high CSF protein level or CSF lymphocytosis should raise suspi-

TABLE 81-2. Indications for Lumbar Puncture and Cerebrospinal Fluid (CSF) Analysis in Patients with Syphilis

Neurologic or opthalmologic signs or symptoms
Other signs or symptoms of tertiary syphilis (e.g., gummas, aortitis)
Failure of treatment for early syphilis
VDRL or RPR titer greater than or equal to 1:32 (unless infection is known to be of less than 1 year's duration)
HIV-positive status
Planned nonpenicillin therapy

RPR = rapid plasma reagin; VDRL = Veneral Disease Research Laboratory.

cion of neurosyphilis even if the CSF VDRL test is negative.
   (b) **Non-neurologic tertiary syphilis.** The diagnosis is established on the basis of the clinical examination.
3. **Treatment**
   a. **Primary, secondary,** or **early latent phase**
      (1) **Penicillin G benzathine,** 2.4 million units administered intramuscularly once, is the treatment of choice.
      (2) **Doxycycline** (100 mg orally twice daily for 14 days) may be used for patients who are allergic to penicillin.
   b. **Late latent phase**
      (1) **Penicillin G benzathine,** 2.4 million units by intramuscular injection weekly for 3 weeks is the treatment of choice.
      (2) **Doxycycline** (100 mg orally twice daily for 4 weeks) may be used for patients who are allergic to penicillin.
   c. **Tertiary syphilis.** In patients with tertiary syphilis but no neurologic or ophthalmologic manifestations, the treatment is the same as for late latent disease.
   d. **Neurosyphilis, syphilitic eye disease, syphilis in a pregnant patient,** or **syphilis in an HIV-infected patient** should be treated in consultation with an infectious disease specialist.
4. **Follow-up and referral**

    a. Follow-up serologic testing is mandatory. All patients should have VDRL or RPR testing 6, 12, and 24 months after treatment. If titers fail to fall four-fold after 12–24 months, or if they increase four-fold at any time, patients should be tested for HIV and have a lumbar puncture before another round of therapy is initiated (unless new reinfection is certain).

    b. Treatment of partners

        (1) A sex partner of a patient with syphilis in the primary, secondary, or early latent phase who was exposed within 90 days of the diagnosed partner's presentation for evaluation should be treated presumptively for primary syphilis.

        (2) An asymptomatic partner who was exposed more than 90 days after the diagnosed partner presented for evaluation should be evaluated with serologic testing and treated accordingly.

IV GENITAL WARTS (CONDYLOMATA ACUMINATA) are caused by **human papillomavirus (HPV).**

A. Clinical manifestations. Genital warts are soft, fleshy, painless growths that can grow to be several centimeters in size if they are left untreated. Certain viruses cause flat warts, which are harder to detect.

B. Approach to the patient. The diagnosis is established through the clinical appearance of the lesion.

C. Treatment eradicates warts in most patients, although recurrences are common. No therapy removes HPV from the tissues.

    1. Provider-administered treatments include **cryotherapy** with topical liquid nitrogen and **podophyllin resin,** which is applied, allowed to dry completely, and then washed off by the patient in 1–4 hours. Pregnant women should not receive podophyllin resin.

    2. Patient-administered treatments include **podofilox 0.5% solution** or **imiquimod 5% cream** for external lesions, and **trichloracetic acid** for lesions on the mucous membranes. Pregnant women should not use podofilox or imiquimod.

        a. Podofilox is applied to the lesions twice daily for 3 days. Treatment is followed by 4 days without treatment, and the cycle is repeated 3–4 more times. There is no need to wash off the podofilox.

    b. **Imiquimod** is applied 3 times per week at bed-time, and washed off 6–10 hours later. Imiquimod may be used for as long as 16 weeks.

    c. **Trichloracetic acid** may be applied weekly for up to 6 weeks.

D. Follow-up and referral

  1. Follow-up

    a. All patients should be seen 1 week after receiving provider-administered treatment, or every few weeks if the treatment is self-administered.

    b. Sex partners should be counseled regarding the risk of infection with continued exposure and the importance of using condoms.

HOT KEY

Women with genital warts (and female partners of infected patients) should have **annual pap smears** because HPV infection is associated with cervical cancer.

---

  2. Referral. Patients with extensive warts or warts on the cervix or in the rectum should be referred to a gynecologist or surgeon.

V   URETHRITIS IN MEN. Urethritis may be gonococcal or non-gonococcal. *Neisseria gonorrhoeae* causes **gonococcal urethritis (gonorrhea).** *Chlamydia trachomatis* is the cause of **nongonococcal urethritis** in approximately 50% of cases, and is the most important organism to identify and treat. Non-gonococcal urethritis can also be caused by *Ureaplasma urealyticum, Trichomonas vaginalis,* and HSV; the cause is unknown in as many as 50% of cases.

A. Clinical manifestations

  1. Gonococcal urethritis. The incubation period is 2–5 days. Symptoms include urethral tingling or discomfort, dysuria, or a mucopurulent discharge.

  2. Nongonococcal urethritis. The incubation period is 1–5 weeks. Symptoms are similar to those of gonorrhea, but the discharge may be less pronounced. Gonococcal and nongonococcal urethritis cannot be differentiated on clinical grounds alone.

B. Approach to the patient (Figure 81-3)

  1. Gonococcal urethritis. The diagnosis can be made by

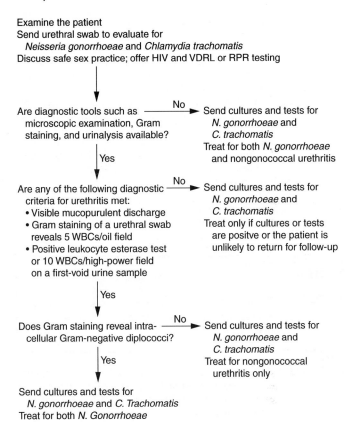

Examine the patient
Send urethral swab to evaluate for
  Neisseria gonorrhoeae and *Chlamydia trachomatis*
Discuss safe sex practice; offer HIV and VDRL or RPR testing

Are diagnostic tools such as ————No———► Send cultures and tests for
  microscopic examination, Gram   *N. gonorrhoeae* and
  staining, and urinalysis available?   *C. trachomatis*
                                            Treat for both *N. gonorrhoeae*
                    │Yes   and nongonococcal urethritis

Are any of the following diagnostic ——No——► Send cultures and tests for
  criteria for urethritis met: *N. gonorrhoeae* and
  • Visible mucopurulent discharge   *C. trachomatis*
  • Gram staining of a urethral swab   Treat only if cultures or tests
    reveals 5 WBCs/oil field   are positve or the patient is
  • Positive leukocyte esterase test   unlikely to return for follow-up
    or 10 WBCs/high-power field
    on a first-void urine sample

                    │Yes

Does Gram staining reveal intra- ————No———► Send cultures and tests for
  cellular Gram-negative diplococci?   *N. gonorrhoeae* and
                                               C. trachomatis
                    │Yes   Treat for nongonococcal
                                               urethritis only

Send cultures and tests for
  N. gonorrhoeae and *C. Trachomatis*
Treat for both *N. Gonorrhoeae*
  and nongonococcal urethritis

FIGURE 81-3. Evaluation of urethritis in men. *RPR* = rapid plasma reagin; *VDRL* = Venereal Disease Research Laboratory; *WBC* = white blood cell.

finding **Gram-negative intracellular diplococci** on **Gram staining** of a urethral swab. All patients should have a **culture** sent for *N. gonorrhoeae* because gonorrhea is a reportable disease.

2. **Nongonococcal urethritis** can be diagnosed by finding 5 white blood cells (WBCs) per oil field on Gram staining of a urethral swab but no intracellular Gram-negative diplococci. A test for *C. trachomatis* (see VI B 2 c) and a culture for *N. gonorrhoeae* should be sent for each patient.

C. **Treatment** is dictated by the clinical situation and the results of laboratory testing (see Figure 81-3).
   1. Because it is not uncommon for patients to have both gonococcal and nongonococcal urethritis, patients with gonococcal urethritis must be treated for both infections (Table 81-3).
   2. Patients who have been definitively shown (by Gram staining) to have nongonococcal urethritis need not be treated for gonorrhea as well. Note that the treatment for nongonococcal urethritis is directed at *C. trachomatis,* but also covers most of the non-chlamydial causes of nongonococcal urethritis.
D. **Follow-up and referral**
   1. Patients should be seen in 1–4 weeks so that the physician can document resolution of symptoms and provide additional counseling regarding safe sex practices.

HOT **KEY**   Persistent or recurrent nongonococcal urethritis may be caused by resistant *U. urealyticum* or *T. vaginalis.* These patients should be treated with metronidazole (2 g orally in one dose) and erythromycin (500 mg four times daily for 7 days).

---

   2. If the patient is symptomatic, partners who may have been exposed within the past 30 days need to be treated; the window increases to 60 days for partners of asymptomatic patients.

VI **CERVICITIS** may or may not be associated with a mucopurulent cervical exudate. If a cervical exudate is present, the condition is called **mucopurulent cervicitis (MPC).** MPC may be caused by *N. gonorrhoeae* or *C. trachomatis,* but in most cases, no organism is identified. Although chlamydial infection can cause MPC, most women with chlamydial cervicitis are asymptomatic and have no cervical exudate.

HOT **KEY**   Chlamydial cervicitis is important to diagnose and treat because it can lead to pelvic inflammatory disease (PID), infertility, and ectopic pregnancy. Screening for *C. trachomatis* is recommended for all sexually active adolescents and young women up to the age of 24 years.

TABLE 81-3. Antibiotic Therapies for *Neisseria gonorrhoeae* infection and *Chlamydia trachomatis* infection

N. gonorrhoeae	C. trachomatis*
Ceftriaxone, 125 mg intramusculary once	Doxycycline, 100 mg orally, twice daily for 7 days
Cefixime, 400 mg orally once	Azithromycin, 1 g orally once†
Ciprofloxacin, 500 mg orally once	Erythromycin, 500 mg orally four times daily for 7 days
Ofloxacin, 400 mg orally once	Ofloxacin, 300 mg orally twice daily for 7 days

*Note that these therapies are effective against most of the other causes of nongonococcal urethritis as well.
†Doubling the dose of azithromycin (2 g given orally once) effectively treats both *N. gonorrhoeae* and *C. trachomatis,* but often causes nausea and abdominal pain.

A. **Clinical manifestations.** Patients may have vaginal discharge, postcoital bleeding, dyspareunia, dysuria, or lower abdominal pain, or they may be completely asymptomatic.

B. **Approach to the patient**

1. **Physical examination.** A clinical diagnosis of mucopurulent cervicitis is established if a cotton swab inserted into the cervical canal reveals a yellow or green exudate. Remember that cervicitis may be present, even if the physical examination is normal.

2. **Laboratory testing**

   a. A **Gram stain** of the exudate can be obtained to look for Gram-negative intracellular diplococci, but the sensitivity is lower than in urethritis.

   b. A **culture** should be sent for *N. gonorrhoeae.*

   c. **Diagnostic tests for *C. trachomatis*** include culture, immunoassays (e.g., Chlamydiazyme) and DNA amplification tests (e.g., ligase chain reaction). DNA amplification tests are very sensitive and specific, even on first-catch urine samples, and are the tests of choice when available.

   d. A **RPR test** should be sent to screen for syphilis.

   e. An **HIV test** should be offered.

C. **Treatment.** Patients with MPC should be treated empirically for both *N. gonorrhoeae* and *C. trachomatis* infection (see Table 81-3) if the prevalence of disease is high in the local population or the patient is unlikely to return for follow-up. Otherwise, treatment should be guided by test results.

D. Follow-up and referral

1. Patients should return in 1–4 weeks so that the physician can document clearing of infection, offer additional counseling regarding safe sex practices, and ensure that the patient has had a pap smear within the past year. If the patient is not up-to-date, a pap smear should be done when the infection is resolved.

2. If the patient is symptomatic, partners who may have been exposed within the past 30 days need to be treated; the window increases to 60 days for partners of asymptomatic patients.

VII **PELVIC INFLAMMATORY DISEASE (PID)** is discussed in Chapter 47.

VIII **VAGINAL INFECTIONS** are discussed in Chapter 48.

IX **EPIDIDYMITIS** is discussed in Chapter 42.

X **HEPATITIS.** Infection with **hepatitis A, B,** or **C virus** may occur through sexual contact. Patients classically present with fever, jaundice, and right upper quadrant abdominal pain and tenderness. Nausea, vomiting, diarrhea, and generalized malaise are also common.

A. Hepatitis A is transmitted by the fecal-oral route. Although it is not usually a sexually transmitted disease, outbreaks may occur in homosexual men.

1. **Clinical manifestations.** The incubation period is 2–6 weeks, and fulminant hepatitis is rare. Initially, symptoms are nonspecific and flu-like. As the disease progresses, the patient may develop jaundice, hepatomegaly, and right upper quadrant tenderness. There is no chronic carrier state.

2. **Approach to the patient.** Liver enzymes and bilirubin levels are elevated. The diagnosis can be made by detecting IgM antibodies to the hepatitis A virus in the patient's serum.

3. **Treatment.** Most patients improve without specific

treatment. Hydration and antiemetics are occasionally required.

4. **Follow-up and referral**

   a. Patients should be seen in 1–4 weeks to ensure that their symptoms have resolved and that liver function has returned to normal.

   b. Partners of patients with hepatitis A can receive postexposure prophylaxis therapy (i.e., an intramuscular injection of immune globulin). Prophylactic therapy is only effective when administered within 2 weeks of exposure.

B. **Hepatitis B.** Sexual transmission accounts for one third to one half of cases of hepatitis B.

1. **Clinical manifestations.** The clinical features are similar to those of hepatitis A, although the patient's symptoms may be more nonspecific.

   a. Fulminant hepatitis occurs in fewer than 1% of patients. The severity of symptoms depends on the viral dose.

   b. Following acute infection, 1%–2% of patients develop chronic hepatitis B, which predisposes to cirrhosis and hepatocellular carcinoma.

2. **Approach to the patient**

   a. Liver enzymes may be markedly elevated.

   b. Patients with acute infection will have IgM antibodies to hepatitis B core antigen (anti-HB_c). IgG antibodies to hepatitis B surface antigen (anti-HB_s) indicate a past, resolved infection and denote immunity.

   c. Persistence of hepatitis B surface antigen (HBsAg) indicates chronic infection.

3. **Treatment**

   a. Patients with fulminant hepatitis must be hospitalized and should be seen by a liver specialist.

   b. Most patients with acute hepatitis require only rest and oral hydration. Hepatotoxic agents (e.g., alcohol, acetaminophen) should be avoided.

   c. Patients with chronic hepatitis B may respond to α-interferon and other antiviral drugs.

4. **Follow-up and referral**

   a. **Follow-up**

      (1) Following an acute infection, patients should be seen every few weeks until the symptoms resolve. These patients should be advised to seek medical attention promptly if their symptoms worsen.

578

Chapter 81

(2) Sex partners of patients with acute hepatitis B should receive the hepatitis B immune globulin and the hepatitis B vaccine (three doses given at 0, 1–2 months, and 4–6 months). Abstinence is recommended until the vaccination is completed. Partners of patients with chronic hepatitis B should also receive the vaccine.

b. Referral. Patients with chronic hepatitis B should be referred to a liver specialist for ongoing care.

HOT

Hepatitis A and B are preventable by vaccination (see Chapter 4). Patients who present with another STD should receive the hepatitis B vaccine.

KEY

C. Hepatitis C. The risk for sexual transmission is thought to be small, but may occur in a subset of patients.
1. **Clinical manifestations.** Most infections are asymptomatic. More than 50% of infected patients develop chronic hepatitis; these patients tend to be asymptomatic until the complications of chronic hepatitis develop (e.g., hepatocellular carcinoma, cirrhosis).
2. **Approach to the patient.** The diagnosis is established by finding antibodies to hepatitis C virus in the patient's serum.
3. **Treatment**
   a. **Acute infection.** Treatment is symptomatic.
   b. **Chronic infection.** Patients may benefit from α-interferon therapy.
4. **Follow-up and referral**
   a. **Follow-up**
      (1) Patients should be seen every few weeks after an acute infection until symptoms resolve. They should be advised to seek medical attention promptly if their symptoms worsen.
      (2) Partners should be counseled regarding the risk of infection and about how to prevent transmission.
   b. **Referral.** Patients with chronic hepatitis C should be referred to a liver specialist.

XI **HIV** is discussed in Chapter 82.

References
1998 Guidelines for treatment of sexually transmitted diseases. Centers for Disease Control and Prevention. *MMWR Morb Mortal Wkly Rep* 47(RR-1):1–11, 1998.
Drugs for sexually transmitted diseases. *Med Lett Drugs Ther* 37(964):117–122, 1995.

82. Acquired Immunodeficiency Syndrome (AIDS)

I **INTRODUCTION.** Care of the patient with HIV infection, a complex and rapidly changing field, has evolved into its own specialty at many centers. Nevertheless, patients benefit from having a primary provider who is knowledgeable in this area.

II **DIAGNOSIS**

A. Patients who have recently been exposed to the virus may present with symptoms of an acute viral infection (e.g., fever, myalgias, lymphadenopathy, pharyngitis, a viral exanthem, and general malaise). More often, routine blood testing or manifestations of late-stage immunodeficiency disease lead to the diagnosis. **HIV antibody tests** are a reliable means of detecting established HIV infection. False-negative results can occur in patients who have been infected within 6 months of testing.

B. A history of exposure (e.g., needle sharing, an unsafe sexual encounter, or a needle stick in a healthcare worker) combined with a suggestive constellation of symptoms may allow diagnosis of HIV infection within weeks or months of the exposure. It is worthwhile to test these patients with **viral load measurements** or **assays for p24 antigen,** which will demonstrate the presence of the virus, as well as with **HIV antibody tests** (which are frequently negative in this setting).

III **APPROACH TO THE PATIENT**

A. **Newly diagnosed HIV.** Several things must be done for a patient who has been newly diagnosed with HIV infection.

1. **Inform the patient of the diagnosis.** Learning that one has been infected with HIV can be emotionally devastating. Physicians must offer emotional support and should arrange supportive psychotherapy where indicated.

   a. It is important to question a patient at the time of

disclosure about the ability of family and friends to offer support.

b. Patients should be screened for suicidal ideation or intent.

HOT

It important to inform patients that HIV disease is a chronic illness that can be managed effectively.

KEY

---

2. Provide counseling regarding necessary lifestyle modifications.
   a. Sexual activity
      (1) Patients should **use latex condoms** during every act of sexual intercourse to prevent the transmission of HIV and to prevent exposure to pathogens such as cytomegalovirus (CMV), herpes simplex virus (HSV), and human papillomavirus (HPV).
      (2) Patients should **avoid oral-anal contact** in order to reduce the risk of intestinal infections (e.g., cryptosporidiosis, shigellosis, *Campylobacter*-associated gastroenteritis, amebiasis, giardiasis, hepatitis A).
   b. Injection drug use
      (1) Discontinuation of drug use. Patients should be encouraged to discontinue injection drug use; motivated heroin users may benefit from referral to a **methadone detoxification program.**
      (2) Needle-exchange program information. Many patients with HIV are infected by sharing needles or drug paraphernalia with others who have the disease. In order to limit the spread of HIV, patients who cannot stop using intravenous drugs should be given information regarding needle-exchange programs.
   c. Diet. Patients should **avoid raw or undercooked eggs and meat.**
   d. Pets
      (1) HIV-positive patients should **avoid acquiring pets younger than 6 months of age** because

young animals are more likely to harbor diarrheal pathogens.

   (2) In order to reduce the patient's exposure to *Toxoplasma gondii,* **litter boxes should be cleaned daily** (but not by the patient). In addition, **cats should not be allowed to eat raw meat.**

3. **Order baseline laboratory studies.** The following studies are helpful for identifying associated disease conditions (e.g., hepatitis) and establishing a baseline for future comparisons when monitoring medication side effects:

   a. **Complete blood count (CBC)**
   b. **Serum electrolyte panel**
   c. **Creatinine, aspartate aminotransferase (AST),** and **alkaline phosphatase (AP) levels**
   d. **Chest radiograph**

4. **Perform appropriate screening tests.**

   a. **Tuberculosis screening**
      (1) All patients with HIV infection should have a **purified protein derivative (PPD) skin test.** In HIV-infected patients, **5 mm of induration** is considered a positive result.
      (2) Any patient with a positive result on PPD testing should have a **chest radiograph** (and, if abnormal, **sputum acid-fast stains)** to assess for active tuberculosis.

HOT **KEY**

Patients with exposure risk (e.g., travel to endemic areas, homelessness, imprisonment, injection drug use) should be screened for tuberculosis annually.

---

   b. **HPV screening.** Cervical and anal cancers as a result of HPV infection are common and rapidly progressive in HIV patients.
      (1) HIV-positive women should have a **pap smear** every 6 months for the first year after diagnosis, and then annually if no abnormal results are obtained. Patients with an abnormal pap smear require referral for **colposcopy.**
      (2) Currently, although there are no formal rec-

ommendations for anal HPV screening via **anoscopy,** many physicians do offer this option to their patients.

c. **Syphilis screening.** A rapid plasma reagin **(RPR)** or **Venereal Disease Research Laboratory (VDRL) test** is recommended yearly to screen for syphilis, which is both more common and more severe in HIV patients.

d. **Hepatitis screening. Hepatitis serologies** should be obtained to identify patients who require vaccination or treatment for active disease.

e. **Toxoplasmosis screening.** A *T. gondii* **serology** should be obtained when HIV infection is diagnosed.

   (1) If the serology is positive, prophylactic therapy should be prescribed when the patient's CD4 count falls below 100 cells/μl.

   (2) If the results are negative, the test should be repeated when the patient's CD4 count falls below 100 cells/μl or if the patient develops neurologic symptoms.

5. **Ensure that the patient is up-to-date on his vaccinations.**

   a. A **pneumococcal vaccine** (to protect against streptococcal pneumonia) is recommended every 6 years and is more effective if given early in the disease.

   b. The **hepatitis B vaccine** is given at 0, 1, and 6 months for patients not already infected with hepatitis B.

   c. The **hepatitis A vaccine** is recommended for patients engaging in anal-oral sexual contact. It should be given at 0 and 6 months.

   d. An annual **influenza vaccine ("flu shot")** is recommended.

   e. The **diphtheria-tetanus vaccine** is indicated every 10 years.

B. **Established disease**

1. **Ongoing monitoring.** Patients with HIV infection should have two measures of disease activity followed at regular intervals (i.e., every 3–4 months).

   a. **Viral load measurements,** obtained using either reverse transcriptase polymerase chain reaction (PCR) or branched DNA assays, are direct measurements of the patient's viral burden. Viral load measurements are **predictors of disease pro-**

gression and are **used to guide treatment decisions related to antiretroviral agents.**
  b. **CD4 counts** can be used to help **predict potential infectious and malignant complications** of HIV disease (Table 82-1) and are **used as the basis for selecting antibiotic prophylaxis.** Table 82-2 summarizes the usual presenting features and accepted treatment regimens for the most common HIV-related diseases.
  2. **Addressing end-of-life issues.** Despite the benefits of combination antiretroviral therapy, no cure for HIV infection has been found. Therefore, end-of-life issues need to be addressed before a patient is too ill to participate meaningfully in making important decisions. Providers should encourage patients to designate a durable power of attorney for health care, to express the degree of medical intervention desired in various circumstances, and to explore options for hospice care.

TABLE 82-1. Summary: CD4 Counts and Likely Infections and Malignancies in HIV-Infected Patients

CD4 Count (cells/μl)	Likely Infections and Malignancies
<800	Bacterial pneumonia, tuberculosis, lymphoma, Kaposi's sarcoma
<500	Coccidioidomycosis, histoplasmosis, candidiasis
<200	*Pneumocystis carinii* pneumonia (PCP), toxoplasmosis, *Cryptococcus* infection
<100	*Mycobacterium avium* complex infection, cytomegalovirus (CMV) infection, primary CNS lymphoma, bacillary angiomatosis
Any CD4 count	Hepatitis, syphilis, herpes virus infection, influenza virus infection

CNS = central nervous system.

TABLE 82-2. Presentation and Treatment of Common Infections and Complications in Patients with HIV Infection

Infection or Malignancy	Presentation	Accepted Treatment Regimens*
Pneumocystis carinii pneumonia (PCP)	Cough, fever, dyspnea, occasionally sputum production	Trimethoprim–sulfamethoxazole, 2 double-strength tablets orally every 8 hours for 21 days†
Mycobacterium tuberculosis infection	Fever, productive cough, night sweats, weight loss	Isoniazid, 5 mg/kg/day (to a maximum dose of 300 mg/day) and rifampin‡, 10 mg/kg/day (to a maximum dose of 600 mg/day) given orally for 6 months **plus** pyrazinamide, 25 mg/kg/day (to a maximum dose 2 g/day) given orally for 2 months (for sensitive organisms only)
Mycobacterium avium complex infection	Fever, anorexia, night sweats, weight loss, diarrhea	Clarithromycin, 500 mg orally twice daily; ethambutol, 15–25 mg/kg/day; and rifabutin§, 300 mg/day given orally‖
Bacterial pneumonia	Productive cough, fever, dyspnea, pleuritic chest pain	Same as for HIV-negative patients
Candidiasis	Oral or esophageal: white plaques on the mucosa, odynophagia. Vaginal: genital pruritis, cheesy discharge	Topical clotrimazole, miconazole, or nystatin; if topical agents are not effective, oral fluconazole can be used (200 mg on the first day, followed by 100 mg daily until improvement occurs)
Cryptococcal meningitis	Fever and headache; less commonly, photophobia, neck stiffness, and altered mental status	Fluconazole, 400 mg orally daily for 6–10 weeks#‖

continued

TABLE 82-2. Presentation and Treatment of Common Infections and Complications in Patients with HIV Infection

Infection or Malignancy	Presentation	Accepted Treatment Regimens*
Cytomegalovirus (CMV) retinitis	Painless visual blurring, scotomata	Ganciclovir, 5 mg/kg intravenously every 12 hours for 14–21 days‖
Herpes simplex virus (HSV) infection	Painful oral or genital ulcers; esophageal ulcers	Acyclovir, 400 mg orally five times daily for 14–21 days‖
Varicella zoster virus infection	Cutaneous vesicles in a dermatomal distribution	Acyclovir, 800 mg orally five times daily for 7 days***
Non-Hodgkin's lymphoma	Fever, night sweats, rapid lymph node enlargement	Combination chemotherapy in consultation with a specialist
Kaposi's sarcoma	Skin most common site, with purple, red, or brown lesions; lower extremity edema frequently occurs	Chemotherapy, radiation, and/or cryotherapy in consultation with a specialist

*Other treatment regimens are also acceptable and, in some circumstances, may be preferred.
†If the patient's PaO₂ is less than 70 mm Hg or the alveolar–arterial PaO₂ gradient is greater than 30 mm Hg also treat with steroids and strongly consider hospitalization.
‡Rifampin should not be used with protease inhibitors.
§Rifabutin should be used with caution in patients who are taking protease inhibitors.
‖Chronic suppressive therapy may be required.
#Patients with more severe disease require hospitalization and intravenous antibiotic therapy with amphotericin B (and possibly flucytosine as well).
***Patients with systemic dissemination or involvement of several dermatomes must be hospitalized.

IV TREATMENT

A. Antiretroviral therapy. Because they can significantly slow disease progression, antiretroviral regimens should be prescribed for almost every patient with HIV infection. Although it is currently recommended that treatment be initiated when the **viral load** reaches **5,000–10,000 copies/ml,** it is probably appropriate to offer treatment to any patient with a detectable viral load.

1. **Compliance.** All antiretroviral regimens are complex, costly, and likely to have some toxic effects. Because resistance to newer antiretroviral drugs develops quickly in patients who do not take the medications regularly, it is important to discuss compliance with the patient before initiating any regimen.

2. **Initial regimen.** The dosages and side effects of agents commonly used in the treatment of HIV infection are given in Table 82-3.

   a. A **three-drug combination** is the most beneficial and limits the development of drug resistance. All recommended drug combinations include two **nucleoside reverse transcriptase inhibitors** and either a **protease inhibitor** (for the strongest effect) or a **non-nucleoside reverse transcriptase inhibitor** (Table 82-4).

   b. A **two-drug combination** (i.e., two nucleoside reverse transcriptase inhibitors) can be used for patients who cannot accept a three-drug regimen.

3. **Adjustments to the initial regimen**

   a. **When to change the regimen**

      (1) **Treatment failure.** An appropriate initial drug regimen results in an undetectable viral load in most patients. If a substantial drop in viral load has not occurred after 6 weeks of therapy, or if the viral load is increasing in a compliant patient with a previously effective drug combination, treatment failure should be assumed, and the drug combination should be changed.

      (2) **Toxicity** that is unacceptable to the patient or that causes the patient to be noncompliant necessitates a change in therapeutic regimen.

      (3) **Suboptimal regimen.** Patients who began therapy before the use of three-drug combinations became widespread may benefit from an update in their regimen.

TABLE 82-3. Agents Used in the Treatment of HIV Infection

Agent	Dosage	Side Effects
Nucleoside reverse transcriptase inhibitors		
Zidovudine (azidodideoxythymidine, AZT)	200 mg three times daily or 300 mg twice daily	Anemia, neutropenia, headache, myositis, hepatitis, nausea
Didanosine (dideoxyinosine, ddI)	200 mg twice daily	Pancreatitis, neuropathy, myositis
Zalcitabine (dideoxycytidine, ddC)*	0.75 mg three times daily	Oral ulcers, neuropathy, pancreatitis
Lamivudine (3TC)	150 mg twice daily	Neutropenia, nausea, pancreatitis
Stavudine (D4T)	40 mg twice daily	Peripheral neuropathy, hepatitis
Protease inhibitors		
Saquinavir	600 mg every 8 hours with a high-fat meal	Diarrhea, nausea, abdominal pain, drug interactions, elevated creatinine kinase levels, hypoglycemia, rash
Ritonavir	600 mg every 12 hours with food; medicine must be refrigerated	Nausea, diarrhea, paresthesias, metallic taste, hepatitis, drug interactions, asthenia
Indinavir	800 mg every 8 hours on an empty stomach	Nephrolithiasis, hyperbilirubinemia, drug interactions
Nelfinavir	750 mg three times daily with food	Diarrhea, loose stools
Non-nucleoside reverse transcriptase inhibitors		
Nevirapine	200 mg daily for 14 days, then 200 mg twice daily	Stevens-Johnson syndrome (rash), headache, nausea, hepatotoxicity
Delavirdine	400 mg three times daily	Under study

*Zalcitabine appears to be less effective than other nucleoside reverse transcriptase inhibitors.

TABLE 82-4. Acceptable Initial Antiretroviral Regimens*

Zidovudine + lamivudine + protease inhibitor
Stavudine + lamivudine + protease inhibitor
Zidovudine + didanosine + protease inhibitor
Stavudine + didanosine + protease inhibitor
Zidovudine + didanosine + non-nucleoside reverse transcriptase
  inhibitor

*Combining zidovudine and stavudine is not recommended due to possible antagonism.

    b. How to change the regimen
       (1) Include a minimum of two drugs that are new to the patient in order to avoid resistance.
       (2) Always change the protease inhibitor in a failing regimen (because resistance to protease inhibitors develops especially quickly). Indinavir and ritonavir often demonstrate cross resistance.
       (3) Consider which agents caused toxicity in the previous regimen when selecting drugs for the new regimen.
  4. Considerations in pregnancy. Care of the mother should be given primary importance.
    a. Three-drug combinations are often used, although safety data for the fetus is limited.
    b. At a minimum, **zidovudine** (which helps prevent vertical transmission of HIV to the infant) should be prescribed. The dose is 100 mg, five times daily throughout the pregnancy. During labor, 2 mg/kg should be administered intravenously for 1 hour, followed by 1 mg/kg until delivery.
B. Prophylactic antimicrobial therapy to protect against several common opportunistic infections is currently considered to be standard of care. The Centers for Disease Control and Prevention (CDC) recommendations for prophylaxis in patients who have not had a first episode of opportunistic disease are given in Table 82-5.

TABLE 82-5. Prophylactic Antimicrobial Therapy

Infection	Clinical Indications for Initiating Therapy	Best Regimen	Sample Alternative Regimens
Pneumocystis carinii pneumonia (PCP)	CD4 count < 200 cells/μl	Trimethoprim–sulfamethoxazole, 1 double-strength tablet daily **or** Trimethoprim–sulfamethoxazole, 1 single-strength tablet daily	Trimethoprim–sulfamethoxazole, one double-strength tablet orally triweekly **or** Dapsone, 100 mg orally daily
Mycobacterium tuberculosis infection	More than 5 mm induration on a PPD test **or** a prior positive PPD test without treatment **or** exposure to a person with active tuberculosis	Isoniazid, 300 mg orally daily and pyridoxine, 50 mg orally daily for 12 months **or** Isoniazid, 900 mg orally biweekly and pyridoxine, 50 mg orally biweekly for 12 months (observed)	Rifampin, 600 mg orally daily for 12 months

Infection	Indication		
Mycobacterium avium complex infection	CD4 count < 50 cells/μl	Clarithromycin, 500 mg orally twice daily **or** Azithromycin, 1200 mg orally weekly	Rifabutin, 300 mg orally daily
Toxoplasma gondii infection	CD4 count < 100 cells/μl and positive IgG antibody to Toxoplasma	Trimethoprim–sulfamethoxazole, 1 double-strength table orally daily	Trimethoprim–sulfamethoxazole, 1 single-strength tablet orally daily **or** Dapsone, 50 mg orally daily **plus** weekly pyrimethamine, 50 mg orally, and leucovorin, 25 mg orally
Varicella zoster virus infection	Exposure to a patient with chicken pox or shingles in patients with no history of varicella zoster virus infection and negative varicella zoster antibody	Varicella zoster immune globulin, 5 vials intramuscularly within 96 hours of exposure	Acyclovir, 800 mg orally five times daily for 3 weeks

HOT

KEY

The CD4 count may not remain as predictive of infectious complications if the count improves as a result of effective antiretroviral therapy. Therefore, most experts recommend that suspicion for particular pathogens and prophylaxis for opportunistic infections be based on the patient's lowest recorded CD4 count.

C. **Postexposure prophylaxis.** Treatment with antiretroviral medications has been proven to reduce transmission of HIV to **healthcare workers following occupational exposure.** The practice of providing antiretroviral medications following high-risk sexual behavior or intravenous drug use is controversial. Clinical trials have begun to examine this area more closely.

V   FOLLOW-UP AND REFERRAL. Management of patients in conjunction with an **AIDS expert** is generally recommended. Most patients should be seen by a **dentist,** an **ophthalmologist,** and a **dietitian.** Other specialty referrals (e.g., to a **dermatologist** or **psychiatrist)** may be helpful, depending on the clinical situation.

References

1997 USPHS/IDSA guidelines for the prevention of opportunistic infections in persons infected with human immunodeficiency virus. *Ann Intern Med* 127(10):922–946, 1997.

Carpenter CC, Fischl MA, Hammer SM, et al: Antiretroviral therapy for HIV infection in 1998: updated recommendations of the International AIDS Society— USA Panel. *JAMA* 280(1):78–86, 1998.

Gold JWM, Telzak EE, White DA: Management of the HIV-infected patient, part II. *Med Clin North Am* 81(2):299–583, 1997.

Kocurek K: Primary care of the HIV patient: standard practice and new developments in the era of managed care. *Med Clin North Am* 80(2):375–410, 1996.

83. Tuberculosis

I INTRODUCTION

A. Incidence. Tuberculosis is considered the most common infectious disease. It is estimated that one third of the world's population is infected with *Mycobacterium tuberculosis*.

1. In the United States, 10–15 million people are infected.
2. Since 1985, a number of factors have led to a steady increase in the number of tuberculosis cases each year:
   a. An increase in the incidence of HIV infection
   b. An increase in the elderly population
   c. Increased immigration from countries where tuberculosis is very common
   d. The development of resistant strains of *M. tuberculosis*

B. Transmission. *M. tuberculosis* is acquired via inhalation of organism-containing aerosolized particles ("droplet nuclei"), spread by coughing. The aerosolized particles spread throughout the lungs (and other sites in the body) and are ingested by macrophages.

C. Clinical stages

1. **Primary tuberculosis.** Initially, infection usually involves the lungs. Most otherwise healthy people control the initial infection when granulomas form around the organism-containing macrophages.
2. **Active tuberculosis** may develop as a progression of primary infection, or as a reactivation of latent infection.
   a. **Progressive primary tuberculosis** develops in patients who are unable to control the initial infection. Patients most at risk include infants, children, older adolescents, the elderly, and immunosuppressed patients.
   b. **Reactivation tuberculosis.** Dormant organisms can live in walled-off granulomas for years, but they may reactivate, especially if host immunity is suppressed.
      (1) In healthy adults, the risk of reactivation is 5%–15%.
      (2) Risk of reactivation is highest within 1–2 years of primary infection.

II APPROACH TO THE PATIENT WITH ACTIVE TUBERCULOSIS

A. Diagnosis

1. **Patient history.** Patients with active tuberculosis most commonly present with:

   a. **Constitutional symptoms** (i.e., fatigue, weight loss, fevers, night sweats)

   b. A **cough,** which may progress from dry to productive

   c. **Symptoms of disseminated disease**

HOT KEY

M. tuberculosis infection is sometimes called the "great mimicker" because it can cause almost any symptom, depending on where in the body infection has occurred. For example, *M. tuberculosis* infection may present with symptoms of meningitis, arthritis, cystitis, epididymitis, gastrointestinal ulcers, pericarditis, or spondylitis (Pott's disease).

---

2. **Physical examination.** Patients often appear chronically ill and have evidence of weight loss. The lung examination may reveal crackles or decreased breath sounds from an effusion, or it may be entirely normal.

3. **Chest radiograph.** If the clinical findings suggest active tuberculosis, the patient should have a chest radiograph. Fibrocavitary disease, nodules, and pneumonic infiltrates are all common radiographic findings.

   a. **Primary progressive tuberculosis** usually involves the **middle** or **lower lung fields.**

   b. **Reactivation tuberculosis** usually involves the **apical** or **posterior segments** of the **upper lobes,** although many patients have disease in other locations of the lung.

4. **Sputum testing**

   a. **Acid-fast staining.** If radiographic findings suggest active tuberculosis, three separate sputum samples should be examined for *M. tuberculosis* (which stains red with acid-fast staining).

   b. **Cultures** for *M. tuberculosis* should be sent. Typically, results are not available for 6–8 weeks, although rapid culture techniques and DNA-probe testing are available in some laboratories.

5. **Bronchoscopy** (with staining and culture of bronchial washings) should be considered for patients when the

clinical suspicion for active tuberculosis is high but sputum examination is negative.

B. **Therapy**

1. **General considerations**

    a. **Complicating factors.** Therapy for active tuberculosis is complicated by many factors, including **drug resistance, medication side effects,** and **poor patient compliance** as a result of the complicated regimen. Treatment can be especially challenging for patients with HIV infection who may be taking multiple medications, and for patients who are homeless or transient.

        (1) Patients with active tuberculosis should be treated by an **infectious disease specialist** or a physician experienced in managing the many factors that can complicate therapy for tuberculosis.

        (2) **Directly observed therapy (DOT)** may be used when patients are having difficulty adhering to medication schedules. Patients undergoing DOT are required to come to their provider's office or a tuberculosis clinic two or three times weekly to receive treatment.

    b. **Reporting.** All cases of suspected or confirmed active tuberculosis must be reported to the **state** or **local health department.**

2. **Regimen.** Accepted initial regimens for treating active tuberculosis generally involve four drugs for at least 2 months, followed by two drugs for an additional 4 months. An example of an appropriate regimen for an adult with active tuberculosis is given in Table 83-1.

3. **Monitoring.** All patients older than 35 years should have a baseline laboratory assessment [including liver function tests, a renal panel, and a complete blood count (CBC) with platelets] before therapy is initiated. In addition, patients should undergo visual acuity and red-green color perception testing. Once therapy has been initiated, monitoring for side effects and therapy effectiveness should take place at regular intervals.

    a. **Impaired hepatic function** may result from isoniazid therapy.

        (1) **Elevated liver enzymes.** If the patient's liver enzyme levels are more than five times the upper limit of normal or there is more than a

TABLE 83-1. Sample 4-Drug Regimen for the Initial Treatment of Active Tuberculosis in an Adult*

Drug	Dose	Schedule	Side Effects	Monitoring
Isoniazid	5–10 mg/kg, to a maximum dose of 300 mg	Once daily for 6 months[†]	Hepatitis, peripheral neuropathy[‡]	Liver function tests monthly for patients older than 35 years (optional for younger patients) Neurologic examination Monitoring of blood levels of other medications
Rifampin	10 mg/kg, to a maximum dose of 600 mg	Once daily for 6 months[†]	Hepatitis, rash, gastrointestinal upset, purpura	Monitoring of blood levels of other medications Liver function tests
Pyrazinamide[§]	15–30 mg/kg, to a maximum dose of 2g	Once daily for 2 months	Hepatitis, arthralgias, hyperuricemia	Liver function tests Serum uric acid level (if gout occurs)

| Ethambutol | 5–25 mg/kg, to a maximum dose of 1 g | Once daily for 2 months | Optic neuritis, rash | Visual acuity and red–green color perception testing should be performed before starting ethambutol therapy; question patient about visual changes monthly |

*This regimen assumes no drug resistance. Consult with local tuberculosis expert or the health department to ensure that this regimen is in accordance with your local resistance patterns.

†After 2 months of daily therapy, it is acceptable to change to directly observed therapy with isoniazid and rifampin administered two or three times per week.

‡Consider pyridoxine (25 mg orally) to prevent neuropathy in patients at high risk (i.e., those older than 65 years; those with diabetes, alcoholism, or chronic renal failure)

§Pyrazinamide must not be used in pregnant women.

three-fold increase from the baseline level, isoniazid therapy should be stopped. Any elevation in liver enzymes necessitates more frequent monitoring.

   (2) Symptoms of hepatitis. If the patient develops symptoms of hepatitis during treatment, isoniazid therapy must be stopped immediately.

   b. **Drug interactions.** Both isoniazid and rifampin interact with many other drugs (e.g., phenytoin, warfarin, oral contraceptives, digoxin, oral hypoglycemic agents, corticosteroids, methadone). Therefore, monitoring of blood drug levels of these medications is necessary.

   c. **Vision problems.** Ethambutol may cause optic neuritis and other vision problems; therefore, the patient should be questioned monthly about any visual changes.

   d. **Response to therapy.** All patients should have serial sputum examinations and culture to ensure that the organism is being cleared from the sputum. If drug resistance is detected, or the sputum cultures remain positive after 2 months of treatment, a tuberculosis specialist should be consulted.

III TUBERCULOSIS SCREENING AND PREVENTION

A. **Screening** is performed with the **purified protein derivative (PPD) skin test.** The goal of tuberculosis screening is to identify asymptomatic patients who have been infected, so that they can receive drug therapy to kill the dormant organisms and prevent reactivation of disease.

   1. **Candidates for screening.** Tuberculosis screening is indicated for patients at high risk for the disease:

      a. Household members and close contacts of patients with active tuberculosis

      b. HIV-infected patients and patients with risk factors for HIV infection and an unknown HIV status

      c. Foreign-born patients from countries where the incidence of tuberculosis is high

      d. Patients living in medically underserved, low-income areas

      e. Injection drug users and patients with alcoholism

      f. Homeless patients

      g. Residents of long-term care facilities (e.g., prisons, nursing homes, psychiatric institutions)

h. Patients with medical conditions associated with a high risk for reactivation of tuberculosis (e.g., diabetes, chronic renal failure)

i. People who work in facilities where infection would put a large number of people at risk (e.g., hospitals, daycare centers)

HOT KEY Prior to performing a PPD test, always question the patient to ensure that he has not been previously treated for active tuberculosis or received prophylactic therapy against *M. tuberculosis* infection. These patients have known prior infection, and therefore do not require skin testing.

2. **Performing the test.** PPD solution (0.1 ml) is injected intradermally (not subcutaneously) into the volar surface of the forearm, using a 27-gauge needle or tuberculin syringe. A wheal measuring 5–10 mm in diameter should form. The patient returns in 48–72 hours so that the amount of induration (not erythema) at the injection site can be measured.

3. **Interpretation of test results.** The "cut-off" for determining a positive test depends on the likelihood of disease in a given patient. High-risk patients are considered to have a positive test with lower levels of induration than low-risk patients (Table 83-2).

4. **Follow-up**
   a. **Positive test.** All patients with a positive PPD test should have a chest radiograph.
      (1) If the chest radiograph shows signs of pulmonary tuberculosis, a full medical evaluation should be performed (see II A).
      (2) If the chest radiograph is negative, preventive therapy should be considered (see III B). Be sure to confirm that the patient has not been adequately treated for active tuberculosis in the past, or given preventive therapy.
   b. **Negative test.** There are two potential causes for a false-negative test result: loss of sensitivity to PPD and anergy.
      (1) **Loss of sensitivity to PPD.** Consider repeating a negative test in 1 week to rule out the possibility that the patient has been previously infected with *M. tuberculosis* but has lost her sensitivity to PPD. In these patients,

TABLE 83-2. Interpretation of Purified Protein Derivative (PPD) Test Results

Size of Induration	Patients in Whom This Result is Considered Positive
≥ 5 mm	Household members and close contacts of patients with active tuberculosis
	HIV-infected patients and patients with risk factors for HIV infection and an unknown HIV status
	Patients with fibrotic lesions on a chest radiograph
≥ 10 mm	Foreign-born patients from countries where the incidence of tuberculosis is high
	Patients living in medically underserved, low-income areas
	Injection drug users and patients with alcoholism
	Homeless patients
	Residents of long-term care facilities
	Patients with medical conditions associated with a high risk for reactivation of tuberculosis*
	People who work in facilities where infection would put a large number of people at risk (e.g., hospitals, correctional facilities, daycare centers)
≥ 15 mm	All other patients

*Conditions that place a patient at high risk for reactivation tuberculosis include diabetes, chronic renal failure, malignancy, silicosis, prior gastrectomy, body weight more than 10% below the ideal, and therapy with corticosteroids or other immunosuppressive drugs.

sensitivity to PPD is regained only after exposure to PPD; therefore, the second test should be positive (this is called the **"booster phenomenon").** If the test is again negative, the patient is either uninfected or anergic.

(2) **Anergy** results in a suppressed host response to the PPD antigen in a patient with active or

past *M. tuberculosis* infection. The "booster phenomenon" does not occur in patients with anergy. Although it is possible to test for anergy by testing for other antigens that the patient should react to (e.g., *Candida,* tetanus), anergy testing is not routinely recommended because a full panel of testing requires exposure to more than 12 antigens.

B. Prophylactic therapy

   1. Indications. Preventive therapy is indicated for certain patients who have a positive PPD and a negative chest radiograph in order to prevent reactivation of the disease.

   a. All of the following patients should receive prophylactic therapy, regardless of their age, if they have positive results on PPD skin testing:

   (1) Patients with HIV infection, or risk factors for HIV infection and an unknown HIV status

   (2) Patients who have had close contact with a patient who has active tuberculosis

   (3) Patients who have a positive result on a PPD test within 2 years of having a negative result (these patients are known as "recent converters")

   (4) Patients with medical conditions that increase the risk of reactivation tuberculosis (see Table 83-2)

   (5) Injection drug users

   b. Patients younger than 35 years should receive prophylactic therapy if they demonstrate an induration of 10 mm or more on the PPD skin test and they meet one or more of the following conditions:

   (1) They were born in a country when the incidence of tuberculosis is very high

   (2) They live in a medically underserved, low-income area

   (3) They live in a long-term care facility

HOT KEY Initiating preventive therapy with a single agent in a patient with active tuberculosis promotes drug resistance. Therefore, if the chest radiograph shows any signs of active tuberculosis, the patient should be started on drug therapy for active tuberculosis until the sputum cultures are negative (which takes at least 2 months). If in doubt, consult an expert.

2. **Regimen. Isoniazid** (5–10 mg/kg up to 300 mg/day maximum) is administered orally daily for 6 months. The duration of therapy should be extended to 12 months for patients with HIV infection or a chest radiograph showing evidence of healed tuberculosis.

   a. **Contraindications.** Isoniazid should not be used in the following patients:

      (1) Those with hepatic injury as a result of previous isoniazid therapy

      (2) Those who experienced a severe reaction to isoniazid in the past (e.g., fever, rash, arthritis)

      (3) Those with current acute or progressive hepatic disease (patients with chronic inactive viral hepatitis may be treated cautiously)

      (4) Those who are pregnant (although harmful effects to the fetus as a result of isoniazid therapy have not been observed, preventive treatment should be delayed until after delivery)

   b. **Monitoring.** Patients should have their liver enzymes monitored periodically. Monthly monitoring is advised for the following patients:

      (1) Those who are older than 35 years

      (2) Those currently using a medication known to interact with isoniazid

      (3) Those with alcoholism

      (4) Those who have a condition that predisposes to neuropathy (e.g., diabetes, alcoholism, chronic renal insufficiency)

      (5) Those who use intravenous drugs

References

Bass JB Jr, Farer LS, Hopewell PC, et al: Treatment of tuberculosis and tuberculosis infection in adults and children. *Am J Respir Crit Care Med* 149(5):1359–1374, 1994.

Drugs for tuberculosis. *Med Lett Drugs Ther* 37(954):67–70, 1995.

84. Approach to Fever

I INTRODUCTION

A. Normal body temperature. The normal oral temperature is 36°C-37.4°C (average = 36.7°C).

1. The range includes 95% of the population. Any temperature higher or lower is considered abnormal.

2. The average rectal temperature is 0.5°C higher and the average axillary temperature is 0.5°C lower than the oral temperature.

HOT

KEY

Think of the three temperatures (axillary, oral, and rectal) in alphabetical order to remember which is lowest and which is highest: A < O < R.

B. Causes. Fever (an elevated temperature) may be a manifestation of infection, malignancy, connective tissue disorders, drug reactions, central nervous system (CNS) disorders, or other diseases.

HOT

KEY

Remember:
- Patients who are elderly, immunocompromised, or taking steroids or nonsteroidal anti-inflammatory drugs (NSAIDs) may not mount a fever, even in the presence of a severe infection.
- The degree of fever is of little predictive value in assessing the severity of an underlying illness in a given patient.
- Hypothermia often signals the presence of an overwhelming infection, and should therefore be evaluated as thoroughly as hyperthermia.

II APPROACH TO THE PATIENT.
In many cases, the cause of the fever is clinically obvious; other times, fever can be the initial manifestation of an elusive illness. This chapter will provide you with a way to approach patients with recent onset of fever from an obscure source.

Chapter 84

A. **Patient history**
   1. **Immune status.** Is the patient immunocompromised (e.g., as a result of leukemia, chemotherapy, steroid use)?
   2. **Medical history.** Patients with a known illness may have a fever caused by their underlying illness (e.g., tumor fever from a lymphoma or a fever from a lupus flare); however, these patients often have superimposed infections, which always need to be systematically ruled out.
   3. **Medication history.** What prescription drugs is the patient taking? The medication history is aimed at discovering drugs that cause immunosuppression (e.g., steroids) and those that may result in drug fever (e.g., neuroleptics, anticholinergics, anesthetics, antibiotics).
   4. **Social history.** What is the patient's travel and sexual history? Is there a history of illicit drug use or other HIV risk factors? Positive answers may trigger a search for parasites, sexually transmitted diseases (STDs), abscesses or endocarditis, or HIV-related diseases.

HOT

Fever should be presumed to be secondary to an infection until proven otherwise, because infections cause the majority of fevers and can be life-threatening.

KEY

B. **Top to bottom approach.** One way of determining the infectious cause of a fever is to start at the patient's head and work your way down. Characteristic signs and symptoms (shown in parentheses) may increase your suspicion for the following disorders:
   1. **Meningitis** (headaches, neck stiffness, photophobia)
   2. **Sinusitis** (sinus tenderness)
   3. **Otitis** (ear pain, diminished hearing)
   4. **Pharyngitis** (sore throat, lymphadenopathy)
   5. **Pneumonia** (cough, pleurisy, dyspnea)
   6. **Endocarditis** (recent dental or other procedure, new skin lesions)
   7. **Abdominal processes** (pain, change in bowel habits, nausea or vomiting)
   8. **Urinary tract infection (UTI)** or **pyelonephritis** (dysuria, frequency, suprapubic or costovertebral angle tenderness)

9. **Pelvic infection** (discharge, dysuria)
10. **Prostatitis** (lower abdominal pain, tender prostate)
11. **Perirectal abscess** (pain, tenderness, swelling)
12. **Cellulitis** (erythema, pain, swelling)
13. **Joint infections** (pain, warmth, swelling)
14. **Local intravenous catheter site infection** (pain, pus)

HOT

In patients who have had broad-spectrum antibiotics and present with diarrhea, always consider *Clostridium difficile* colitis.

KEY

C. **Physical examination.** A complete physical examination is necessary. Pelvic and rectal examinations are useful for evaluating the possibility of pelvic inflammatory disease (PID), prostatitis, and perirectal abscesses as potential causes of fever.

D. **Laboratory studies.** The history and physical examination may provide you with enough information to make a diagnosis. Quite commonly, however, you may remain unsure about the etiology of the fever. The following laboratory tests will help you assess the likelihood of an infection, and may also help to localize the source.

1. **Complete blood count (CBC) with platelets**

   a. **Neutropenia** with fever is a medical emergency, and requires hospitalization and broad-spectrum antibiotics.

   b. **A leftward shifted white blood cell (WBC) count** often implies significant bacterial infection.

   c. **A low WBC count** may be just as worrisome as a high one. Patients with alcoholism, elderly patients, and immunocompromised patients may not have an elevated WBC count, even in the presence of a serious infection. On the other hand, African-American patients normally have WBC counts slightly below the given "normal" range.

2. **Electrolytes with blood urea nitrogen (BUN) and creatinine.** The presence of an anion gap may indicate sepsis.

3. **Prothrombin time (PT) and partial thromboplastin time (PTT).** Abnormal coagulation studies may indicate disseminated intravascular coagulation (DIC), a sign of serious infection.

4. Liver tests [e.g., bilirubin, alkaline phosphatase (AP), and transaminase levels] help evaluate the possibility of hepatobiliary disease (e.g., cholecystitis, ascending cholangitis, liver abscess, hepatitis).

5. Amylase levels may be helpful if pancreatitis is suspected.

6. Urinalysis should always be done to evaluate the possibility of UTI.

7. Urine pregnancy test. A pregnancy test should be considered in all women of childbearing age.

8. Cultures

    a. **Blood cultures** provide the gold standard for diagnosing endocarditis and bacteremia, and are therefore always required in intravenous drug users presenting with fever. Patients who require blood cultures are usually admitted for close follow-up.

    b. **Urine cultures** should be obtained whenever the fever is unexplained.

    c. **Sputum evaluation** may be useful for all patients with respiratory tract symptoms.

    d. **Throat culture** may be useful in patients with pharyngitis.

    e. **Cerebrospinal fluid (CSF) analysis** and **culture** is necessary in patients with meningeal symptoms or signs, altered mental status, or HIV infection and an unexplained fever.

    f. **Body fluid analysis** and **culture.** Patients with a fever accompanied by ascites, a pleural or joint effusion, or any other type of fluid collection need a diagnostic tap.

HOT

Patients who present with fever and rash should have a skin biopsy unless the diagnosis is straightforward.

KEY

E. Radiographs

    1. Chest. Posterior-anterior (PA) and lateral views should be taken on all patients with unexplained fever.

    2. Abdomen. Flat and upright views are useful when the patient has a fever and abdominal pain. Make sure to look for air-fluid levels, bowel distention, kidney stones, and free air.

F. **Ancillary studies.** If a diagnosis still has not been made, you need to consider the **easiest place for an infection to hide**—the **abdomen** and **pelvis.**

1. **Computed tomography (CT).** A CT scan is the best radiographic test in this situation. It provides a thorough evaluation of the intra-abdominal organs, and is more sensitive than ultrasound for detecting occult abscesses.

2. **Ultrasound.** Abdominal ultrasound is often inadequate for ruling out intra-abdominal abscesses and other pathology, but may be better than a CT scan for evaluating the gallbladder and bile ducts (e.g., for cholecystitis or ascending cholangitis).

3. **Other tests** (e.g., **bone marrow biopsy, indium** or **gallium scans, bone scans)** may be obtained if the cause of the fever is still in question.

 III **TREATMENT**

A. **General measures**

1. **Fluids.** Patients should be encouraged to increase their fluid intake to compensate for increased insensible losses.

2. **Discontinuation of medications.** Discontinuing medications that may be responsible for a fever can be both diagnostic and therapeutic.

3. **Antipyretic therapy. Acetaminophen** (325–650 mg every 4 hours) is the usual first-line therapy for a fever.

4. **Antibiotic therapy** is initiated when an infection is diagnosed. Empiric antibiotic therapy and close follow-up may also be indicated for patients with suspected infection.

HOT

If blood cultures are required (e.g., for a patient with suspected endocarditis), blood samples should be obtained before antibiotic therapy is initiated.

KEY

B. **Hospital admission** may be warranted when:

1. A potentially dangerous infection is suspected

2. The patient is elderly, immunocompromised, or has a complicating medical condition

3. The patient is dehydrated

IV FOLLOW-UP AND REFERRAL

A. **Follow-up.** Extremely close follow-up is required for out-patients with a fever.

B. **Referral**

1. **Infectious disease specialist.** Consultation with an infectious disease specialist should be considered at the start of an investigation for unexplained fever. All patients with an unexplained fever of 3 weeks duration should be evaluated by an infectious disease expert.

2. **Other specialists.** Referral to other specialists may be helpful, depending on the location of a known or suspected infection.

References

Arnow PM, Flaherty JP: Fever of unknown origin. *Lancet* 350(9077):575–580, 1997.

Dermatology

Dermatology

85. Approach to Skin Diseases

....

I **DESCRIBING DERMATOLOGIC LESIONS.** Using a systematic, 3-step approach to describe a dermatologic lesion enables classification of the lesion (thereby limiting the differential diagnosis) and facilitates communication with consultants and colleagues.

- **A.** First, classify the primary lesion, using Table 85-1. Major types of primary lesions include:
  1. **Macules** and **patches**
  2. **Papules** and **plaques**
  3. **Vesicles** and **bullae**
  4. **Pustules** and **cysts (abscesses)**
  5. **Nodules** and **tumors**
- **B.** Next, note any secondary changes (i.e., changes that occur after the primary lesion has appeared). Examples of secondary changes include:
  1. **Scale**
  2. **Crust**
  3. **Excoriation**
  4. **Erosion** (loss of the epidermis)
  5. **Ulceration** (loss of the epidermis and dermis)
- **C.** Once you have identified the type of lesion and noted any secondary changes, enhance the description by detailing the lesion's:
  1. **Size**
  2. **Color**
  3. **Shape**
  4. **Location on the body**
  5. **Distribution** (i.e., how the lesions are situated with respect to each other—grouped, linear, or dermatomal)

II **DIAGNOSIS AND TREATMENT OF COMMON DERMATOLOGIC LESIONS.** The causes, clinical findings, and treatments of common dermatologic lesions are summarized according to primary lesion type in Tables 85-2 through 85-8.

References
Fitzpatrick TB, Johnson RA, Polano MK, et al: *Color Atlas and Synopsis of Clinical Dermatology,* 3rd ed. New York, McGraw-Hill, 1996.
Lookingbill DP, Marks JG Jr: *Principles of Dermatology,* 2nd ed. Philadelphia, WB Saunders, 1993.

TABLE 85-1. Classification of Primary Dermatologic Lesions		
Appearance of Lesion	If the lesion is < 0.5 cm in diameter, then it is a:	If the lesion is > 0.5 cm in diameter, then it is a:
Flat and nonpalpable	Macule	Patch
Elevated and palpable	Papule	Plaque
Collection of clear fluid	Vesicle	Bulla
Collection of white or yellow fluid	Pustule	Cyst or abscess
Elevated and deep (subcutaneous)	Nodule	Tumor

TABLE 85-2. Causes, Clinical Findings, and Treatments for the Major Causes of Macules and Patches

Lesion	Cause	Clinical Findings	Treatment
Drug eruption	Side effect of various medications	Lesions are often maculo-papular, distributed on the truck, bright red, and confluent; lesions on the palms, soles, or mucosal surfaces are worrisome for severe reactions	Withdrawal of causative agent; oral antihistamines, topical steroids, or Sarna or calamine lotion for pruritus; hospitalization may be necessary for patients with severe reactions
Viral exanthem	Skin reaction to circulating virus	Erythematous macules and papules (usually less red and less confluent than those seen in drug reactions); systemic signs and symptoms of illness are also present	Sarna or calamine lotion or oral antihistamines for pruritus
Lentigo ("liver spots")	Sun exposure	Hyperpigmented or brown macules	Sunscreen; bleaching agents of limited benefit

continued

TABLE 85-2. Causes, Clinical Findings, and Treatments for the Major Causes of Macules and Patches

Lesion	Cause	Clinical Findings	Treatment
Urticaria ("hives")	Reaction to drugs, foods, physical agents (e.g., cold, sun, pressure), or stress	Transient but often recurrent wheals	Avoidance of causative agent; oral antihistamines
Erythema multiforme	HSV, drugs, Mycoplasma infection	"Target" lesion (dark center with a clear halo); dark ring often on palms	Acyclovir suppression for HSV; withdrawal of offending drug
"Toxic" erythema	Group A steptococci, Staphylococcus aureus, other (unknown) agents	Confluent, erythematous macules and fine ("sandpaper") papules, accentuated in skin folds, often involving the mucous membranes and usually not pruritic; patient appears ill	Antibiotic therapy for underlying bacterial infection

HSV = herpes simplex virus.

TABLE 85-3. Causes, Clinical Findings, and Treatments for the Major Causes of Papules*

Lesion	Cause	Clinical Findings	Treatment
Basal cell cancer	Sun exposure, radiation	Pearly, translucent papules, often with a rolled border[†] Often accompanied by telangiectasias	Biopsy or referral for excision
Squamous cell cancer	Sun exposure, toxic exposure	Face is a common location Indurated papules with scale or crust; nonhealing ulcers are also suspicious[‡] Sun-exposed surfaces are common locations	Biopsy or referral for excision
Scabies	*Sarcoptes scabiei* infection	Burrows in finger webs and on genitals; penile itching (in men) or breast itching (in women) is very suspicious; face is usually spared, except in immuno-compromised patients Eggs or mites on microscopic examination of a deep scraping of the papule confirms the diagnosis	Permethrin 5% cream applied to entire body from the neck down overnight and repeated in 1 week (treat close contacts as well) Oral antihistamines and topical steroids (itching often persists even after adequate treatment) Laundering of clothes and bedding in hot water or isolation in a plastic bag

*Drug eruption, viral exanthem, and "toxic" erythema can also be papular but are discussed in Table 85-2.
[†]Basal cell cancer may also be associated with nodules.
[‡]Squamous cell cancer may also be associated with plaques or nodules.

TABLE 85-4. Causes, Clinical Findings, and Treatments for the Major Causes of Plaques

Lesion	Cause	Clinical Findings	Treatment
Actinic (solar) keratosis*	Sun exposure	Rough, dry, "sandpaper-like" lesions; sometimes easier to palpate the lesion than to see it	Liquid nitrogen; if lesions are extensive, consider flourouracil 5% cream twice daily for 1–2 weeks (lesions will become eryhematous, then gradually resolve)
Atopic dermatitis	Unclear; associated with a history of hay fever, asthma, allergic rhinitis, or stress	Pruritic inflammation of the skin (excoriation can place patients at risk for developing staphylococcal or viral skin infections) Erythema and scale usually occur on the flexor surfaces of the skin Skin lines become accentuated or lichenified	Topical steroids, oral antihistamines, moisturizers, and avoidance of soap and hot water
Contact dermatitis	External allergen	Travel and work history may be significant; inquire about toiletries and exposure to common cleaning solutions	Avoidance of causative agent Topical steroids; if the lesions are extensive, consider a short course of oral steroids (7–10 days)
Psoriasis	Unknown; believed to be hereditary	Silver scale, commonly located on the extensor surfaces, in the gluteal fold, and at sites of minor trauma Nail pitting Arthritis may be present	Topical steroids, tar solutions, or vitamin D preparations (e.g., calcipotriene) Refer to dermatologist for oral agents or light therapy if psoriasis is extensive

Seborrheic dermatitis	Unknown	Chronic scaling and erythema; most active in the distribution of the sebaceous glands of the face	Combined therapy with a low-potency steroid cream and an antifungal cream can be tried; Anti-dandruff shampoo for scalp
Seborrheic keratosis†	Unknown	Benign skin growth with a "stuck on" appearance; incidence increases with age†	Curettage or liquid nitrogen
Tinea	Fungal infection (dermatophytes)	Annular lesions with raised borders and central clearing; Fine scale at edge (or border) of lesion; Scrapings of scale from the border of the lesion show hyphae or budding cells on KOH preparation	Topical antifungal agents; a systemic antifungal agent (e.g., griseofulvin, 500 mg orally daily for 4–6 weeks) may be used for severe or extensive infections and infections of the scalp or face
Xerosis (severe dry skin)	Aging skin, various oral medications (especially anticholesterol drugs)	Common in the elderly and during the winter; skin is often scaly, itchy, and erythematous; often seen on the legs	Moisturizers, low-potency steroids, and avoidance of hot water and soap

KOH = potassium hydroxide.
*Actinic keratosis may also be associated with papules; it may be a precursor to squamous cell cancer.
†Seborrheic keratosis may also be associated with pigmented lesions.

TABLE 85-5. Causes, Clinical Findings, and Treatments for the Major Causes of Vesicles and Bullae

Lesion	Cause	Clinical Findings	Treatment
Impetigo	*Streptococcus, Staphylococcus*	Honey-colored crust	Appropriate systemic antibiotic (e.g., dicloxacillin, first-generation cephalosporin), or topical mupirocin
Herpes simplex	Herpes simplex virus (HSV), types 1 and 2	Multinucleated giant cells on a Tzanck smear confirms the diagnosis	Oral acyclovir (400 mg three times daily, or 200 mg five times daily, for 10 days) for first episodes and the early treatment of recurrent disease; consider intravenous acyclovir for patients with disseminated disease and immunocompromised patients
Herpes zoster	Varicella zoster virus	Dermatomal distribution is classic	Acyclovir (800 mg orally five times daily for 7–10 days, if given within 3 days of the appearance of the lesion); consider intravenous acyclovir for immuno-compromised patients with severe disease

TABLE 85-6. Causes, Clinical Findings, and Treatments for the Major Causes of Pustules and Cysts

Lesion	Cause	Clinical Findings	Treatment
Acne (disorder of the pilosebaceous units leading to increased sebum production, follicular obstruction, bacterial proliferation, and inflammation)	Multifactorial (abnormal keratinization, overgrowth of *Propionibacterium acnes*, hormones, abnormal inflammatory response to *P. acnes*)	Noninflammatory lesions (i.e., comedones, also known as "whiteheads," and "blackheads") Inflammatory lesions (i.e., pustules, papules, nodules, and cysts); may lead to scarring Hirsutism and irregular menses in women may indicate an endocrine abnormality Medication history may reveal corticosteroid use	Noninflammatory/ comedonal acne: Benzoyl peroxide 5% and/or retin A 0.025% cream to start (retin A should be used at night to avoid photosensitivity); topical antibiotic may be added if the patient has mild inflammatory lesions Inflammatory acne: Oral antibiotics (e.g., tetracycline or erythromycin, 500 mg twice daily or minocycline, 50–100 mg twice daily) Nodulocystic acne: Referral to a dermatologist for isotretinoin (Accutane) therapy

continued

TABLE 85-6. Causes, Clinical Findings, and Treatments for the Major Causes of Pustules and Cysts

Lesion	Cause	Clinical Findings	Treatment
Folliculitis (inflammation of the hair follicle)	*Staphylococcus* infection most common cause *Pseudomonas* infection ("hot tub" folliculitis)	Follicularly based pustules, commonly in areas of friction	Systemic antibiotics (e.g., dicloxacillin, 250 mg four times daily or cefazolin, 500 mg four times daily)
Rosacea (inflammation of the sebaceous glands of the face)*	Unknown	Telangiectasias, inflammatory papules and pustules Seen in middle-aged and elderly patients Symptoms are worsened by flushing, alcohol, and spicy foods	Topical metronidazole gel or clindamycin twice daily Systemic tetracycline or erythromycin, 500 mg twice daily

*Can lead to rhinophyma.

TABLE 85-7. Causes, Clinical Findings, and Treatments for the Major Causes of Nodules			
Lesion	Cause	Clinical Findings	Treatment
Calluses (thickening of the epidermis)	Friction and pressure	Skin lines seen across the lesion	Relieve pressure and friction
Keloid (excessive tissue growth or repair)	Trauma	Core visible when the lesion is pared Young African-Americans affected most often	Intralesional corticosteroid injections (e.g., triamcinolone, 10 mg/ml) may help lesions regress
Warts	Papillomavirus infection	Skin lines not seen across the lesion Red-brown or black dots visible when the lesion is pared	Liquid nitrogen, salicylic acid, podophyllin

TABLE 85-8. Causes, Clinical Findings, and Treatments for the Major Causes of Pigmented Lesions

Lesion	Cause	Clinical Findings	Treatment
Malignant melanoma	Malignant transformation and growth of melanocytes	**A**symmetry **B**order irregular **C**olor irregular **D**iameter greater than 0.6 cm (but any enlarging lesion is suspicious)	Referral to a dermatologist for excision
Nevi (moles)	Unknown	< 5 mm well circumscribed defined border, single shade (beige to brown)	No treatment necessary

86. Pruritus

I **INTRODUCTION.** Itching can be caused by a variety of dermatologic and non-dermatologic disorders.

A. **Dermatologic disorders.** Itching is a very common symptom of dermatologic disorders. Skin lesions are usually present when a dermatologic disorder is the cause of the itching.

B. **Systemic disorders.** When no lesions are present, the itching is often caused by a systemic disorder. Fifteen percent of patients with itching but without skin lesions have a systemic disorder diagnosed at initial presentation.

II **CAUSES OF PRURITUS**

A. **Dermatologic disorders**

1. **Xerosis (dry skin)** is a very common cause.
2. **Infestation** (e.g., scabies, pediculosis) and **insect bites** cause pruritus.
3. Other causes include **urticaria, atopic** or **contact dermatitis, superficial fungal infections, drug reactions, sunburn, dermatitis herpetiformis, fiberglass dermatitis, lichen planus,** and **folliculitis.**

B. **Systemic disorders**

1. **Uremia** is the most common cause of pruritus when lesions are not present.
2. **Total bilirubin elevation** as a result of primary biliary cirrhosis, extrahepatic biliary obstruction, and cholestatic drugs can cause pruritus.
3. **Cancer.** Neoplasms that cause pruritus include lymphoma (especially Hodgkin's disease) and breast, lung, and stomach cancer.
4. **Hematologic disorders.** Polycythemia vera (and the other myeloproliferative disorders) and iron deficiency anemia can cause pruritus.
5. **Endocrine disorders** (e.g., diabetes mellitus, hyper- and hypothyroidism, carcinoid syndrome) can cause pruritus.

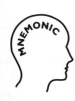

Causes of Pruritus ("ITCHED")

Infestation (e.g., scabies)
Total bilirubin elevation (e.g., primary biliary cirrhosis)
Chronic renal failure (uremia) or **C**ancer
Hematologic disorders
Endocrine disorders
Dry skin or other dermatologic disorders

III APPROACH TO THE PATIENT

A. Patient history. A detailed history focusing on medications, other medical conditions, travel, hobbies, occupation, and the presence of constitutional symptoms (e.g., weight loss, fever) is very useful.

1. The itching associated with Hodgkin's disease is often described as a "burning" sensation, especially on the lower extremities.

2. Patients with scabies usually describe worsening of their pruritus at night.

3. Polycythemia vera is often associated with a "prickly" itch that usually occurs as the patient cools off after bathing.

4. Xerosis is common in the elderly, especially when the heater is turned on during the winter months.

B. Physical examination

1. A thorough dermatologic examination, focusing on the presence of burrows (due to scabies), plate-like scaling (due to xerosis), or any other dermatologic lesions should be performed.

HOT KEY

The dermatologic lesions are often missed on examination of patients with scabies, insect bites, dermatitis herpetiformis, or chronic urticaria.

2. If no obvious skin cause is found, examination of the abdomen (to look for hepatosplenomegaly) and the peripheral lymph nodes is necessary.

C. Laboratory and imaging studies. If the history and examination are not revealing, a **complete blood count (CBC)**

with **platelets; alkaline phosphatase (AP), bilirubin, thyroid-stimulating hormone (TSH),** and **creatinine levels;** and a **chest radiograph** should be considered. **Biopsy** of the pruritic skin should also be considered for those with persistent symptoms without an obvious cause.

IV **TREATMENT** of the specific cause is, of course, the optimal management.

A. **Discontinue** drugs that may cause the release of histamine [e.g., opiates, nonsteroidal anti-inflammatory drugs (NSAIDs)] if possible.

B. **Antihistamines.** Hydroxyzine (25–50 mg orally every 4–6 hours) or loratadine (10 mg orally daily) may provide symptomatic relief.

C. **Doxepin cream 5%** may be applied to the affected areas as needed.

D. **Ultraviolet light B** (at suberythema doses, 2–3 times per week for 4 weeks) may be helpful for patients with renal failure or biliary obstruction.

E. If the cause of the pruritus is not evident, try treating for xerosis by prescribing a 2-week course of **emollients** (e.g., Aquaphor) and the use of a **mild soap** (e.g., Dove).

V **FOLLOW-UP AND REFERRAL**

A. Patients who have pruritus of unknown cause and who do not respond to treatment for xerosis or symptomatic treatment should be referred to a dermatologist.

B. Patients who continue to itch despite extensive evaluation should be seen 2–4 times per year. Pay particular attention to the dermatologic examination (look for evidence of lesions) and examination of the lymph nodes, liver, and spleen (look for enlargement, which could indicate malignancy).

References

Kam PC, Tan KH: Pruritus—itching for a cause and relief? *Anaesthesia* 51(12):1133–1138, 1996.

Millikan LE: Treating pruritus. What's new in safe relief of symptoms? *Postgrad Med* 99(1):173–176, 179–184, 1996.

87. Palpable Purpura

··

I | **PALPABLE PURPURA** represents blood that is no longer confined to the vessel; therefore, this rash is raised (palpable) and does not blanch with pressure (purpura). Palpable purpura is usually confined to the lower extremities and is usually caused by one of two disorders:

A. **Severe thrombocytopenia** (i.e., a platelet count less than 20,000 cells/μl)

B. **Vasculitis** (i.e., a diverse group of diseases characterized by inflammation of the blood vessel wall, leading to ischemia and tissue necrosis)

II | **VASCULITIS.** This chapter focuses on the vasculitic causes of palpable purpura, which are usually more difficult to diagnose than the thrombocytopenic causes. (see chapter 71)

A. **Pathogenesis.** The pathogenesis of vasculitis is shown in Figure 87-1.

B. **Classification.** The classification of vasculitis is confusing and controversial because there is considerable overlap among the different vasculitides, and because the underlying cause of the vasculitis is usually unknown. One useful and clinically oriented classification scheme is based on determining the predominant clinical manifestations of the disease.

    1. If **systemic manifestations predominate,** the patient probably has a predominantly **systemic vasculitis** (Table 87-1). The systemic vasculitides can be grouped into five major categories.

        a. **Systemic necrotizing vasculitides**

            (1) **Classic polyarteritis nodosa (PAN).** The musculoskeletal system, kidneys, central and peripheral nervous systems, gastrointestinal system, skin, and heart are affected, but the lungs are usually spared.

            (2) **Churg-Strauss syndrome** is similar to PAN, except the lungs are usually involved and peripheral eosinophilia is present. Churg-Strauss syndrome is often associated with asthma.

        b. **Wegener's granulomatosis** is a granulomatous vasculitis of the upper and lower respiratory tracts combined with glomerulonephritis.

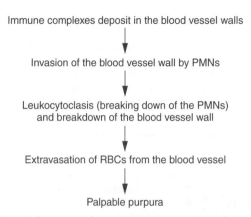

Immune complexes deposit in the blood vessel walls

⬇

Invasion of the blood vessel wall by PMNs

⬇

Leukocytoclasis (breaking down of the PMNs)
and breakdown of the blood vessel wall

⬇

Extravasation of RBCs from the blood vessel

⬇

Palpable purpura

FIGURE 87-1. Pathogenesis of vasculitis. *PMNs* = polymorphonuclear
neutrophils; *RBCs* = red blood cells.

TABLE 87-1. Systemic Manifestations of Vasculitides

Constitutional symptoms (e.g., fever, fatigue, weight loss, anorexia)
Musculoskeletal symptoms (e.g., arthritis, arthralgias, proximal
muscle pain)
Symptoms from organ ischemia (e.g., abdominal pain)
Symptoms suggestive of pulmonary, renal, or nervous system
involvement (e.g., hemoptysis, dyspnea, dark urine, peripheral
edema, peripheral neuropathy)

c. **Temporal arteritis** usually involves the temporal
artery or another branch of the carotid artery and
is seen in patients older than 50 years. Headache,
jaw claudication, and an elevated erythrocyte sedimentation rate (ESR) are characteristic. Temporal arteritis may be associated with polymyalgia
rheumatica.

d. **Takayasu's aortitis** primarily involves the aortic
arch and its branches. The typical patient is a
young Asian woman. Pulselessness on examination is classic.

e. **Miscellaneous systemic vasculitides** include
Kawasaki syndrome and Behçet's syndrome.
Some authors include Schönlein-Henoch purpura

(especially when it occurs in pediatric patients) in this category.

2. If **cutaneous manifestations predominate,** the patient probably has predominantly **cutaneous vasculitis** (also known as hypersensitivity vasculitis, leukocytoclastic vasculitis, or secondary vasculitis). Predominantly cutaneous vasculitis is associated with many diseases or agents (hence the name "secondary vasculitis").

Secondary Causes of Vasculitis ("VASCULITIS")

Various drugs
Autoimmune disorders
Serum sickness
Cryoglobulinemia
Ulcerative colitis
Low complement
Infections
Tumor
IgA deposition
Smoking-related (thromboangiitis obliterans)

---

a. **Various drugs.** Allopurinol, sulfa drugs, penicillins are just a few of many drugs that can cause a hypersensitivity vasculitis.

b. **Autoimmune disorders.** Systemic lupus erythematosus (SLE) and rheumatoid arthritis may cause a vasculitis.

c. **Serum sickness** occurs approximately 1 week after exposure to an antigen and is characterized by fever and arthralgias.

d. **Cryoglobulinemia** is characterized by immunoglobulins that precipitate in cold temperatures. Clinical manifestations may include arthralgias, hepatosplenomegaly, and glomerulonephritis.

e. **Ulcerative colitis** is occasionally associated with a secondary vasculitis.

f. **Low complement (hypocomplementemic urticarial vasculitis)** occurs most often in young women. All serum complement levels are low.

g. **Infections.** Endocarditis, meningococcemia, *Neisseria gonorrhoeae* infection, infectious mononucleosis, hepatitis B or C, and Rocky Mountain spotted fever may be associated with a vasculitis.

TABLE 87-2 Evaluation of Various Vasculitides

Type of Vasculitis	Diagnostic Studies
Predominantly systemic	
Classic PAN	p-ANCA, angiogram, biopsy of involved organs
Churg-Strauss syndrome	p-ANCA, eosinophil count, lung biopsy
Wegener's granulomatosis	c-ANCA, biopsy of involved organs
Temporal arteritis	ESR, temporal artery biopsy
Takayasu's aortitis	Arteriogram
Predominantly cutaneous	
Various drugs	History, resolution on discontinuation of drug
Auto-immune	ANA, RF
Serum sickness	Serum complement levels
Cryoglobulinemia	Cryoglobulin levels
Ulcerative colitis	Colonoscopy with biopsy
Low complement	Serum complement levels
Infection	Blood cultures, hepatitis B and C serologies
Tumor	Serum protein electrophoresis, CT scan, biopsy of node or bone marrow
IgA deposition	Biopsy of skin or kidney (IgA staining)
Smoking-related	History, resolution on smoking cessation

ANA = antineutrophil antibody; c-ANCA = cytoplasmic staining antineutrophil cytoplasmic antibody; p-ANCA = perinuclear staining antineutrophil cytoplasmic antibody; CT = computed tomography; ESR = erythrocyte sedimentation rate; PAN = polyarteritis nodosa; RF = rheumatoid factor.

---

   h. **Tumor. Lymphoma** and **multiple myeloma** are the malignancies most often associated with vasculitis.

   i. **IgA deposition** may result in Schönlein-Henoch purpura or IgA nephropathy. Schönlein-Henoch purpura is rare in adults (peak age is 6 years) and is characterized by palpable purpura (present in almost 100% of patients), arthralgias, gastrointestinal symptoms (e.g., nausea, vomiting, pain, bleeding), and renal findings (e.g., hematuria, proteinuria).

    j. Smoking-related. Thromboangiitis obliterans occurs predominantly in men younger than 40 years who are heavy smokers.

C. Approach to the patient with vasculitis

    1. Obtain skin biopsy results to confirm that a vasculitis is present. Usually, patients are referred emergently to a dermatologist for a skin biopsy.

    2. Determine the underlying cause. After obtaining a complete patient history (including a review of systems and medications) and performing a thorough physical examination, order routine laboratory tests [i.e., a complete blood count (CBC), a serum chemistry panel, and urinalysis]. Further testing can help diagnose a particular disease (Table 87-2).

D. Treatment of vasculitis depends on the underlying disorder.

E. Follow-up and referral. Palpable purpura usually represents a medical emergency. Often, patients are admitted to the hospital for expeditious evaluation. Follow-up depends on the underlying disease and the recommendations made by the consultants (i.e., a dermatologist, rheumatologist, or both). In general, patients should be seen frequently until symptoms abate or the underlying cause is determined.

References

Decleva I, Marzano AV, Barbareschi M, et al: Cutaneous manifestations in systemic vasculitis. *Clin Rev Allergy Immunol* 15(1):5–20, 1997.

Hunder G: Vasculitis: diagnosis and therapy. *Am J Med* 100(2A):37S-45S, 1996.

Watts RA, Scott DG: Vasculitis. *Baillieres Clin Rheumatol* 9(3):529–554, 1995.

PART XIV

Psychiatry

88. Depression

I INTRODUCTION

A. Depression is **extremely common:** the lifetime incidence of major depression is 10% in men and 20% in women.

B. In the medical setting, the **diagnosis** of depression is **missed in 30%–50% of patients.**

C. **Risk factors** for depression include:
1. Age 35–45 years in women, or greater than 55 years in men
2. Female gender
3. Personal or family history of depression
4. Presence of a serious medical condition
5. Presence of social stressors and a lack of social support
6. Substance abuse (e.g., alcoholism)

II CLINICAL MANIFESTATIONS OF DEPRESSION.
Patients may present in many different ways, which may account for the high incidence of missed diagnoses. The following findings may suggest depression:

A. **Weight loss** (especially common in elderly patients)
B. **Unkempt appearance**
C. **Irritable or depressed affect**
D. **Vagueness**
E. **Anxiety**
F. **Multiple somatic complaints**
G. **Failure of appropriate treatment regimen for a medical illness**

III DIFFERENTIAL DIAGNOSIS

HOT

KEY

Depression may coexist with most of the conditions in the differential diagnosis.

A. **Psychiatric disorders**
1. Other mood disorders, such as dysthymia or bipolar disorder

  2. Anxiety disorder
  3. Personality disorder, especially borderline or obsessive-compulsive disorder
B. Normal bereavement. Approximately 5% of patients with normal bereavement may develop a mood disorder.
C. Neurologic disorders
  1. Parkinson's disease
  2. Cerebrovascular disease
  3. Seizure disorder
  4. Dementia
  5. Head trauma
D. Substance abuse
E. Endocrine disorders (e.g., thyroid or adrenal disorders)
F. Medications
  1. Corticosteroids or hormone replacement therapy (HRT)
  2. Antihypertensives
  3. Analgesics, especially narcotics
  4. Any drugs acting on the central nervous system (CNS)

IV APPROACH TO THE PATIENT

A. Establish the diagnosis
  1. The diagnosis of depression is made using the *Diagnostic and Statistical Manual of Mental Disorders,* 4th edition (DSM-IV) diagnostic criteria. The mnemonic "1, 2, 3, 4, 5" can help you remember how to diagnose depression.

Diagnosis of Depression ("1, 2, 3, 4, 5")

1 of the following **2** criteria must be present:
    Depressed mood
    Anhedonia
3 thought disturbances
    Suicidal ideation
    Decreased concentration
    Guilt
4 physical symptoms
    Insomnia
    Decreased energy or fatigue
    Psychomotor agitation or retardation
    Weight loss or gain
5 total criteria must be present

2. Make sure to rule out other psychiatric and medical conditions and evaluate whether certain medications or substance abuse may be contributing to the illness.

B. Assess the patient's risk factors for suicide

1. **Most patients who complete suicide do so on their first or second attempt.** Patients who have a history of attempting suicide (e.g., more than 4 or 5 previous attempts) are more likely to attempt suicide in the future, but are much less likely to succeed. This pattern may indicate an underlying personality disorder.

2. **Asking patients about suicidal ideation does not lead patients to commit suicide; rather, it identifies patients at risk.** The risk factors for committing suicide can be remembered by the mnemonic, "SAD PERSONS."

Risk Factors for Committing Suicide ("SAD PERSONS")

Sex (male:female ratio = 4:1)
Age (older white men at greatest risk)
Depression (70% of suicides follow a depressive episode)

Previous attempts
ETOH use
Rational thinking loss (cognitive slowing, psychotic depression, pre-existing organic brain disease)
Social support deficit
Organized plan
No spouse
Sicknesses (especially post-myocardial infarction)

V **TREATMENT.** Seventy percent of patients with major depression improve with initial treatment. However, a single episode may last for 2 years or longer, and relapses occur in most patients.

A. Selective serotonin reuptake inhibitors (SSRIs) are the most commonly prescribed medications for major depression, given their relatively benign side effect profiles, and few untoward effects in patients who attempt to overdose.

1. **Agents** (Table 88-1). Although fluoxetine has been around the longest, sertraline and paroxetine have

TABLE 88-1. Selective Serotonin Reuptake Inhibitors (SSRIs)

Generic Name	Brand Name	Advantages	Disadvantages	Dosing
Paroxetine	Paxil	Most sedating Shortest half-life	May cause withdrawal symptoms if discontinued abruptly	**Starting dose:** 10 mg daily in elderly patients, 20 mg daily otherwise **Maximum dose:** 40 mg daily
Sertraline	Zoloft	Less activating than fluoxetine; less sedating than paroxetine Least inhibition of cytochrome p-450 system	Most gastrointestinal side effects	**Starting dose:** 25 mg daily in elderly patients; 50 mg daily otherwise **Maximum dose:** 150–200 mg daily
Fluoxetine	Prozac	Most activating May decrease appetite	May cause insomnia or jitteriness Long half-life Most inhibition of the cytochrome P-450 system	**Starting dose:** 10 mg daily in elderly patients; 20 mg daily otherwise **Maximum dose:** 40 mg daily

fewer side effects and drug interactions and are therefore preferred.

    a. **Sertraline** is the best-tolerated SSRI.

    b. **Paroxetine,** which has sedating properties, can be used in patients whose predominant symptoms include agitated depression or insomnia.

  2. **Side effects.** The most common side effects of SSRIs include **gastrointestinal problems** (e.g., nausea, vomiting, diarrhea) and **sexual dysfunction** (e.g., decreased libido, erectile dysfunction). SSRIs also inhibit the cytochrome P-450 system and therefore **may affect warfarin, phenytoin,** and **tricyclic antidepressant levels.**

HOT KEY

Achieving the maximal antidepressive effect may take 4–6 weeks with SSRIs. Patients should be made aware of this delayed effect so that they do not stop taking the medication prematurely.

B. **Tricyclic antidepressants,** which are inexpensive and very effective, have been available for many years. Patients who have agitated depression or concomitant neuropathic pain may benefit the most from tricyclic antidepressants.

  1. **Agents** (Table 88-2)

    a. **Amitriptyline** is the most well-recognized of the tricyclic antidepressants, but its anticholinergic side effects are poorly tolerated.

    b. **Nortriptyline** and **desipramine** are equally as efficacious as amitriptyline, both for use as antidepressant as well as for the treatment of neuropathic pain. These agents should be used in favor of amitriptyline.

  2. **Side effects.** Because the side effect profile is daunting (especially in elderly patients) and there is a narrow therapeutic index, tricyclic antidepressants are generally favored less than SSRIs for the treatment of depression.

C. **Atypical antidepressants** are summarized in Table 88-3.

TABLE 88-2. Tricyclic Antidepressants

Generic Name	Brand name	Advantages	Disadvantages	Dosing
Nortriptyline	Pamelor	Associated with least orthostasis	Anticholinergic effects	**Starting dose:** 25 mg daily **Maximum dose:** 150–200 mg daily
Desipramine	Norpramin	Twice as potent as other tricyclic antidepressants Least sedating Least anticholinergic	Can be activating; can cause insomnia	**Starting dose:** 50 mg daily **Maximum dose:** 200–300 mg daily
Amitriptyline	Elavil	. . .	Highly anticholinergic	**Starting dose:** 50 mg daily **Maximum dose:** 200–300 mg daily

TABLE 88-3. Atypical Antidepressants

Generic Name	Brand Name	Mechanism	Advantages	Disadvantages	Dosing
Trazodone	Desyrel	Serotonin reuptake inhibitor	Highly sedating Well-tolerated by elderly patients and patients with post-traumatic stress disorder Difficult to overdose	Can cause orthostasis or priapism Therapeutic levels difficult to achieve due to sedative qualities	**Starting dose:** 50 mg at bedtime **Maximum dose:** 400–600 mg daily divided doses
Bupropion	Wellbutrin	Weak dopamine and norepine-phrine inhibitor	No anticholinergic side effects Good for patients older than 65 years Few side effects	Contraindicated in patients with organic brain disease or seizure disorder	**Starting dose:** 75 mg twice daily (150 mg once daily if using slow-release formula) **Maximum dose:** 150 mg three times daily (150 mg twice daily if using slow-release formula)

continued

TABLE 88-3. Atypical Antidepressants

Generic Name	Brand Name	Mechanism	Advantages	Disadvantages	Dosing
Nefazodone	Serzone	Serotonin receptor antagonist and reuptake inhibitor	Low incidence of sexual side effects Less sedation and orthostasis than with trazodone Difficult to overdose	Inhibition of the cytochrome P-450 system	**Starting dose:** 100 mg twice daily **Maximum dose:** 150–250 mg twice daily
Venlafaxine	Effexor	Serotonin and norepinephrine reuptake inhibitor	Can be activating Mild side effect profile Low incidence of sexual side effects	Can cause dose-dependent increases in blood pressure	**Starting dose:** 37.5 mg twice daily **Maximum dose:** 375 mg daily in divided doses

HOT

KEY

Bupropion has also been approved by the Food and Drug Administration (FDA) as an aid for smoking cessation.

D. **Monoamine oxidase (MAO) inhibitors** are rarely used in the primary care setting because of the absolute need for adherence to the regimen and the possibility of causing a hypertensive crisis in the presence of sympathomimetics. MAO inhibitors include isocarboxazid (Marplan), tranylcypromine (Parnate), and phenelzine (Nardil).

E. **Psychostimulants** are typically prescribed by psychiatrists for terminally ill patients. These agents include dextroamphetamine (Dexedrine) and methylphenidate (Ritalin).

VI FOLLOW-UP AND REFERRAL

A. **Follow-up**
   1. Patients receiving pharmacologic therapy should be seen every 1–4 weeks. Medication should be maintained for 9–12 months; at this point, tapering of the dose may be tried.
   2. Most patients eventually relapse; if this occurs, a second 1-year trial can be undertaken. A second relapse usually indicates the need for lifelong medical therapy.

B. **Referral** to a psychiatrist is indicated for patients with an unclear diagnosis or psychotic features, and for patients who fail treatment or may require atypical therapy. Patients who may be at risk for suicide should undergo immediate psychiatric evaluation.

References

Lebowitz BD, Pearson JL, Schneider LS, et al: Diagnosis and treatment of depression in late life: consensus statement update. *JAMA* 278(14):1186–1190, 1997.

Preskorn SH, Baker BS: Outpatient management of the depressed patient. *Dis Mon* 41(2):73–140, 1995.

89. Alcohol Abuse and Dependence

I INTRODUCTION

A. Alcohol abuse and dependence are extremely common, with a lifetime prevalence approaching 15%.
   1. One hundred thousand Americans die each year from complications of alcohol use.
   2. Almost 25% of Americans say that drinking has been a source of trouble in their families.
B. Alcohol abuse and dependence are often underdiagnosed and undertreated, despite the fact that effective treatment is available.

II CLINICAL MANIFESTATIONS.

The patient, or one of his family members or friends, may express concern about health or behavioral problems related to drinking. Often, however, the discussion is not patient-initiated; therefore, the physician should be aware of social issues and medical complications that may become apparent during the office visit and could suggest alcohol abuse.

A. **Social issues**
   1. Arrests for driving while intoxicated, fighting, or other behaviors associated with alcohol use
   2. Absence from work or loss of jobs due to drinking
   3. Relationship problems
   4. Repeated bouts of intoxication and "blackouts"
B. **Medical complications.** Many medical complications can result from excessive alcohol use. Some of the most common are:
   1. **Gastrointestinal disorders** (e.g., gastritis, hepatitis, cirrhosis, esophageal varices, hepatoma, pancreatitis, malabsorption)
   2. **Neurologic disorders** (e.g., ataxia, peripheral neuropathy, Wernicke's encephalopathy, dementia)
   3. **Cardiovascular disorders** (e.g., hypertension, tachycardia, cardiomyopathy)
   4. **Hematologic disorders** (e.g., anemia, thrombocytopenia)
   5. **Endocrine disorders** (e.g., hypoglycemia, ketoacidosis, hypokalemia, hyponatremia)
   6. **Trauma** (e.g., automobile accidents, falls, domestic violence)

PATTERNS OF USE. A drink is defined as 1 ounce (30 ml) of distilled alcohol (e.g., brandy, gin, rum, vodka, whiskey), 4 ounces of wine, or 12 ounces of beer.

   A. Low-risk. These patients have fewer than 1–2 drinks per day (less than 1 drink per day in women and people older than 65 years) and no more than 3–4 drinks per occasion. They practice abstinence in high-risk situations (e.g., when pregnant, before driving, or when taking medications that should not be taken with alcohol).

   B. High-risk. For men, "high risk" is defined as more than 14 drinks per week, or more than 4 drinks per occasion. For women, the definition is more than 7 drinks per week, or more than 3 drinks per occasion.

   C. Alcohol abuse. A patient can be said to have a "drinking problem" if any of the following criteria are met:
      1. The patient has been arrested for driving while intoxicated
      2. The patient has experienced impaired social functioning or disrupted relationships with friends and family as a result of alcohol use
      3. The patient has lost a job as a result of alcohol use

   D. Alcohol dependence. These patients are dependent on alcohol and meet at least three of the following seven *Diagnostic and Statistical Manual of Mental Disorders,* 4th edition (DSM-IV) criteria for substance dependence:
      1. They drink more than they intend
      2. They have a persistent desire to drink, or have been unsuccessful in attempts to stop drinking
      3. They spend a significant amount of time procuring alcohol
      4. They have given up social and occupational activities because of alcohol
      5. They drink despite physical or psychological problems
      6. They exhibit tolerance (a sign of physical dependence)
      7. They exhibit withdrawal (a sign of physical dependence)

 APPROACH TO THE PATIENT. All patients should be screened for alcohol use, given the high prevalence of alcohol use and the proven effectiveness of intervention. All three of the following screening techniques should be implemented:

A. **Engage the patient in a discussion regarding his use of alcohol** with questions such as "Do you drink alcohol? If not, what made you decide not to drink?" or "Please tell me about your use of alcohol."

B. **Use the CAGE questionnaire,** a simple and well-validated screening tool for the detection of alcohol abuse.

Screening Questions for the Detection of Alcohol Abuse ("CAGE")

Cut down on your drinking?
Annoyed by others?
Guilty about drinking?
Eye-opener to counteract a hangover?

1. Have you ever felt that you should cut down on your drinking?
2. Have people annoyed you by criticizing your drinking?
3. Have you ever felt guilty about drinking?
4. Have you ever needed an eye-opener in the morning to calm your nerves or to get rid of a hangover?

C. **Ask questions about the patient's pattern of use.**
   1. How many drinks do you have in an average week?
   2. On a typical day, how many drinks do you have?
   3. What is the maximum number of drinks that you have had on any occasion in the past month?

HOT

Because alcohol abuse and dependence are highly associated with depression and anxiety, care should be taken to diagnose and initiate treatment for depression.

KEY

 V TREATMENT

HOT

Much of the strategy used to help patients reduce or quit drinking applies to patients with other types of substance abuse disorders as well.

KEY

A. Counseling. Although not all patients with a positive screening test have an alcohol abuse disorder, all patients with a positive screening test should receive counseling about alcohol use and its associated problems. Brief counseling interventions (e.g., lasting 5–15 minutes) are associated with a two-fold decrease in alcohol consumption by heavy drinkers. Counseling "FRAMES" an effective cessation program.

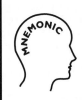

Counseling for Heavy Drinkers ("FRAMES")

Feedback about screening results
Responsibility for change with patient
Advice regarding consumption goals
Menu of options for reducing alcohol consumption
Empathy
Self-efficacy (patient empowerment)

---

1. **Provide feedback about screening results**
   a. Be straightforward and nonjudgmental.
   b. State your concerns about the potential or actual detrimental effects of drinking on the patient's health.
   c. Use neutral, nonstigmatizing language (e.g., avoid labels such as "alcoholic" or "addict").
2. **Educate the patient about safe consumption limits (or abstinence).** Most high-risk or heavy drinkers do not realize that they are using alcohol abnormally. Clearly state your recommendations regarding consumption goals (e.g., "I recommend that you limit your alcohol use to 1–2 drinks per day" or "I don't think it is safe for you to drink any alcohol.")
3. **Provide a "menu" of options for reducing alcohol consumption.** Ask the patient what measures she thinks will work. Possibilities include:
   a. Set a date to quit drinking or reduce the amount of alcohol consumed
   b. Keep a diary
   c. Make a written agreement
   d. Enlist help from an alcohol or substance abuse counselor
   e. Attend group counseling sessions
   f. Join a self-help program, such as Alcoholics Anonymous
   g. Enroll in an inpatient detoxification program

    4. Provide empathy and encouragement. Support the patient's efforts by letting him know that you understand the difficulties involved. Empower the patient by helping him to realize that he can change (e.g., "I'm impressed by your motivation to stop drinking. Your resolve will help you reach this goal.")

B. Outpatient pharmacotherapy

  1. General considerations

    a. Eligibility for outpatient treatment. Patients may exhibit impaired short-term memory, poor judgement, and decreased motor skills while undergoing detoxification. In order for patients to be successful with outpatient treatment, they should have all of the following:

      (1) A network of family and friends to provide psychological support

      (2) No history of severe withdrawal symptoms, severe alcohol dependence, or other drug use

      (3) A willingness to avoid driving and operating heavy machinery

      (4) The ability to attend a day treatment program or an intensive outpatient substance abuse treatment program

    b. Contraindications to outpatient treatment include the following:

      (1) A history of hallucinations, seizures, or delirium as a result of alcohol withdrawal

      (2) A documented history of very heavy alcohol use and tolerance

      (3) Concomitant abuse of other drugs

      (4) Pregnancy

      (5) A high risk for suicide

      (6) A lack of a reliable social support system

  2. Detoxification can be achieved using benzodiazepines, carbamazepine, or phenobarbital.

    a. Benzodiazepines

      (1) Contraindications. Relative contraindications include age greater than 60 years and chronic obstructive pulmonary disease (COPD).

      (2) Side effects include decreased consciousness, ataxia, impaired short-term memory, slurred speech, and agitation.

      (3) Agents (Table 89-1)

        (a) Chlordiazepoxide is the drug of choice because of its long-acting, "self-tapering"

TABLE 89-1. Dosing Regimens for Outpatient Pharmacologic Detoxification Therapy with Benzodiazepines*

Drug	Dosing Regimen
Chlordiazepoxide	Give 25–50 mg every 6 hours until tremulousness decreases, the pulse rate is lowered to less than 100 beats/min, and withdrawal symptoms have resolved.
	Decrease the dose to 25 mg every 6 hours on the second and third days, and taper the dose by approximately 20% each subsequent day until withdrawal is complete.
Oxazepam	Give 30 mg every 6 hours on day 1; hold for sedation.
	Decrease the dose by 20% daily until withdrawal is complete.
Lorazepam	Give 2 mg every 6 hours on day 1; hold for sedation.
	Decrease the dose by 20% daily until withdrawal is complete.

*If symptoms of withdrawal cannot be controlled with these doses of medication, hospital admission should be considered.

nature; however, it is contraindicated in patients with liver disease.

   (b) Oxazepam or **lorazepam** are used for patients with liver disease.

  b. Carbamazepine is widely used in Europe, but may not prevent withdrawal seizures or delirium. In short treatment protocols, carbamazepine has not been shown to cause significant hematologic or hepatic toxicity. The dosing regimen is 200–400 mg orally twice daily for 7 days.

    c. **Phenobarbital** is not recommended as an initial choice because there is less evidence of its efficacy. The abuse for potential is low, but there is a greater risk of respiratory depression than with benzodiazepines, and the margin of safety may be lower than that of benzodiazepines when high doses are required.

3. Adjunctive therapy

    a. **Adrenergic agents** (e.g., atenolol, 50 mg daily for 3–7 days or clonidine, 0.1 mg twice daily for 3–7 days) may be useful as adjunctive therapy in patients with high heart rate or blood pressure. These agents do not treat alcohol withdrawal.

    b. **Nutritional support** should be provided, as well as replenishment of vitamins:

        (1) Thiamine, 100 g orally daily

        (2) Folic acid, 1 mg orally daily

        (3) Multivitamins that include pyridoxine and ascorbic acid

4. Relapse prevention

    a. **Disulfiram** interferes with the metabolism of acetaldehyde, which accumulates in the blood after alcohol use. If alcohol is used while on the medication, the patient will experience unpleasant symptoms (e.g., flushing, vasodilation, headache, tachycardia, diaphoresis, hyperventilation, nausea, vomiting) for 1–3 hours.

        (1) Dosing regimen. Initiate therapy after the patient is alcohol-free for 4–5 days with a dose of 0.5 g orally daily for 1–3 weeks. The maintenance dosage is 0.25–0.5 g daily. The effects of disulfiram may last for 3–7 days after the last dose.

        (2) Side effects include optic neuritis, peripheral neuropathy, rash, and hepatitis (rare). Psychotic reactions, which are also rare, are associated with a high dosage or combined drug toxicity (particularly metronidazole or isoniazid use).

        (3) Contraindications include acute hepatitis, significant cardiac disease, pregnancy, severe chronic lung disease, schizophrenia or bipolar affective disorder, suicidal ideation, rubber allergy, occupational exposure to solvents or alcohol, and the concurrent use of metronidazole or isoniazid.

b. **Naltrexone** interferes with the pleasurable effects of both alcohol and opiates. The best candidates for naltrexone therapy are patients with high levels of alcohol dependence or craving or a family history of alcoholism.

(1) **Dosing regimen.** Initiate therapy as soon as withdrawal symptoms have resolved. The dose is 25 mg daily with food early in the day; this dose may be increased to 50 mg daily.

(2) **Side effects.** Naltrexone is generally well tolerated, although nausea or abdominal cramping may occur about 1 hour after taking the medicine. Anxiety, malaise, and insomnia are less common.

(3) **Contraindications**. The following patients are not candidates for naltrexone therapy:

(a) Patients who are dependent on opioids, or who have stopped opioid use within the past 2 weeks

(b) Patients who require opioid analgesics for pain

(c) Patients with acute hepatitis

(d) Pregnant patients

VI FOLLOW-UP AND REFERRAL

A. **Follow-up.** Patients who begin a trial of alcohol use reduction or abstinence should be followed closely (i.e., once a week to once a month) during the initial phases so that the physician can provide support and encouragement, and assess continued drinking.

B. **Referral.** Patients who fail to respond to a brief intervention session or who meet the criteria for alcohol dependence should be strongly considered for referral to a substance abuse treatment program.

References

National Institute on Alcohol Abuse and Alcoholism: *The Physician's Guide to Helping Patients with Alcohol Problems.* (NIH/NIAAA Publication No. 95–3769). Bethesda, MD, 1995.

Barnes HN, Samet JH: Brief interventions with substance-abusing patients. *Med Clin North Am* 81(4):867–879, 1997.

O'Connor PG, Schottenfeld RS: Patients with alcohol problems. *N Engl J Med* 338(9):592–602, 1998.

90. Psychosis

....

I **INTRODUCTION.** The defining feature of psychosis (i.e., the inability to distinguish what is real from what is not) is **impaired reality testing** (i.e., an inability to test subjective ideas and experiences against objective facts of the external world).

II **CLINICAL MANIFESTATIONS OF PSYCHOSIS.** The most common symptoms are:

A. Disorders of thought content (delusions)
B. Disorders of perception (hallucinations)
C. Bizarre forms of speaking and behavior

III **CAUSES OF PSYCHOSIS.** All psychoses are ultimately organic and fall within the realm of both general medicine and psychiatry. However, there are two general categories of psychoses: **primary** and **secondary.**

A. Primary psychosis is not caused by another condition.
   1. **Schizophrenia** is a lifelong disease characterized by psychotic symptoms with intermittent exacerbations and a deterioration in social functioning.
      a. The **prevalence** is estimated at 1%.
      b. The **cause** remains unknown, although evidence suggests a strong genetic component and excessive activity of the dopamine systems.
      c. **Phases**
         (1) The **prodromal phase** typically starts between adolescence and early adulthood and may persist for years before the first acute psychotic episode occurs. Patients withdraw from social relationships, become indifferent to grooming, develop suspicious attitudes, and have a gradual deterioration in scholastic and vocational abilities.
         (2) **Acute psychotic episodes** are marked by delusions, hallucinations, a flattened or inappropriate affect, disorganized speech, bizarre posturing or behavior, and an inability to carry out goal-directed behavior. Between episodes, the psychosis may resolve com-

pletely, although impaired social and occupational function often persists.

2. **Mood disorder with psychotic features.** Psychosis occurs only during episodes of the mood disorder (i.e., depression or mania).

3. **Schizoaffective disorder.** Psychosis occurs at times where there are no prominent mood symptoms, as well as during episodes of the mood disorder.

4. **Schizophreniform disorder** is identical to schizophrenia, except that the disorder only lasts for 1–6 months, and there may not be a decline in social functioning.

5. **Brief psychotic disorder.** The duration of illness is less than 1 month and there is no prodromal phase.

6. **Delusional disorder** is characterized by one or more non-bizarre (i.e., conceivable) delusions (e.g., "someone is stealing my clothes").

7. **Schizotypal personality disorder.** Prominent symptoms include magical thinking, paranoia, and odd behavior.

8. **Psychosis not otherwise specified.** The psychosis cannot be categorized.

HOT **KEY** Familiarity with the primary psychoses is important to the generalist for two principal reasons: these patients often present to a generalist first, and the generalist can provide much of the care for patients with chronic psychiatric disorders.

B. **Secondary psychosis** is caused by the presence of another condition. Key features include disturbances in consciousness (i.e., delirium); disorientation of person, place, or time; and impaired intellectual function (e.g., impaired calculation or memory).

1. **Psychosis resulting from a medical condition** (e.g., hypercalcemia, hypoxia, tumor). In this situation, the psychosis is a direct physiologic effect of the medical condition.

2. **Psychosis in association with dementia.** Severe dementia can cause an individual to lose complete touch with reality, but even mild forms of dementia can induce psychosis. Features of psychosis in dementia often include suspiciousness, paranoia, or persecutory delusions.

3. **Substance-induced psychosis** (e.g., delirium tremens) can occur in association with intoxication or withdrawal from a drug.

IV APPROACH TO THE PATIENT

A. **Perform a mental status examination.** The mental status examination is crucial for two reasons: it helps to establish the cause of the psychosis, and it can be used as a tool for monitoring the patient's condition over hours, days, or months. Pay careful attention to the following areas:
   1. **Speech.** For example, is the patient's speech unusually rapid or slow?
   2. **Affect** is the observed emotional state of the patient during the interview. Words used to describe affect include "depressed," "euphoric," and "flat."
   3. **Mood** is the patient's emotional state over the past few days, weeks, or months.
   4. **Thought process.** Words used to describe the patient's thought process include "linear," "tangential," and "loose."
   5. **Thought content.** Is the patient experiencing delusions or hallucinations?
   6. **Cognitive function** is assessed using the Mini Mental State Examination (see Chapter 65, Table 65-1).

B. **Attempt to determine whether the psychosis is secondary or primary.**
   1. **Patient history.** With the exception of psychosis in association with dementia, secondary psychosis often presents with delirium (see Chapter 65 III A). The hallmark features of secondary psychosis include clouding of consciousness, inattentiveness, cognitive impairment, and rapid fluctuations in mental state. If hallucinations or delusions are present, they are fleeting and poorly systemized, unlike those of primary psychosis.
   2. **Physical examination and laboratory studies.** Perform a complete physical examination and obtain appropriate laboratory and imaging studies to evaluate for delirium or dementia (see Chapter 65 IV A 2, B 2–3).

C. **Assess the urgency of the situation.** Clearly, more than one 15-minute session may be required to determine the cause and nature of the patient's psychosis. Is it safe to send the patient home? If any of the following features are present, the patient needs immediate psychiatric consultation or hospitalization, regardless of the cause of the psychosis:

1. The patient has significant suicidal or homicidal ideation.
2. The patient inadvertently is a danger to himself or others.
3. The patient cannot provide food, shelter, or clothing for himself.

D. **Consult with a psychiatrist if the psychosis is primary.** In nearly all cases of new-onset primary psychosis, consultation with a psychiatrist is indicated.

V **TREATMENT.** Patients should be managed in consultation with a psychiatrist.

A. **Primary psychosis**
   1. **Acute therapy.** Consultation with a psychiatrist should be obtained for patients with acute psychotic episodes.
   2. **Chronic therapy** may be handled by a generalist. The goal is to minimize the patient's psychosis using the lowest dose of neuroleptic possible. "Atypical" neuroleptics should be tried first (to minimize side effects). The equivalent of 1–2 mg/day of risperidone often suffices.

   a. **Specific situations**
      (1) **Mood disorder with psychotic symptoms**. Add an antidepressant (to treat depression) and a mood stabilizer (to treat mania), as indicated. Taper the dose of the neuroleptic when the psychotic symptoms have resolved.
      (2) **Dementia.** Use a low dose of neuroleptics (e.g., risperidone, 0.5–1.0 mg once or twice daily) only if a specific symptom (e.g., delusions, aggression, hallucinations) is causing distress or presents a danger to the patient or others.

   b. **Ensuring patient compliance.** Noncompliance with psychiatric medications may be the greatest factor leading to repeat hospitalizations. The following strategies may improve patient compliance:
      (1) Schedule frequent follow-up visits (at least one per month).
      (2) Educate the patient and her family members about the disease.
         (a) Schedule a meeting with the family.
         (b) Recommend resources, such as Torrey:

> *Surviving Schizophrenia: A Manual for Families, Consumers, and Providers,* 3rd edition.

    (3) Recruit family members and friends to aid the patient.

    (4) Adjust therapy to minimize side effects.

    (5) Try a long-acting intramuscular neuroleptic (e.g., fluphenazine, 25–50 mg every 2–4 weeks) instead of oral medications.

B. Secondary psychosis. The general approach is to diagnose and treat the underlying condition. Often, these patients require hospitalization. The treatment of psychosis in association with dementia is similar to that of primary psychosis (see V A).

C. Treatment of side effects from neuroleptic agents

    1. Early side effects include sedation, anticholinergic symptoms (e.g., dry mouth, stuffy nose), orthostatic hypotension, drug-induced Parkinson's syndrome, acute dystonias (contractures), akathisia (motor restlessness), and neuroleptic malignant syndrome (characterized by muscle rigidity and a high fever). Early side effects often decrease or resolve after 1–2 months.

HOT

KEY

Low-potency neuroleptics (e.g., chlorpromazine) are more likely to cause sedation and less likely to cause extrapyramidal symptoms; the reverse is true for high-potency agents (e.g., haloperidol).

---

    2. Late side effects include tardive dyskinesia (involuntary movements of a choreiform nature), Parkinsonian syndrome, and akathisia.

    3. Motor disorders can be treated with the following measures:

        a. Anticholinergic agents (e.g., benztropine, 1 mg twice daily or diphenhydramine, 25–50 mg four times daily)

        b. Anti-Parkinson agents

        c. Reduction of the neuroleptic dose

        d. Switching from a conventional to an "atypical" neuroleptic, such as olanzapine or risperidone

VI **FOLLOW-UP AND REFERRAL.** A variety of programs and professionals are available to assist the psychotic patient, including:

A. Vocational rehabilitation programs, sheltered workshops, or day treatment programs

B. Psychotherapists (may help the patient to focus on behavior modification and compliance)

C. Occupational therapists

D. Social workers (may help locate sources of financial support)

References

Diagnostic And Statistical Manual of Mental Disorders, 4th ed. American Psychiatric Association, Washington, DC, 1994.

Jenike MA: Psychiatric illness in the elderly: a review. *J Geriatr Psychiatry Neurol* 9(2):57–82, 1996.

Summary of Mnemonics

PART I: GENERAL CARE OF THE AMBULATORY PATIENT

Enhancing the Patient-Provider Relationship
("WE CARE") .... Chapter 1

Warmly greet the patient (e.g., address her by the name she prefers)
Equalize the relationship by avoiding condescension
Care for the patient as a person, not just as a patient (e.g., express an interest in the patient's family, job, or hobbies)
Allow the patient to tell her story without frequent interruptions
Resist using jargon to explain things
Encourage questions by asking "What questions can I answer?" after every visit

Potential Etiologies ("CHOPPED MINTS") .... Chapter 1

Congenital
Hematologic or vascular
Organ disease
Psychiatric or **P**sychogenic
Pregnancy-related
Environmental
Drugs (prescription, over-the-counter, herbal, illicit)
Metabolic or endocrine
Infectious, **I**nflammatory, **I**atrogenic, or **I**diopathic
Neoplasm-related (and paraneoplastic syndromes)
Trauma
Surgical or procedure-related

PART II: OPHTHALMOLOGY AND OTOLARYNGOLOGY

Common Causes of Singultus ("SINGULTUS") . . . . . Chapter 10

Surgery (post-surgical status) or lesions of the abdomen, chest, or neck

Infections adjacent to the diaphragm (e.g., lower lobe pneumonia, subphrenic abscess, peritonitis, pericarditis, cholecystitis, hepatitis)

Nervous system disorders (e.g., stroke, meningitis, brain tumor, multiple sclerosis)

Gastric distention (a very common cause, usually self-limited)

Uremia

Low serum calcium, sodium, or potassium

Tumor of the pancreas or stomach

Psychogenic and idiopathic

Steroids and other drugs (e.g., alcohol, benzodiazepines, barbiturates)

History and Physical Examination Findings in Sinusitis
    ("TAP TAP") . . . . Chapter 11

Toothache (maxillary)
Abnormal or poor response to decongestants
Purulent nasal discharge in history
Tenderness to palpation
Abnormal transillumination
Purulent nasal discharge on examination

PART III: CARDIOLOGY

Causes of Syncope ("SYNCOPE") . . . . Chapter 15

Situational
Vasovagal (the "V" looks like a "Y")
Neurogenic
Cardiac
Orthostatic hypotension
Psychiatric
Everything else

Causes of Secondary Hypertension (CENT) .... Chapter 16

One anatomic cause
Two renal causes
Three adrenal causes
Four CENTs
    Calcium (hypercalcemia)
    Ethanol abuse or Estrogen (oral contraceptives)
    Neurologic disease
    Thyrotoxicosis

Classes of Drugs Used to Control Blood Pressure
    ("ABCDE") .... Chapter 16

ACE inhibitors and Angiotensin II receptor blockers
β blockers
Calcium channel antagonists
Diuretics
Everything else (i.e., central α agonists, α blockers, combination
    therapy)

Risk Factors for CAD ("Start Helping CAD Fast") .. Chapter 17

Smoking
Hypertension
Cholesterol (hyperlipidemia)
Age
Diabetes mellitus
Family history of CAD

Tertiary Prevention of CAD ("ABCs") .... Chapter 17

Aspirin and Angiotensin-converting enzyme (ACE) inhibitors
β Blockers
Cholesterol reduction

Causes of Cardiomyopathy ("PIPED") .... Chapter 18

Post-myocarditis
Idiopathic
Peripartum
Ethanol
Drugs (cocaine and heroin)

Factors that Can Exacerbate CHF
("FAILURE") .... Chapter 18

Forgot meds
Arrhythmia or **A**nemia
Infections, **I**schemia, or **I**nfarction
Lifestyle (e.g. increased sodium intake, stress)
Upregulators (e.g., thyroid disease, pregnancy)
Rheumatic valve or worsening of other valvular diseases
Embolism (pulmonary)

Causes of Atrial Fibrillation
("WATCH ATRIAL Ps") .... Chapter 19

WPW syndrome
Alcohol (intoxication, withdrawal, "holiday heart")
Thyrotoxicosis
CHF, **C**oronary artery disease (CAD), or **C**ardiomyopathy
Hypertension

Atrial septal defect (ASD)
Theophylline and other drugs (β agonists)
Rheumatic and other valve disease
Infections (e.g., myocarditis, endocarditis)
Amyloid and other infiltrative diseases
Lone (idiopathic) atrial fibrillation

Pulmonary or **P**ericardial disease
Sick sinus syndrome or **S**tress

Risk Factors for Stroke in Patients with Atrial Fibrillation
("CHASED") .... Chapter 19

CHF (within 3 months)
Hypertension
Age > 65 years
Stroke in past
Echocardiographic abnormalities (left atrial size > 5 cm, left ventricular dysfunction)
Diabetes

PART IV: PULMONOLOGY

Causes of wheezing other than Asthma
("CARES") .... Chapter 25

Cardiac asthma (i.e., CHF) or **C**hurg-Strauss syndrome
Allergic bronchopulmonary aspergillosis
Reflux esophagitis
Exposures (irritants, medications) or **E**mbolism (pulmonary)
Sinusitis or **S**trongyloides infection

Treatment for Acute Asthma ("ASTHMA") .... Chapter 25

Albuterol and **A**trovent
Steroids
Theophylline
Humidified oxygen
Magnesium
Antibiotics

Criteria for Hospital Admission of Patients with
Community-Acquired Pneumonia
("ADMIT NOW") .... Chapter 29

Age > 65 years (depending on individual situation)
Decreased immunity (e.g., cancer, diabetes, AIDS, splenectomy)
Mental status changes
Increased A-a gradient or increased respiratory rate
Two or more lobes involved

No home (i.e., homeless patients)
Organ system failure (increased creatinine, bone marrow suppression, systolic blood pressure < 90 mm Hg, liver failure)
WBC count greater than 30,000/mm^3 or less than 4000/mm^3

PART V: GASTROENTEROLOGY

Systemic and Metabolic Causes of Abdominal
     Pain ("Puking My Very BAD LUNCH") .... Chapter 32

Porphyria
Mediterranean fever
Vasculitis

Black widow spider bite
Addison's disease or **A**ngioedema
Diabetic ketoacidosis

Lead poisoning
Uremia
Neurogenic (impingement on spinal nerves or roots, diabetes, syphilis)
Calcium (hypercalcemia)
Herpes zoster

Major Types of Chronic Diarrhea
     ("SOME MD FUNCTION") .... Chapter 33

Secretory diarrhea
Osmotic diarrhea
Motility disorder
Exudative diarrhea

Malabsorption
Decreased immunity

FUNCTIONal diarrhea

Causes of Constipation ("DUODENUM") .... Chapter 34

Diet
ψsychiatric conditions
Obstruction
Drugs
Endocrine or metabolic disorders
Neurologic disorders
Unknown
Miscellaneous

Conditions That Can Exacerbate GERD
("ACIDS") .... Chapter 39

Acid hypersecretion (e.g., Zollinger-Ellison disease) or **A**lcohol
   abuse
Connective tissue disease (e.g., scleroderma)
Infections of the esophagus (e.g., cytomegalovirus, herpes, candidiasis)
Diabetic gastroparesis or **D**rug therapy (e.g., calcium channel
   blockers, β agonists, α blockers, theophylline, narcotics, progestins)
Smoking

Indications for Upper Endoscopy ("DANGER") .... Chapter 36

Drop in weight
Anemia or **A**bdominal mass
New onset of pain and age > 40 years
Guaiac-positive stool
Endemic risk (patient from area with endemic gastric cancer, such
   as Japan)
Response to treatment inadequate

PART VI: NEPHROLOGY AND UROLOGY

Causes of Hematuria ("GREEN PIS") .... Chapter 39

Glomerulonephritis
Renal cyst or trauma
Exercise
Embolism or infarction
Neoplasm

Prostate hypertrophy
Infection
Stones

Characteristics of the Nephrotic Syndrome
("PALE") .... Chapter 40

Proteinuria (> 3.5 grams/24 hours)
Albumin (low)
Lipids (elevated)
Edema

Causes of Nonrenal Proteinuria
("PROTEIN") .... Chapter 40

Pulmonary edema or congestive heart failure (CHF)
Relative lordotic position
Orthostatic proteinuria (i.e., proteinuria when sitting upright but not in the supine position)
Temperature increase (i.e., fever)
Exercise (following vigorous exercise)
Injury to the head or cerebrovascular accident (CVA)
Idiopathic (diagnosis of exclusion)
Norepinephrine excess (emotional stress)

Secondary Causes of Nephrotic Syndrome
("THIS LAD HAS nephrotic syndrome") .... Chapter 40

Tumors
Heroin, **H**eavy metals, and toxins
Infection
   Hepatitis B and C
   AIDS
   Subacute bacterial endocarditis, **S**yphilis, and **S**chistosomiasis
Systemic disorders
   Lupus
   Amyloid
   Diabetes

PART VII: GYNECOLOGY

7 Major Causes of Secondary Amenorrhea
("3 + 2 + 1 + 1") .... Chapter 45

3 Endocrine (hypothalamic or pituitary dysfunction, hyperpro-lactinemia, thyroid disorder)
2 Ovarian (polycystic ovary syndrome, premature ovarian failure)
1 Uterine (Asherman's syndrome)
1 Obstetric (pregnancy)

Causes of Acute Urinary Incontinence
  ("DAMN DRIPS") .... Chapter 49

Delirium
Atrophic urethritis or vaginitis
Medications—e.g., sedative-hypnotics, diuretics, anticholinergics,
  α-adrenergic agonists or antagonists
Neurologic disorders—e.g., cord compression, cauda equina syn-
  drome

Diabetes mellitus or insipidus
Restricted mobility
Infection—urinary tract infection (UTI)
Psychiatric disorders—e.g., depression
Stool impaction

Birth Control Methods ("COITUS") .... Chapter 50

Condoms and other barrier methods
Oral contraceptives and other hormonal methods
Intrauterine device (IUD)
Timing methods
Unprotected (coitus interruptus)
Surgical methods

PART VIII: ORTHOPEDICS AND RHEUMATOLOGY

Treatment of an Acute Ankle Sprain ("PRICE") .... Chapter 52

Protection of the area
Rest
Ice
Compression
Elevation

Anatomy of the Shoulder Joint ("4–3–2–1") .... Chapter 54

4 muscles—supraspinatus, infraspinatus, teres minor, subscapularis
  (rotator cuff)
3 joints—acromioclavicular, sternoclavicular, glenohumeral
2 tendons—supraspinatus, biceps
1 bursa—subacromial

Muscles of the Shoulder Joint ("SITS") .... Chapter 54

Supraspinatus
Infraspinatus
Teres minor
Subscapularis

Causes of Monoarticular Arthritis
("If I Make The Diagnosis, No More Harm") ..... Chapter 59

Infection of the joint
Inflammatory disease
Metabolic disorders
Trauma
DJD
Neoplasia
Miscellaneous causes (foreign body synovitis, avascular necrosis)
Hemarthrosis

Criteria for the Diagnosis of Rheumatoid Arthritis
("AMASS RX") .... Chapter 60

Arthritis in 3 or more joint areas
Morning stiffness lasting 1 hour or more
Arthritis of the hand joints
Symmetric arthritis
Serum rheumatoid factor (RF) present

Rheumatoid nodules
X-ray changes consistent with rheumatoid arthritis (e.g., erosions)

Criteria for the Diagnosis of SLE ("P-MOAD") ..... Chapter 60

Positive antineutrophil antibody (ANA) test: seen in 95% of patients
Positive other immunologic test [antibody (Ab) to double-stranded DNA, Ab to Smith, lupus erythematosus (LE) cell preparation, or false-positive syphilis serology]
Psychosis, seizures, or other neurologic abnormalities
Photosensitivity rash
Polyserositis (pleuritis, pericarditis, or peritonitis)
Proteinuria or renal involvement
Pancytopenia or single-cell line "penia" (anemia, thrombocytopenia, leukopenia)
Malar rash
Oral ulcers
Arthritis
Discoid rash

PART IX: NEUROLOGY

Differential Diagnosis for Headache ("Take Care to Diagnose
My Symptoms; I don't want to be MAIMED") .... Chapter 62

Tension headache
Cluster headache
Drugs or **D**ental pain
Migraine headache
Sinusitis or **S**ystemic illness

Mass lesion
Arteritis or **A**cute angle glaucoma
Ischemia
Meningitis
Encephalitis or **E**levated intracranial pressure (ICP)
Dural venous sinus thrombosis

Worrisome Symptoms Associated with Headache ("NEW
FEARS") .... Chapter 62

NEW or different headache (especially in patients older than 40
years)

Fever
Exertional headache (e.g., headache with exercise, cough, sexual
activity)
Abnormal mental status or personality changes
Recent history of trauma
Severe symptoms

Causes of Central Vertigo ("SPIN") .... Chapter 63

Sclerosis (i.e., multiple sclerosis)
Pretty bad migraine (especially basilar)
Ischemia or CNS lesions [especially basilar transient ischemic at-
tack (TIA)]
Neuroma (i.e., acoustic neuroma)

Common Causes of Peripheral Vertigo
   ("AMPLITUDE") .... Chapter 63

Acoustic neuroma
Meniere's disease (endolymphatic hydrops)
Positional vertigo
Labyrinthitis
Infection of the middle or inner ear
Trauma (head)
ψsychogenic
Drugs
Endocrine disorders

Reversible Dementias ("DEMENTIA") .... Chapter 65

Drug effects
Emotional disorders
Metabolic or endocrine disorders
Ear or **E**ye dysfunction
Nutritional deficiencies or **N**eurologic disorders
Trauma or **T**umor
Ischemia or **I**nfection
Alcohol

Causes of Polyneuropathy ("DANG
   THERAPIST") .... Chapter 66

Diabetes (and other metabolic disorders)
Alcohol abuse
Nutritional deficiency (e.g., vitamin B_{12}, thiamine, pyridoxine, fo-
   late)
Guillain-Barré syndrome and other idiopathic causes

Tumor-related (i.e., paraneoplastic syndrome)
Hereditary disorders (e.g., Charcot-Marie-Tooth disease)
Endocrine disorders (e.g., hypothyroidism, acromegaly)
Renal disease (i.e., uremia)
Amyloidosis
Porphyria or **P**olycythemia
Infections and **I**mmune-mediated disorders (e.g., AIDS, leprosy,
   Lyme disease, syphilis, vasculitis)
Sarcoidosis
Toxins and drugs (e.g., alcohol, heavy metals, pesticides)

Secondary Causes of Carpal Tunnel Syndrome
("WRIST PAIN") .... Chapter 67

Work-related
Rheumatoid arthritis
Infiltrative disorders (e.g., amyloidosis)
Sarcoidosis
Thyroid dysfunction (i.e., hypothyroidism) and other endocrine
disorders (e.g., diabetes mellitus)

Pregnancy
Acromegaly
Inflammatory tenosynovitis (caused by Reiter's syndrome, gout,
soft tissue infection, disseminated gonococcal infection)
Neoplasm (primarily leukemia)

Causes of Facial Paresis ("MR FaCIaL SaG") .... Chapter 68

Mononucleosis or **M**ultiple Sclerosis
Ramsay Hunt syndrome

Fracture of the facial bones
Cancer of the ear or parotid gland
Idiopathic (Bell's palsy)
Lyme disease

Sarcoidosis
Guillain-Barré syndrome

PART X: HEMATOLOGY AND ONCOLOGY

Causes of DIC ("MOIST") .... Chapter 69

Malignancy
Obstetric complications
Infection
Shock
Trauma

Causes of Absolute Polycythemia ("Hypoxia Can Cause
Polycythemia Every Time") .... Chapter 70

Hypoxia (chronic)
Carboxyhemoglobinemia
Cushing's syndrome or **C**orticosteroids
Polycythemia vera
Erythropoietin-secreting **T**umors

Causes of Decreased Platelet Production
("PANYTO") .... Chapter 71

Paroxysmal nocturnal hemoglobinuria (PNH)
Aplasia
Neoplasms and **N**ear neoplasms
Vitamin deficiency (the "V" looks like a "Y")
Toxins, drugs, and radiation therapy
Overwhelming infection

Causes of Eosinophilia ("PHILIA CAN
ACT FAST") .... Chapter 72

Pulmonary disease
Helminthic infections
   Filariasis
   Ascariasis
   Schistosomiasis or *Strongyloides* infection
   Trichinosis
Infections, in general
   Allergic bronchopulmonary aspergillosis
   Coccidioidomycosis
   Tuberculosis (especially chronic)
L-Tryptophan
Immunologic disorders
Addison's disease

Cutaneous disorders
Allergic disorders
Neoplasms

Causes of Generalized Lymphadenopathy
("SHE HAS CUTE LAN") .... Chapter 74

Syphilis
Hepatitis
Epstein-Barr virus

Histoplasmosis
AIDS/HIV
Serum sickness

Cytomegalovirus (CMV)
Unusual drugs (e.g., hydantoin derivatives, antithyroid medications, antileprosy medications, isoniazid)
Toxoplasmosis
Erythrophagocytic lymphohistiocytosis

Leishmaniasis
Arthritis (rheumatoid)
Neoplasm (i.e., leukemia, lymphoma)

PART XI: ENDOCRINOLOGY

Causes of Hypocalcemia ("HIPOCAL") .... Chapter 79

Hypoparathyroidism
Infection
Pancreatitis
Overload States
Chronic renal failure
Absorption abnormalities
Loop diuretics and other drugs

Causes of Hypercalcemia ("My Favorite
    MISHAP") .... Chapter 79

Medications (e.g., lithium, thiazide diuretics)
Familial hypocalciuric hypercalcemia (FHH)

Malignancy
Intoxication (vitamin D or A overdose) or **I**mmobilization
Sarcoidosis (and other granulomatous diseases)
Hyperparathyroidism or **H**yperthyroidism
Addison's disease or milk-**A**lkali syndrome
Paget's disease or **P**heochromocytoma

PART XIII: DERMATOLOGY

Causes of Pruritus ("ITCHED") .... Chapter 86

Infestation (e.g., scabies)
Total bilirubin elevation (e.g., primary biliary cirrhosis)
Chronic renal failure (uremia) or **C**ancer
Hematologic disorders
Endocrine disorders
Dry skin or other dermatologic disorders

Various drugs
Autoimmune disorders
Serum sickness
Cryoglobulinemia
Ulcerative colitis
Low complement
Infections
Tumor
IgA deposition
Smoking-related (thromboangiitis obliterans)

PART XIV: PSYCHIATRY

1 of the following **2** criteria must be present:
    Depressed mood
    Anhedonia
3 thought disturbances
    Suicidal ideation
    Decreased concentration
    Guilt
4 physical symptoms
    Insomnia
    Decreased energy or fatigue
    Psychomotor agitation or retardation
    Weight loss or gain
5 criteria total must be present

Sex (male:female ratio = 4:1)
Age (older white men at greatest risk)
Depression (70% of suicides follow a depressive episode)

Previous attempts
ETOH use
Rational thinking loss (cognitive slowing, psychotic depression,
    pre-existing organic brain disease)
Social support deficit
Organized plan
No spouse
Sicknesses (especially post-myocardial infarction)

Cut down on your drinking?
Annoyed by others?
Guilty about drinking?
Eye-opener to counteract a hangover?

Feedback about screening results
Responsibility for change with patient
Advice regarding consumption goals
Menu of options for reducing alcohol consumption
Empathy
Self-efficacy (patient empowerment)

Index